Pocket
MEDICINE
High-Yield Board Review
Second Edition

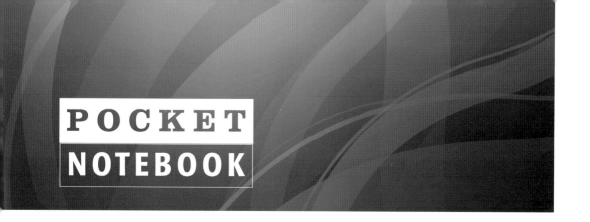

POCKET NOTEBOOK

Pocket MEDICINE
High-Yield Board Review
Second Edition

Editor

Marc S. Sabatine, MD, MPH

Professor of Medicine
Harvard Medical School

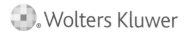

. Wolters Kluwer

Philadelphia • Baltimore • New York • London
Buenos Aires • Hong Kong • Sydney • Tokyo

Acquisitions Editor: Joe Cho
Development Editor: Cindy Yoo
Editorial Coordinator: Vinodhini Varadharajalu
Senior Production Project Manager: Kirstin Johnson
Marketing Manager: Kirsten Watrud
Manager, Graphic Arts & Design: Stephen Druding
Manufacturing Coordinator: Beth Welsh/Lisa Bowling
Prepress Vendor: S4Carlisle Publishing Services

Second Edition

9 8 7 6 5 4 3 2 1

Printed in Mexico

Library of Congress Cataloging-in-Publication Data

ISBN-13: 978-1-975209-81-0
ISBN-10: 1-975209-81-8

Cataloging in Publication data available on request from publisher.

shop.lww.com

QUADM0423

CONTRIBUTORS

Andrew Abboud, MD
Internal Medicine Resident, Massachusetts General Hospital

Andrew S. Allegretti, MD, MSc
Director of ICU Nephrology, Attending Physician, Nephrology Division, and Principal Investigator, Kidney Research Center, Massachusetts General Hospital
Instructor in Medicine, Harvard Medical School

Jillian M. Berkman, MD
Neurology Resident, Mass General Brigham Neurology Residency Program

Michael P. Bowley, MD, PhD
Instructor in Neurology, Massachusetts General Hospital
Associate Program Director, Mass General Brigham Neurology Residency Program

Earllondra R. Brooks, MD
Neurology Resident, Mass General Brigham Neurology Residency

Caitlin Colling, MD
Endocrinology Fellow, Massachusetts General Hospital

Jean M. Connors, MD
Medical Director, Anticoagulation Management Services
Hematology Division, Brigham and Women's Hospital & Dana-Farber Cancer Institute
Associate Professor of Medicine, Harvard Medical School

Ian D. Cooley, MD
Rheumatology Fellow, Massachusetts General Hospital

Daniel J. DeAngelo, MD, PhD
Chief of the Division of Leukemia, Dana-Farber Cancer Institute
Professor of Medicine, Harvard Medical School

Brett J. Doliner, MD
Internal Medicine Resident, Massachusetts General Hospital

Rachel E. Erdil, MD
Infectious Disease Fellow, Massachusetts General Hospital

Rachel C. Frank, MD
Cardiology Fellow, Massachusetts General Hospital

Robert P. Friday, MD, PhD
Chief, Division of Rheumatology, Newton-Wellesley Hospital
Affiliate Physician, Rheumatology Unit, Massachusetts General Hospital
Instructor in Medicine, Harvard Medical School

Lawrence S. Friedman, MD
The Anton R. Fried, MD, Chair, Department of Medicine, Newton-Wellesley Hospital
Assistant Chief of Medicine, Massachusetts General Hospital
Professor of Medicine, Harvard Medical School
Professor of Medicine, Tufts University School of Medicine

Robert Hallowell, MD
Director, Interstitial Lung Disease Program and Pulmonary Ambulatory Clinic, Pulmonary/
 Critical Care Unit, Massachusetts General Hospital
Assistant Professor of Medicine, Harvard Medical School

Daniel S. Harrison, MD
Neurology Resident, Mass General Brigham Neurology Residency Program

Sara Khosrowjerdi, MD
Internal Medicine Resident, Massachusetts General Hospital

Howard J. Lee, Jr., MD
Internal Medicine Resident, Massachusetts General Hospital

Michael Mannstadt, MD
Chief, Endocrine Unit, Massachusetts General Hospital
Associate Professor of Medicine, Harvard Medical School

Zoe N. Memel, MD
Internal Medicine Resident, Massachusetts General Hospital

Louisa A. Mounsey, MD
Internal Medicine Resident, Massachusetts General Hospital

Michelle L. O'Donoghue, MD, MPH
Senior Investigator, TIMI Study Group
Associate Physician, Cardiovascular Division, Brigham and Women's Hospital
Affiliate Physician, Cardiology Division, Massachusetts General Hospital
Associate Professor of Medicine, Harvard Medical School

Jessica C. O'Neil, MD
Internal Medicine Resident, Massachusetts General Hospital

Bradley J. Petek, MD
Cardiology Fellow, Massachusetts General Hospital

Ignacio Portales Castillo, MD
Nephrology Fellow, BWH/MGH Joint Nephrology Fellowship Program

Eric M. Przybyszewski, MD
Gastroenterology Fellow, Massachusetts General Hospital

John Y. Rhee, MD, MPH
Neurology Resident, Mass General Brigham Neurology Residency Program

Thomas J. Roberts, MD
Hematology-Oncology Fellow, Dana-Farber/Mass General Brigham

David P. Ryan, MD
Clinical Director, Massachusetts General Hospital Cancer Center
Chief of Hematology/Oncology, Massachusetts General Hospital
Professor of Medicine, Harvard Medical School

Marc S. Sabatine, MD, MPH
Chair, TIMI Study Group
Lewis Dexter, MD, Distinguished Chair in Cardiovascular Medicine, Brigham and Women's
  Hospital
Affiliate Physician, Cardiology Division, Massachusetts General Hospital
Professor of Medicine, Harvard Medical School

Daria Schatoff, MD
Internal Medicine Resident, Massachusetts General Hospital

MacLean C. Sellars, MD, PhD
Hematology-Oncology Fellow, Dana-Farber/Mass General Brigham

Sarah E. Street, MD
Nephrology Fellow, BWH/MGH Joint Nephrology Fellowship Program

Alison Trainor, MD
Pulmonary and Critical Care Fellow, Massachusetts General Hospital and Beth Israel Deaconess
  Medical Center

Zandra E. Walton, MD, PhD
Internal Medicine Resident, Massachusetts General Hospital

Rebecca L. Williamson, MD, PhD
Neurology Resident, Mass General Brigham Neurology Residency Program

Kimon C. Zachary, MD
Attending Physician, Infectious Disease Division, Massachusetts General Hospital
Assistant Professor of Medicine, Harvard Medical School

To my parents, Matthew and Lee Sabatine, to their namesake grandchildren Matteo and Natalie, and to my wife Jennifer.

Many readers of *Pocket Medicine* have commented that they use that book not only on the wards but also for preparation for their Board exams. To help further address that need, we created *Pocket Medicine High-Yield Board Review*. The very positive response to the 1st edition suggests we crafted a useful product.

In this new, 2nd edition, we have updated prior questions and added new questions to provide readers with over 600 case-based questions across 9 subspecialties. The annotated answers are detailed and review the key diagnostic and therapeutic principles. Readers will see that the cases are based not only on the exceptional medical knowledge and clinical acumen of the teams of authors for each subspecialty for the 8th edition of *Pocket Medicine*, but also reflect the recent experience of the more junior members in taking Board exams. As always, we welcome any suggestions for improvement.

I hope that you find *Pocket Medicine High-Yield Board Review* useful not only for your examination but also to help hone your knowledge of internal medicine.

MARC S. SABATINE, MD, MPH

CONTENTS

1 CARDIOLOGY 1
Andrew Abboud, Brett J. Doliner, Rachel C. Frank, Bradley J. Petek, Marc S. Sabatine, Michelle L. O'Donoghue

2 PULMONARY 58
Louisa A. Mounsey, Alison Trainor, Robert Hallowell

3 GASTROENTEROLOGY 84
Zoe N. Memel, Eric M. Przybyszewski, Lawrence S. Friedman

4 NEPHROLOGY 114
Sarah E. Street, Ignacio Portales Castillo, Andrew S. Allegretti

5 HEMATOLOGY-ONCOLOGY 149
Sara Khosrowjerdi, Howard J. Lee, Jr., Thomas J. Roberts, MacLean C. Sellars, Jean M. Connors, Daniel J. DeAngelo, David P. Ryan

6 INFECTIOUS DISEASES 209
Jessica C. O'Neil, Rachel E. Erdil, Kimon C. Zachary

7 ENDOCRINOLOGY 231
Daria Schatoff, Caitlin Colling, Michael Mannstadt

8 RHEUMATOLOGY 260
Zandra E. Walton, Ian D. Cooley, Robert P. Friday

9 NEUROLOGY 291
Jillian M. Berkman, Earllondra R. Brooks, Daniel S. Harrison, John Y. Rhee, Rebecca L. Williamson, Michael P. Bowley

ABBREVIATIONS 310

CARDIOLOGY

QUESTIONS

1. A 59-year-old man with a history of hypertension (HTN) and hyperlipidemia presents with 1 hour of substernal chest pressure rated an 8 on a scale of 1 to 10 with radiation down the left arm and associated with diaphoresis. Initial vital signs are notable for a blood pressure (BP) of 92/64 mmHg and a heart rate (HR) of 92 beats/min. His electrocardiogram (ECG) is shown below:

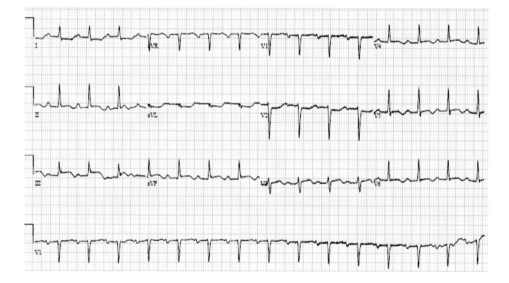

What is the most likely diagnosis?

A. Anterior ST-elevation myocardial infarction (STEMI)

B. Inferior STEMI

C. Pericarditis

D. ST changes not meeting specific ischemic criteria; additional ECGs should be obtained

2. A 72-year-old man with a history of paroxysmal atrial fibrillation (AF) presents with substernal chest pain following 3 days of rhinorrhea and nasal congestion. His initial vital signs are notable for the absence of a fever, HR of 58 beats/min, BP of 102/58 mmHg, and oxygen saturation of 98% on room air. His initial ECG is shown below:

CARDIOLOGY

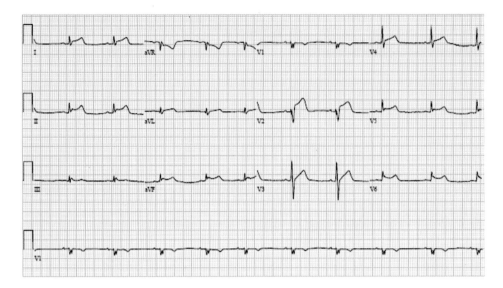

What is the most likely diagnosis?

A. Anterior STEMI

B. Inferior STEMI

C. Pericarditis

D. ST changes not meeting specific ischemia criteria; additional ECGs should be obtained

3. A 78-year-old man with a history of heart failure (HF) with reduced ejection fraction (HFrEF) presents to clinic for posthospitalization follow-up. He reports no current chest pain, anginal equivalents, or dyspnea on exertion. His ECG is shown below:

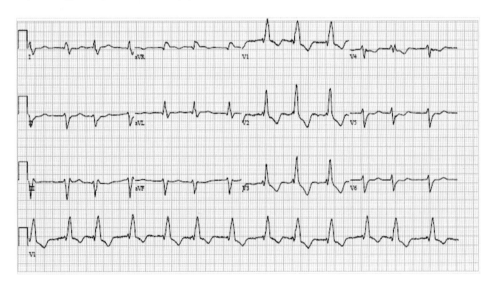

What is the correct interpretation?

A. AF with left bundle branch block (LBBB)

B. AF with right bundle branch block (RBBB)

C. AF with RBBB and left anterior fascicular block

D. Complete heart block (CHB) with RBBB

4. A 72-year-old man with a history of stage 4 chronic kidney disease secondary to HTN presents to the hospital with fatigue and malaise for the past 3 days. He reports no chest pain. His ECG is shown below:

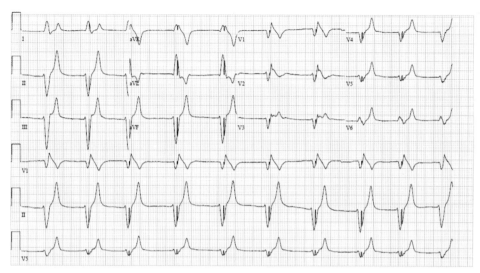

What is the most likely etiology of the ECG changes?

A. Hypercalcemia
B. Hyperkalemia
C. Hypokalemia
D. Ischemia

5. A 39-year-old man with a history of substance use on methadone is admitted with community-acquired pneumonia and started on levofloxacin. His ECG on admission is shown below:

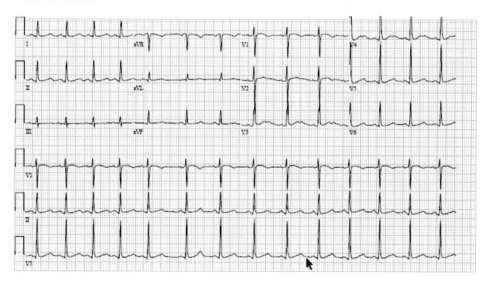

Which of the following would INCREASE his risk of life-threatening arrhythmia?

A. Dose-reducing his methadone
B. Ensuring his electrolytes are replete
C. Initiating β-blocker therapy
D. Transitioning from levofloxacin to doxycycline

6. A 45-year-old woman with a history of tobacco use presents with 20 minutes of new-onset substernal chest pressure. Her vital signs are notable for a HR of 102 beats/min, a BP of 94/68 mmHg, and oxygen saturation of 90% on room air. Her examination is notable for elevated jugular venous pulsations; tachycardia without murmurs, rubs, or gallops; clear lungs; and left greater than right lower extremity edema. Her ECG is shown below:

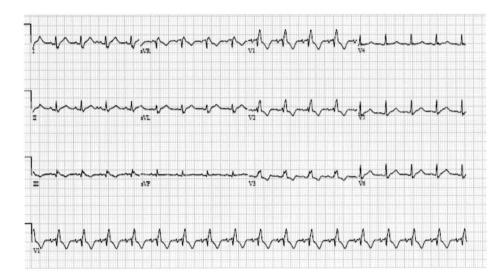

   What is the most likely diagnosis?
   A. Inferior STEMI
   B. Non-ST-elevation MI (NSTEMI)
   C. Pericarditis
   D. Pulmonary embolism

7. A 68-year-old man presents with severe substernal pressure, nausea, and vomiting for the past 30 minutes. He reports the chest pressure started over the course of 10 minutes and has continued to worsen. He is diaphoretic and in moderate distress. Vital signs are notable for a BP of 118/78 mmHg, an HR of 94 beats/min, and oxygen saturation of 98% on room air. Physical examination reveals clear lung fields without any murmurs, rubs, or gallops on cardiac auscultation. ECG is checked and shows an R wave > S wave in V_1 with ST-segment depressions in V_1 to V_3.

   What is the next best step?
   A. Check posterior leads
   B. Rule out pulmonary embolism by computed tomography (CT) of the chest
   C. Start colchicine for pericarditis
   D. Trial of a proton pump inhibitor

8. A 69-year-old man with a history of HTN and hyperlipidemia presents with 90 minutes of substernal chest pain. The pain is described as a pressure sensation with radiation down the left arm and associated with diaphoresis. Initial vital signs are notable for a BP of 92/64 mmHg, a HR of 92 beats/min, and oxygen saturation of 94% on room air. He was given a full-dose aspirin by Emergency Medical Services (EMS) prior to arrival. His ECG is shown below:

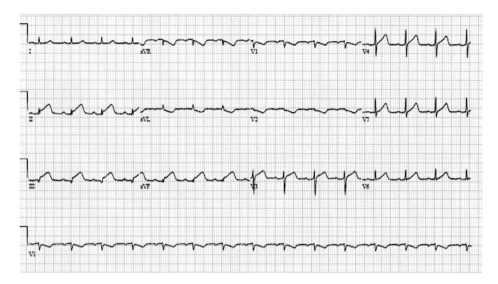

Right-sided leads are obtained that reveal elevation in lead V$_4$R. What is the next best step?

A. Activate the cardiac catheterization lab for urgent revascularization

B. Administer nitroglycerin

C. Obtain posterior ECG leads

D. Perform transthoracic echocardiogram (TTE)

9. A 72-year-old man with a history of HTN presents with new onset of pleuritic and sharp left-sided chest pain radiating to the shoulders. The pain started subacutely and is worsened when lying flat and improved by leaning forward. He has not had any preceding chest pain or dyspnea with exertion. For the past week, he has had rhinorrhea and a dry cough. Vital signs are notable for tachycardia with an HR of 104 beats/min and a BP of 122/78 mmHg. Oxygen saturation is 98% on room air and respiratory rate is 18 breaths/min. His ECG is shown below:

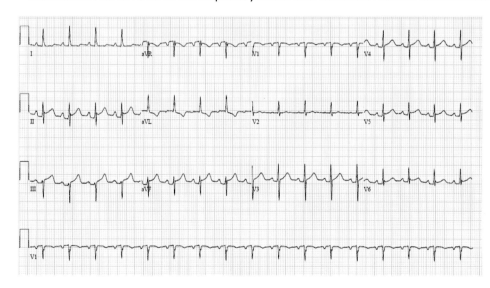

Which of the following is most consistent with the clinical presentation and ECG?

A. Acute pericarditis

B. Acute pulmonary embolism

C. Aortic dissection

D. STEMI

10. A 76-year-old woman with HTN and diabetes mellitus presents with chest pain and is found to have an elevated troponin value. She is brought for cardiac catheterization for presumed type 1 myocardial infarction (MI). At angiography, she is not found to have any evidence of epicardial coronary disease. She has an echocardiogram that shows depressed left ventricular ejection fraction (LVEF) of 35% with global hypokinesis.

What should be considered the next appropriate step in her workup?
  A. Cardiac magnetic resonance imaging (MRI)
  B. Coronary CT angiography (CTA)
  C. Exercise treadmill test with perfusion imaging
  D. Supine bicycle stress echocardiogram

11. A 68-year-old man with a history of HTN, hyperlipidemia, and diabetes presents with shortness of breath on exertion, worsening in the past several weeks. His primary care physician calls you to ask about the optimal stress test to order for him. You review his chart and see that he has a LBBB at baseline and had a left knee replacement 10 months ago. He has limited exercise capacity per primary care physician documentation.

Which test should you recommend?
  A. Dobutamine stress echocardiography
  B. Exercise ECG stress test only
  C. Exercise stress test with perfusion imaging
  D. Pharmacologic stress test with perfusion imaging

12. A 49-year-old man with HTN, hyperlipidemia, chronic knee pain requiring a cane, and family history of early coronary artery disease (CAD) presents to the emergency department (ED) with several days of chest pain. The pain does not reliably occur with exertion. When it does occur with exertion, it does not reliably resolve with rest and is not provoked by more intense exercise. Vital signs are within normal limits. His ECG has no ischemic changes. His serum troponin is below the upper reference limit and his renal function is normal.

Which of the following choices would be the most reasonable first test to order?
  A. Cardiac MRI without stress testing
  B. Coronary angiogram
  C. Coronary CTA
  D. Exercise stress test

13. A 72-year-old man with a remote history of MI, HTN, hyperlipidemia, and diabetes (last hemoglobin A_{1c} of 11.2%) presents with a HF symptoms. He is found to have a reduced LVEF of 34%. He is subsequently taken to the cardiac catheterization lab for coronary angiography and was found to have obstructive disease of the right coronary artery (RCA) and a severe stenosis of the left anterior descending (LAD) artery.

What are the next best steps in management?
  A. Treat heart failure symptoms
  B. Obtain stress test
  C. CABG
  D. Multivessel PCI

14. A 68-year-old man with a history of intermittent substernal exertional chest pain over the past 3 weeks presents for an ECG exercise stress test. He can complete 4 metabolic equivalents (METs) before he stops because of angina. The maximum HR achieved is 112 beats/min, which is 74% of the maximum predicted HR by age. Initial BP is 136/82 mmHg and at peak exercise is 126/80 mmHg. The ECG obtained 7 minutes into recovery is shown below:

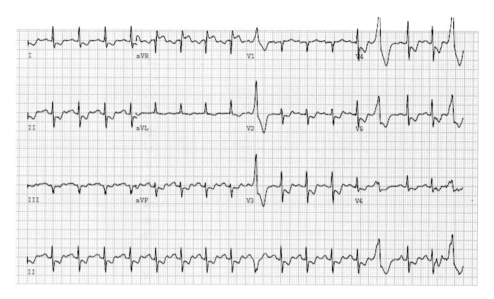

What is the next best diagnostic test?

A. Cardiac MRI
B. Coronary angiography
C. Coronary CTA
D. Repeat pharmacologic stress test with perfusion imaging

15. A 72-year-old man with HTN presented to primary care clinic with complaints of exertional chest pain that subsided at rest. His home medications included aspirin and lisinopril. He was referred for an exercise treadmill test. He achieved 90% of his maximum predicted HR and experienced chest pain at peak exercise. His ECG exhibited nonspecific changes. Perfusion imaging demonstrated mild lateral wall ischemia with an estimated LVEF of 65%.

Which of the following would be the next most appropriate step?

A. Initiate β-blocker and statin
B. Perform a TTE
C. Reassure patient with no change in medical therapy
D. Refer for coronary angiography

16. A 57-year-old man is admitted to the cardiac intensive care unit (ICU) for closer monitoring following uncomplicated placement of a drug-eluting stent to the proximal LAD artery after presenting with an anterior STEMI. The right femoral artery was accessed for the procedure. Three hours after the procedure, the patient feels a "pop" in his groin after coughing. Thereafter, a rapidly expanding mass is observed in the right groin.

Which of the following is the most appropriate first step in his management?

A. Administration of blood products
B. Antiplatelet therapy discontinuation
C. CT of the abdomen
D. Manual compression of the access site

17. A 63-year-old woman with a history of hyperlipidemia and CAD for which she underwent elective placement of a drug-eluting stent for stable ischemic heart disease 7 months ago presents to routine primary care clinic follow-up. She remains adherent to her dual anti-platelet therapy with aspirin and clopidogrel. She strongly wishes to undergo elective right knee replacement, which would require discontinuation of clopidogrel periprocedurally.

Which of the following would you recommend?

A. A pharmacologic stress test with perfusion imaging can guide safety of clopidogrel discontinuation

B. Clopidogrel can be held to permit a knee replacement

C. Elective knee replacement must be deferred until 12 months of dual antiplatelet therapy have been completed

D. The procedure can be performed with an intravenous (IV) cangrelor bridge once clopidogrel has been discontinued

18. A 63-year-old man with no known past medical history presents to the ED with 20 minutes of substernal chest pressure radiating to his left arm and occurring at rest. It resolved spontaneously shortly following his presentation. His ECG shows no ST-segment or T-wave changes. Serial troponin values are undetectable.

Which of the following is the next appropriate step in his management?

A. A conservative strategy of aspirin, β-blocker, and nitrates, as needed, followed by noninvasive risk stratification (stress testing) to help determine if coronary angiography is appropriate, provided the patient remains asymptomatic

B. Discharge the patient home

C. Plan for coronary angiography within 24 to 72 hours of presentation

D. Urgent angiography with the intent to revascularize

19. A 42-year-old woman with no known medical history presented with substernal chest pain for 1 hour. ECG shows diffuse nonspecific ST-segment changes. First troponin is elevated >99th percentile. She is taken for urgent coronary angiography because of ongoing chest pain refractory to medical management. Coronary angiography revealed no obstructive epicardial CAD with 30% mid-LAD disease and 20% distal RCA disease. TTE reveals diffuse hypokinesis with an LVEF of 40%.

The next best step is:

A. Cardiac MRI

B. Dobutamine stress test

C. Transesophageal echocardiogram (TEE)

D. Coronary CTA (CCTA)

20. A 45-year-old man with no past medical history presents with acute-onset substernal chest pain. His physical examination reveals a BP of 98/72 mmHg, a HR of 108 beats/min, and a respiratory rate of 24 breaths/min. His jugular venous pressure (JVP) is elevated. Cardio-vascular examination is notable for tachycardia with an S_3 gallop appreciated. He has basilar rales on posterior auscultation of his lungs and his lower extremities are cool to the touch. His presenting 12-lead ECG demonstrates inferior ST-segment elevations prompting urgent coronary angiography.

At this stage, which of the following medications should be avoided?

A. Aspirin

B. Atorvastatin

C. Metoprolol

D. Ticagrelor

21. A 75-year-old woman presents several hours after symptom onset with an anterior STEMI. She undergoes emergent coronary angiography with placement of a drug-eluting stent to her proximal LAD artery via the right femoral artery. She is admitted to the cardiac ICU for monitoring. On day 3 in the hospital, she becomes acutely hypotensive, requiring escalating vasopressor support. Physical examination reveals a harsh holosystolic murmur best heard at the left lower sternal border with a palpable systolic thrill. Her femoral artery access site is without evidence of a hematoma.

Which of the following is the next best diagnostic step?

A. Measurement of intracardiac pressures by pulmonary artery (PA) catheter
B. Noncontrast CT of the abdomen/pelvis
C. Urgent repeat coronary angiography to assess stent patency
D. Urgent TTE

22. A 65-year-old man presents to a non–percutaneous coronary intervention (PCI)-capable hospital with crushing substernal chest pain that began while shoveling snow. A 12-lead ECG reveals 2-mm ST-segment elevations in the anterior leads. He is initiated on appropriate therapy but requires vasopressor support for evolving cardiogenic shock. Because of the inclement weather, the nearest PCI-capable hospital is >3 hours away.

Which of the following would be the most appropriate management strategies?

A. Administer alteplase within 30 minutes of hospital arrival and proceed with transfer to PCI-capable facility if evidence of failed reperfusion or reocclusion
B. Administer alteplase within 30 minutes of hospital arrival and proceed with urgent transfer to PCI-capable facility
C. Administer alteplase within 30 minutes of hospital arrival and transfer to PCI-capable facility within 3 to 24 hours
D. Initiate immediate transfer to a PCI-capable facility

23. A 36-year-old G1P1 now 5 days postpartum presents with 9/10 substernal burning chest pain and diaphoresis for the past 45 minutes. Initial vitals notable for tachycardia with HR 120 beats/min, BP 90/74 mmHg. ECG is shown below:

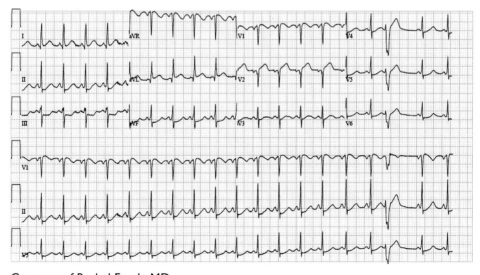

Courtesy of Rachel Frank, MD.

The next best step is:

A. Activate cardiac catheterization lab for coronary angiography
B. Schedule elective stress test
C. Obtain TEE
D. Treat for hyperkalemia

24. A 67-year-old man with a history of HTN, hyperlipidemia, type 2 diabetes, peptic ulcer disease, and ischemic stroke presents to the ED with sudden-onset substernal chest pain. His home medication regimen includes amlodipine, aspirin, atorvastatin, and metformin. Vital signs reveal a HR of 60 beats/min and BP of 169/100 mmHg. His initial ECG is notable for 2 mm ST elevations in the anterior leads (V_2-V_4), so a code STEMI is called. He is at a non-PCI-capable hospital, and the closest hospital with PCI capability is 4 hours away. He recently had an ischemic stroke 1 month prior to admission and has a history of peptic ulcer disease diagnosed in the setting of a gastrointestinal (GI) bleed 9 years prior to the current presentation. Fibrinolytic therapy is contemplated.

Which of the following would be an absolute contraindication for fibrinolytic therapy?

A. BP of 169/100 mmHg
B. History of ischemic stroke <3 months prior to admission
C. Aspirin use
D. Prior history of peptic ulcer disease

25. A 61-year-old man presents with unrelenting substernal chest pain that started 30 minutes ago and is found to have inferior ST-segment elevation and no other ECG changes. He is hemodynamically stable. He is brought for urgent coronary angiography where he is found to have an occluded mid-RCA. He is also found to have an 80% proximal LAD lesion.

In addition to stenting the RCA, what would be the best course of action?

A. Make arrangements to stent the LAD in the next 45 days
B. Make no further plans for revascularization
C. Perform fractional flow reserve on the LAD lesion
D. Schedule an outpatient stress test to evaluate the LAD

26. A 52-year-old man with a history of hyperlipidemia and recently diagnosed colon cancer on FOLFOX presents to the ED with sudden-onset substernal chest pressure at rest with radiation to his left shoulder. His symptoms promptly improved with sublingual nitroglycerin administered by paramedics. His initial ECG is notable for sinus tachycardia with transient inferior ST-segment elevation. High-sensitivity troponin testing reveals mildly elevated serum troponin. He is taken for urgent coronary angiography, which reveals normal coronary anatomy without evidence of significant coronary disease. He is admitted to a cardiac step-down unit for monitoring and remains chest pain free. A repeat echocardiogram shows preserved cardiac function without wall motion abnormality.

What is the most likely cause of this patient's presentation?

A. Leucovorin
B. Oxaliplatin
C. 5-fluorouracil (5-FU)
D. Stress cardiomyopathy

27. A 78-year-old woman with HTN presented with NSTEMI and underwent placement of a drug-eluting stent to her RCA. Her low-density lipoprotein cholesterol (LDL-C) on a high-intensity statin is 105 mg/dL.

    What, if any, changes should be made to her lipid-lowering regimen prior to discharge?
    A. Add a bile sequestrant
    B. Add a fibrate
    C. Add ezetimibe
    D. Continue high-intensity statin alone

28. An 83-year-old woman with a history of hyperlipidemia presented with NSTEMI and declined coronary arteriography. She was managed conservatively and initiated on a high-intensity statin and a β-blocker.

    Her antiplatelet regimen initially should ideally include which of the following drugs?
    A. Aspirin
    B. Prasugrel
    C. Ticagrelor
    D. A and B
    E. A and C

29. A 56-year-old man presents with recurrent episodes of substernal chest pain for 15 minutes at rest accompanied by ST-segment depressions on ECG that resolve after administration of sublingual nitroglycerin. Acute myocardial infarction is demonstrated with a rise and fall of troponin. His serum creatinine is normal.

    In addition to appropriate pharmacotherapy, what is the next best strategy for him?
    A. CT coronary angiography
    B. Inpatient stress test
    C. Invasive coronary angiography
    D. Outpatient stress test

30. You now consider the timing of angiography for the patient in Question 29. What would be the optimal timing?
    A. Immediately
    B. Within 24 hours
    C. Within 72 hours

31. A 45-year-old woman with a history of migraines presents with acute-onset crushing substernal chest pain. ECG demonstrates marked anterior ST-segment elevations. After 10 minutes, the patient's pain abruptly resolves following administration of nitroglycerin and the ECG returns to normal. Coronary angiography is performed and shows minimal evidence of obstructive CAD.

    Which therapy is most likely to help mitigate the risk of the patient experiencing recurrent symptoms?
    A. Aspirin
    B. Clopidogrel
    C. Diltiazem
    D. Metoprolol

32. A 57-year-old man with HTN, hyperlipidemia, and diabetes presents with retrosternal chest pressure radiating to the jaw that began at rest and has now lasted for 1 hour. His presenting troponin is just above the upper limit of normal. The presenting ECG is shown below:

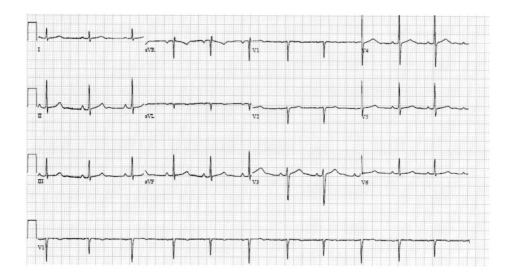

Which of the following would be the first next best step?

A. CT to assess for pulmonary embolism
B. Posterior leads (leads V_7-V_9)
C. Right-sided precordial leads (V_4R-V_6R)
D. Serial troponin measurements

33. A 55-year-old female with past medical history of HTN and hypothyroidism presents to the ED with 2 days of chest pain, present at rest and at exertion. On initial evaluation, her ECG demonstrates ST depressions in all precordial leads and her serum high-sensitivity troponin rises from 4300 to 4457 ng/L. She is administered 325 mg of aspirin and taken emergently to the cardiac catheterization lab, where she is found to have nonobstructive coronary disease. On subsequent TTE, she is found to have globally reduced systolic function, scattered regional wall motion abnormalities, and a small pericardial effusion.

Which of the following is the most likely diagnosis?

A. Coronary artery dissection
B. Myocarditis
C. Microvascular CAD
D. Stress cardiomyopathy

34. A 60-year-old man with diabetes is hospitalized with NSTEMI and undergoes placement of a drug-eluting stent in his RCA. He has no other medical problems and is without complaints. His current medication regimen includes aspirin, clopidogrel, metoprolol, metformin, and atorvastatin. He is at low risk of bleeding. The patient inquires when he can stop clopidogrel.

What would be your recommendation?

A. Stop clopidogrel at 3 months because it is a drug-eluting stent
B. Stop clopidogrel at 6 months because it is a drug-eluting stent
C. Stop clopidogrel now and continue aspirin monotherapy
D. Take clopidogrel for at least 1 year

CARDIOLOGY

35. You are called to the bedside of a 52-year-old man with a history of coronary disease who is in the ICU with hypotension on day 7 of his hospitalization. The patient is intubated and warm on examination. He underwent placement of a PA catheter for worsening hemodynamic instability. As you are waiting for labs, imaging, echo, and ECG, you obtain intracardiac pressures from the PA catheter, which show central venous pressure 4, PA 28/12, and pulmonary capillary wedge pressure (PCWP) 8 (all in mmHg). Cardiac index (CI) by Fick is 4.2 L/min.

What is the most likely etiology of his shock?

A. Cardiogenic shock
B. Distributive shock
C. Hypovolemic shock
D. Obstructive shock

36. A 53-year-old woman with severe symptomatic mitral regurgitation secondary to mitral valve prolapse is admitted to the cardiac ICU. A PA catheter is inserted to understand her intracardiac hemodynamics. Her mean PCWP is 20 mmHg.

What would you expect her mean left atrial pressure and LV end-diastolic pressure (LVEDP) to be in comparison to the wedge pressure?

A. Left atrial—higher; LVEDP—higher
B. Left atrial—higher; LVEDP—same
C. Left atrial—lower; LVEDP—lower
D. Left atrial—same; LVEDP—lower

37. A 61-year-old man with HFrEF (20%) is admitted to the ICU for cardiogenic shock. He is started on dobutamine at 2 μg/kg/min and started on a lasix drip at 10 mg/h based on his clinical examination. His HR is 110 beats/min and his BP is 110/70 mmHg. Later that day, a PA catheter is placed and his relevant filling pressures are: central venous pressure 12, PA 50/26, PCWP 24 (all in mmHg), and systemic vascular resistance (SVR) 1630 dynes/s/cm^{-5}. CI by thermodilution is 1.8 L/min/m^2 (cardiac output 3.5 L/min).

Which of the following changes would you make first?

A. Add norepinephrine
B. Add vasopressin
C. Increase dobutamine
D. Increase lasix drip dose

38. An 88-year-old woman is admitted to the ICU for altered mental status, fever, and poor urinary output. She is found to have a depressed EF with a low cardiac output and is started on dobutamine. Her BP continues to trend downward and a PA line is placed. Her BP is 90/45 mmHg (mean arterial pressure [MAP] 60 mmHg) on low-dose norepinephrine with decreasing urine output. Her lactate is 4.5 mg/dL. Her central venous pressure is 11 mmHg and PCWP 12 mmHg. Her cardiac output on inotropes is 4 L/min, CI 1.8 L/min/m^2, and SVR 1000 dynes/s/cm^{-5}.

How would you classify her shock?

A. Mixed—cardiogenic and distributive
B. Purely cardiogenic
C. Purely distributive
D. Tamponade

39. A 79-year-old woman presented late with an anterior MI and underwent primary PCI. She was in cardiogenic shock; a PA catheter was placed, she was started on medium-dose dobutamine, and was admitted to the cardiac ICU. Her hemodynamics began to slowly improve. On the third day in the hospital, her BP and urine output decreased and her extremities were cooler. Conversely, her mixed venous saturation (MVO_2) markedly increased from 65% to 85%.

What is the next best step?

A. Add norepinephrine
B. Continue to monitor her MVO_2 saturation
C. Decrease the dobutamine
D. Emergent TTE

40. A 54-year-old man transfers his care to your primary care practice and you are seeing him for an initial visit to establish care. He has a history of ischemic cardiomyopathy following an MI 1 year ago and has shortness of breath with exertion. A TTE from 1 year ago revealed an LVEF of 27%. He underwent implantation of an implantable cardioverter-defibrillator (ICD) 10 months ago. You review his medication regimen with him.

Which of the following medications has NOT been shown to reduce mortality in patients with symptomatic HF with reduced LV function?

A. Carvedilol
B. Furosemide
C. Lisinopril
D. Spironolactone

41. A 75-year-old woman with HF with preserved EF and stage 3 chronic kidney disease presents to the ED with 2 weeks of progressive weight gain, increased abdominal girth, and orthopnea. She has been using escalating doses of diuretics at home without relief of her symptoms (original home dose furosemide 20 mg daily, now taking 40 mg twice daily). Vital signs on presentation reveal a HR of 88 beats/min, BP of 146/78 mmHg, and oxygen saturation of 94% on room air. Physical examination is notable for bibasilar crackles and JVD, and lower extremities are warm with edema graded 2+ to the thighs. Laboratory evaluation reveals acute kidney injury (AKI) with a serum creatinine of 1.7 mg/dL (baseline 1.2 mg/dL 2 months prior).

What is the next most appropriate step in care?

A. Administer intravenous crystalloid
B. Administer intravenous furosemide
C. Administer oral furosemide
D. Initiate inotropes in the cardiac ICU, given concern for cardiogenic shock

42. A 60-year-old woman presents to the ED with an acute anterior MI complicated by cardiogenic shock. She has a history of HTN, type 2 diabetes, ischemic cardiomyopathy, AF on warfarin, ascending aortic aneurysm, moderate aortic regurgitation, and severe mitral regurgitation. Vital signs reveal a HR of 102 beats/min, BP of 80/50 mmHg, and oxygen saturation of 86% on room air. Her examination is notable for normal heart sounds, cool distal extremities, and 1+ lower extremity edema. The cardiac catheterization lab is activated and will be ready in 30 minutes. Your intern asks if an intra-aortic balloon pump would be beneficial for temporary support. You review the mechanism of a balloon pump.

Which of the following is NOT a benefit of an intra-aortic balloon pump?

A. Decreased aortic regurgitation
B. Decreased myocardial oxygen demand
C. Increased cardiac output
D. Increased coronary perfusion

43. A 32-year-old man with an idiopathic dilated cardiomyopathy (LVEF 18%) is admitted for shortness of breath. On examination, his JVP is 14 cm, he has bibasilar crackles, and has 2+ pitting edema in his lower extremities. His lower extremities are warm. His lactate is 1.2 mg/dL, liver function tests (LFTs) are normal, creatinine is 0.9 mg/dL, and urine output is 100 mL/h over the past 6 hours. BP is 90/60 mmHg.

Which of the following therapies would you start in him?

A. Diuresis + inotropes
B. Diuresis + vasopressors
C. Diuresis alone
D. Inotropes alone

44. A 73-year-old female with a history of HFrEF, CAD, and diabetes mellitus is seen in outpatient clinic for a follow-up visit. She can ambulate around her home without difficulty and regularly participates in a cardiac rehabilitation program. Her home medications include aspirin, atorvastatin, sacubitril-valsartan, metoprolol succinate, spironolactone, and dulaglutide.

Which medication should be added to her guideline-directed medical therapy (GDMT)?

A. Dapagliflozin
B. Isosorbide mononitrate
C. Diltiazem
D. Glipizide

45. A 70-year-old man with a history of ischemic cardiomyopathy, last EF of 18%, presents to the ED after an episode of acute-onset nausea, chest pain, and syncope. He reports no longer feeling nauseated but feels weak and short of breath. On examination, you notice his extremities are cool to the touch and he has no peripheral edema or JVD; he has no crackles on lung auscultation. Vitals are checked showing a HR of 105 beats/min, BP 95/75 mmHg, respiratory rate 18 breaths/min, and 100% O_2 saturation. His serum lactate is 4.0 mmol/L. A technician comes to interrogate the patient's ICD and notes there was a sustained run of monomorphic ventricular tachycardia (VT) prior to presentation. The patient is transferred to the cardiac ICU and a PA line is inserted for tailored therapy. The pulmonary arterial pressure is measured at 30/15 mmHg and the PCWP is 12 mmHg. Using the thermodilution technique, you note the CI to be low at 1.8 L/min/m² and the SVR to be high at 2000 dynes/s/cm⁻⁵.

Which of the following would be the most helpful intervention to improve CI?

A. Nitroprusside
B. Furosemide
C. Amiodarone
D. Metoprolol

46. A 66-year-old woman with long-standing HTN and obstructive sleep apnea is admitted to the hospital with dyspnea on exertion and a 30 lb weight gain. Physical examination reveals a pulse of 90 beats/min, BP of 175/85 mmHg, JVP of 12 cm, bibasilar crackles, and 2+ lower extremity edema to her shins. Laboratory testing reveals a creatinine of 1.2 mg/dL. TTE reveals a LVEF of 60% without wall motion abnormalities and normal valvular function. She is admitted to the cardiology service and is diuresed. Her BP is effectively treated with amlodipine.

What medication can be started in this patient to reduce the risk of rehospitalization for HF?

A. Aspirin
B. Lisinopril
C. Sildenafil
D. Empagliflozin

47. A 56-year-old man with a newly diagnosed nonischemic cardiomyopathy (LVEF 20%) is discharged. New cardiac medications during this admission include sacubitril/valsartan 24/26 mg PO BID, carvedilol 12.5 mg PO BID, and spironolactone 12.5 mg PO daily. He was previously on torsemide 20 mg PO BID and this is continued at the time of discharge. He is seen 7 days after discharge and reports new dizziness and light-headedness. Vital signs are notable for sinus tachycardia with a HR of 110 beats/min, BP 88/66 mmHg, and he is saturating 98% on room air. His JVP is <5 cm by examination. Labs are notable for creatinine 2.2 mg/dL (baseline 0.9 mg/dL).

Which of the following may have contributed to the aforementioned presentation?

A. Increased sodium intake after discharge
B. Medication noncompliance
C. No reduction in diuretic dosing after starting sacubitril/valsartan
D. Increased fluid intake

48. A 56-year-old man with an idiopathic dilated cardiomyopathy (LVEF 15%) had stopped all his medications because of financial constraints and is admitted for acute decompensated HF with pulmonary edema and elevated serum creatinine and lactate. His BP is 85/50 mmHg. Empiric dobutamine and low-dose norepinephrine are started. A PA line is placed, his filling pressures are high, and his CI on medium- to high-dose dobutamine is 1.5 L/min/m². He is anuric despite diuretics, and his lactate remains elevated.

What is the next best step?

A. Increase the inotropes and diuretics
B. Increase the norepinephrine
C. Insert a percutaneous LV assist device (eg, Impella or TandemHeart)
D. Insert an intra-aortic balloon pump

49. A 21-year-old college student is referred to the ED for generalized fatigue and dyspnea. His presenting systolic BP is 60 mmHg and his lower extremities are cool. A bedside ultrasound reveals severely impaired left and right ventricular function. His high-sensitivity troponin T level is very elevated at 2320 ng/L. A rapid influenza test subsequently returns positive. A PA catheter is inserted and he is initiated on dobutamine, norepinephrine, and vasopressin for hemodynamic support. Over the subsequent 6 hours, the patient's pharmacologic support is escalated to maximal ionotropic and vasopressor support with marginal hemodynamics.

Which of the following would be the next most appropriate step in management?

A. Emergency coronary arteriography
B. Initiation of venoarterial extracorporeal membrane oxygenation
C. Insertion of a percutaneous ventricular assist device
D. Insertion of an intra-aortic balloon pump

50. A 33-year-old man presents to the ED with 1 day of fever, myalgias, and dyspnea. He has a history of a long-standing polysubstance use disorder, including alcohol, cocaine, and intravenous heroin. Over the last 6 months, he has not been able to climb a flight of stairs without experiencing shortness of breath. Vital signs are notable for sinus tachycardia with HRs in the 110 to 120 beats/min range.

A nasal swab returns positive for influenza. A chest radiograph shows interstitial pulmonary opacities and bilateral pleural effusions. A TTE is obtained and shows a dilated cardiomyopathy with an LVEF of 18%. He undergoes a thorough investigation for causes of his cardiomyopathy. Coronary angiography reveals no significant CAD. A cardiac MRI does not suggest acute myocarditis. Laboratory testing results include a negative human immunodeficiency virus (HIV) test, a normal serum protein electrophoresis (SPEP), normal iron studies, an antinuclear antibody (ANA) titer positive at 1:40, and a normal thyroid-stimulating hormone (TSH). He is started on oseltamivir and furosemide with significant improvement in symptoms. He is seen by psychiatry and is committed to abstinence from substance use.

Which of the following is the next best step regarding management of his cardiomyopathy?

A. Discharge on oseltamivir and furosemide with plans to repeat TTE in 1 month; if EF is still depressed, initiate neurohormonal blockade
B. Initiation of angiotensin-converting enzyme (ACE) inhibitor and β-blocker; repeat TTE in 3 months
C. Myocardial biopsy to determine etiology of cardiomyopathy
D. Placement of an ICD prior to discharge

51. A 52-year-old woman with hypertrophic obstructive cardiomyopathy (HOCM) and an LV outflow gradient of 60 mmHg is admitted to the ICU with septic shock. Two liters of intravenous crystalloid and broad-spectrum antibiotics are administered. Central and arterial lines are placed at the bedside. Central venous pressure is now 12 mmHg. The MAP is 55 mmHg and the intensivist recommends initiation of vasopressors for BP augmentation. She is started on norepinephrine, and despite rapid dose escalation, her BP continues to decline.

What is the next best step in this patient's care?

A. Administer additional intravenous crystalloid
B. Discontinue norepinephrine and initiate phenylephrine
C. Start dobutamine in addition to norepinephrine
D. Start trial of diuretics

52. A 44-year-old male was newly diagnosed with hypertrophic cardiomyopathy after a routine ECG was noted to be abnormal. There is no family history of sudden cardiac death, and he reports no personal history of syncope or palpitations. TTE shows LVEF of 65% without LV aneurysm. LV maximal wall thickness is 27 mm.

Which of the following would be a reason to consider primary prevention ICD placement?

A. BP decrease of ≥20 mmHg with exercise
B. 5% late gadolinium enhancement on cardiac MRI
C. LVEF 55%
D. None of the above

53. A 72-year-old man presents to the ED with bilateral leg swelling. He has a history of HTN, AF on warfarin, multiple myeloma, stage 3 chronic kidney disease, and Parkinson disease. Oxygen saturation on room air is 86%, which improves to 94% with 2 L of supplemental oxygen by nasal cannula. Physical examination is notable for JVP to 14 cm and pitting edema to the knees. Cardiac examination reveals a II/VI midsystolic crescendo-decrescendo murmur at the right upper sternal border and an S_4 gallop. Pulmonary examination reveals bilateral crackles at the lung bases.

A chest radiograph reveals interstitial pulmonary opacities and a right pleural effusion. N-terminal b-type natriuretic peptide (NT-proBNP) is 8000 pg/mL (previously 500 pg/mL). An ECG is notable for low voltages and diffuse T-wave abnormalities. A TTE from 1 year ago reveals an LVEF of 66%, biventricular wall thickening, an enlarged left atrium, and evidence of diastolic dysfunction.

What is the most likely etiology of his diastolic HF?

A. Amyloidosis
B. Hypertrophic cardiomyopathy
C. Long-standing HTN
D. Sarcoidosis

54. A 32-year-old man with a history of HOCM presents to your clinic. He feels well today and has no new symptoms. His echocardiogram reveals an LVEF of 75% with increased LV wall thickness of 15 mm (normal 7-11 mm) and systolic anterior motion of his mitral valve. He recently was reading information about his cardiac disease online and is worried about the risk of sudden cardiac death.

Which of the following is NOT a high-risk feature for sudden cardiac death in patients with HOCM?

A. Family history of sudden cardiac death
B. LV wall thickness of 15 mm
C. Nonsustained VT
D. Unexplained syncope

55. A patient with known HOCM presents to clinic for routine follow-up. He has experienced persistent symptoms of shortness of breath and activity intolerance despite maximal uptitration of current medications. His regimen includes metoprolol succinate, verapamil, aspirin, and a multivitamin. You perform an echocardiogram in clinic that shows redemonstration of LV hypertrophy with a disproportionally thick septum and a left ventricular outflow tract (LVOT) gradient at rest of 45 mmHg.

What is the most appropriate next step in management?

A. Add digoxin
B. Start furosemide
C. Make no changes and follow up in 6 months
D. Refer for surgical myomectomy

56. An 80-year-old male presents to the hospital with several months of progressive weight gain, dyspnea on exertion, and leg swelling. He also complains of pins-and-needles sensation in his fingers. An echocardiogram reveals a small LV cavity, biatrial dilation, and thick ventricular walls (interventricular septum thickness = 17 mm). A laboratory evaluation reveals a normal SPEP and serum free light chains (SFLC), normal iron studies, and a normal ANA.

Which of the following is the next best diagnostic evaluation?

A. Technetium-99m pyrophosphate scan
B. Endomyocardial biopsy
C. Cardiac positron emission tomography (PET) scan
D. Fat pad biopsy

57. A 58-year-old woman with HTN and hyperlipidemia presents to the ED with chest pressure and shortness of breath. Her husband died unexpectedly 2 days ago. Her ECG shows ST elevations in leads V_2 to V_6 and her high-sensitivity troponin T is slightly elevated to 28 ng/L. A TTE reveals an akinetic apex with a hyperkinetic base. LVEF is 34%.

Which of the following is the next best step?

A. Coronary angiography
B. Observation for 24 hours with serial troponin and then discharge if no arrhythmias or hemodynamic instability
C. Reassurance, discharge, and repeat TTE in 1 to 2 weeks
D. Trial of antacid and anxiolytic

58. A 56-year-old man presents with focal neurologic deficits and was subsequently found to have a stroke involving the left middle cerebral artery (MCA). As part of his stroke workup, he undergoes a TTE. Echocardiogram reveals severe biventricular dysfunction with LVEF of 25%. There are no regional wall motion abnormalities noted. An ischemia evaluation is unrevealing. On further history, the patient reports drinking six 4-oz alcoholic drinks per night. During the hospitalization, he was found to have paroxysmal AF with rapid ventricular response lasting 5 minutes and terminating spontaneously.

Which of the following is the best advice for the patient regarding his alcohol use?

A. Absolute abstinence from alcohol
B. Limiting alcohol use to <7 drinks per week
C. Limiting alcohol use to <14 drinks per week
D. No limitations on alcohol use

59. You are asked to evaluate a 68-year-old man who presents to the ED with syncope. He has a history of HFrEF, CAD, and type 2 diabetes. He was walking to the bathroom when he felt light-headed and collapsed, awaking seconds afterward. He noted no chest pain or palpitations preceding the event. His initial vital signs include a HR of 64 beats/min, BP of 106/62 mmHg, and oxygen saturation of 96% on room air. His ECG shows normal sinus rhythm and repolarization abnormalities consistent with LV hypertrophy. A TTE is performed, which reveals an LVEF of 30%, thickening and calcification of the aortic valve, valve area of 0.8 cm^2, and mean gradient across the aortic valve of 28 mmHg.

Which of the following is the next best step?

A. Proceed to dobutamine stress echo
B. Proceed to surgical aortic valve replacement
C. Proceed to transcatheter aortic valve replacement
D. Repeat TTE in 1 year

60. A 52-year-old woman with no significant past medical history is seen by her primary care physician and found to have a new murmur. She feels well and maintains an active lifestyle, running 2 to 3 miles every day without symptoms. Her vital signs reveal a HR of 65 beats/min and BP of 100/60 mmHg. Cardiac auscultation reveals a II/VI systolic mid-peaking crescendo-decrescendo murmur. A TTE is obtained, which shows a bicuspid aortic valve with aortic valve area of 1.2 cm^2 and mean gradient of 32 mmHg.

What is the next best step regarding her aortic valve disease?

A. Consult cardiothoracic surgery for aortic valve replacement during this admission
B. Outpatient referral for aortic valve replacement
C. Repeat TEE next month
D. Repeat TTE every 1 to 2 years

61. A 69-year-old man with HTN presents to cardiology clinic with dyspnea on exertion for 1 month. He subsequently undergoes invasive coronary angiography, which shows nonobstructive CAD, and a TTE, which shows severe aortic stenosis. He has a trileaflet aortic valve. His Society of Thoracic Surgery (STS) predicted risk of surgical mortality is 2%.

Which of the following is the next best step in management?

A. Heart team approach to determine recommendation for surgical versus transcatheter aortic valve replacement
B. Referral to cardiothoracic surgery for surgical aortic valve replacement
C. Referral to interventional cardiology for transcatheter aortic valve replacement
D. Trial of medical management prior to aortic valve replacement

62. A 27-year-old man with no past medical history presents to his primary care physician after an episode of syncope while walking up a flight of stairs. He had a TTE performed, which

was notable for an LVEF of 57% and severe aortic stenosis (aortic velocity 4.3 m/s, mean gradient 54 mmHg, and peak gradient 90 mmHg) in the setting of a unicuspid aortic valve. He has no known history of bleeding complications.

What is the best next step in management?

A. Bioprosthetic aortic valve replacement
B. Mechanical aortic valve replacement
C. Aortic balloon valvuloplasty
D. Repeat TTE in 6 months

63. A 62-year-old obese man presents to the ED with acute onset of dyspnea. He has a history of smoking, HTN, and hyperlipidemia. He reports that 3 days prior to admission, he had substernal chest pain lasting hours that he thought was heartburn, although it was not alleviated with over-the-counter antacids. Vital signs are notable for HR of 120 beats/min, BP of 70/50 mmHg, and oxygen saturation of 84% on room air. Physical examination is notable for elevated jugular venous pulsations and normal heart sounds with a II/VI holosystolic murmur at the apex without thrill. Pulmonary auscultation reveals bilateral crackles halfway up the lung fields. ECG shows Q waves in II, III, and aVF.

What is the most likely etiology of his presentation?

A. LV dysfunction
B. Mitral regurgitation
C. Pulmonary embolism
D. Ventricular septal rupture

64. An 81-year-old woman presents to the hospital after a mechanical fall and is found to have a hip fracture. She has a history of mechanical aortic valve replacement 10 years ago, AF diagnosed 3 years ago, hypothyroidism, and HTN. Home medications include warfarin, amlodipine, and levothyroxine. She has a history of cardiac thromboembolism 6 years ago, after which her international normalized ratio (INR) goal was increased to 2.5 to 3.5. Vital signs reveal HR of 60 beats/min and BP of 120/60 mmHg. Physical examination is remarkable for left leg external rotation, abduction, and shortening compared to the right leg. You are consulted for perioperative management of her anticoagulation. She is on coumadin and has been taking her anticoagulation regularly. INR on presentation is 2.7.

Which of the following would be recommended?

A. Stop coumadin 2 days prior to surgery and restart 12 to 24 hours afterward without any heparin bridge
B. Stop coumadin indefinitely given fall risk
C. Stop coumadin now and bridge with unfractionated heparin
D. Switch from coumadin to dabigatran

65. A 69-year-old female with a history of HTN and aortic regurgitation presents for follow-up in outpatient clinic. Her last TTE 1 year prior showed a normal EF (LVEF 60%), severe aortic regurgitation, a left ventricular end-systolic diameter (LVESD) of 44 mm, and an aortic root diameter of 39 mm. Today, she had a repeat TTE that showed an LVEF of 51%, severe aortic regurgitation, a LVESD of 46 mm, and an aortic root diameter of 40 mm. She has remained asymptomatic and is very active walking 3 to 5 miles/day without any significant limitations. Her current medication regimen includes atorvastatin and lisinopril.

What is the best next step in management?

A. Repeat a TTE in 6 months
B. Dobutamine stress echocardiogram
C. Referral for aortic valve replacement
D. Cardiac magnetic resonance angiography

66. A 52-year-old woman presents to your clinic for evaluation of a heart murmur. She has a history of HTN that is well treated with amlodipine. She reports that she continues to live an active lifestyle and enjoys running for exercise. She denies any dyspnea or angina on exertion. Vital signs are notable for HR of 80 beats/min, BP of 110/60 mmHg, and oxygen saturation of 99% on room air. Physical examination is notable for a regular rate, normal heart sounds with a II/VI holosystolic murmur at the apex without a thrill. Echocardiogram reveals an LVEF of 55%, anterior mitral valve prolapse with severe mitral regurgitation, and a left ventricular end-systolic diameter (LVESD) of 41 mm.

What is the next best step in management?

A. Initiate furosemide
B. Order ambulatory ECG monitoring to screen for AF
C. Refer for mitral valve surgery
D. Repeat TTE in 6 months

67. A 69-year-old woman with a history of mitral valve prolapse with mechanical mitral valve replacement presents to the ED after she was found to have an INR of 9.1 on routine lab testing. Her previous INR goal has been 2.5 to 3.5. Vital signs reveal HR of 60 beats/min and BP of 120/80 mmHg. Her hemoglobin is 12.1 (previously 12.9). There are no obvious signs of bleeding.

What is the best next step in management?

A. Administer IV vitamin K
B. Administer prothrombin complex concentrate
C. Hold the warfarin and monitor
D. Administer fresh frozen plasma

68. A 32-year-old woman in the 22nd week of her first pregnancy presents to your clinic for evaluation of a heart murmur. She has a history of rheumatic mitral stenosis. Prior to her pregnancy, she felt well and had no limitations to exercise or daily activity. Over the past 2 weeks, she has had progressive dyspnea with minimal exertion. Vital signs are notable for HR of 60 beats/min, BP of 120/70 mmHg, and oxygen saturation of 99% on room air. Physical examination is notable for a regular rate, normal heart sounds with a high-pitched early diastolic sound followed by a mid-diastolic rumble heard at the apex. Echocardiogram reveals an LVEF of 55%, rheumatic mitral stenosis with mitral valve area of 1.2 cm², and mean gradient of 11 mmHg.

What is the next best step in management?

A. Initiate metoprolol
B. Initiate warfarin
C. Refer for mitral valve surgery
D. Refer for percutaneous mitral balloon commissurotomy as anatomy allows

69. A 45-year-old female with HTN, hyperlipidemia, and prediabetes is evaluated for sharp chest pain that started 8 hours ago. She is afebrile and normotensive with sinus tachycardia. Her lungs are clear to auscultation and her cardiovascular examination reveals no rubs, murmurs, or gallops, no peripheral edema or JVD. Laboratory work reveals normal serial high-sensitivity troponin and an elevated C-reactive protein. ECG shows diffuse ST-segment elevation with PR-segment depression. A TTE shows preserved cardiac function without wall motion or acute valvular abnormality, and a small pericardial effusion.

Which of the following is the most appropriate next step in management?

A. Pericardiocentesis
B. Pharmacologic stress testing
C. Emergent cardiac catheterization
D. High-dose aspirin and colchicine

70. A 58-year-old woman with a history of breast cancer presents with shortness of breath. She reports progressive shortness of breath over the past 3 days that has steadily worsened. Initial vital signs are notable for a HR of 104 beats/min, a BP of 88/64 mmHg, and a respiratory rate of 28 breaths/min. Physical examination reveals jugular venous pulsation at 12 cm and muffled heart sounds. You check for a pulsus paradoxus and find that it is 18 mmHg.

What is the next best step in treatment?

A. Consult cardiothoracic surgery for pericardial window
B. Consult interventional cardiology for pericardiocentesis
C. Give 500 mL fluid bolus
D. Obtain a CT scan to evaluate for pulmonary embolism

71. A 72-year-old woman with a history of HTN, AF, and breast cancer treated with resection and radiation presents with abdominal pain, lower extremity edema, weight gain, and shortness of breath. She reports no chest pain. Her vital signs are notable for a HR of 106 beats/min, a BP of 98/64 mmHg, a respiratory rate of 20 breaths/min, and oxygen saturation of 92% on room air.

Examination is notable for lungs that are clear to auscultation bilaterally. The jugular venous pulsation is noted to rise with inspiration. Cardiac auscultation reveals an irregularly irregular rhythm without murmurs, rubs, or gallops. Abdominal examination reveals hepatomegaly with shifting dullness concerning for ascites and bilateral lower extremity edema.

The 12-lead ECG demonstrates low voltages. TTE reveals increased inspiratory flow across the tricuspid valve with decreased inspiratory flow across the mitral valve. No effusion is present. The patient is sent for simultaneous left and right heart catheterization and is found to have discordant LV and RV peaks during the respiratory cycle as well as equalization of the RV end-diastolic pressure and LVEDP.

What are these findings most consistent with?

A. Acute viral pericarditis
B. Constrictive pericarditis
C. Restrictive cardiomyopathy
D. Severe pulmonary HTN

72. A 32-year-old man presents with sharp 8/10 substernal chest pain. The pain started a few hours ago and is worse with inspiration. He reports a prodromal episode of rhinorrhea and cough about 7 days prior to presentation. Vital signs are notable for a HR of 88 beats/min, a BP of 120/74 mmHg, and an oxygen saturation of 100% on room air. A troponin test is drawn and in process. A 12-lead ECG is shown below:

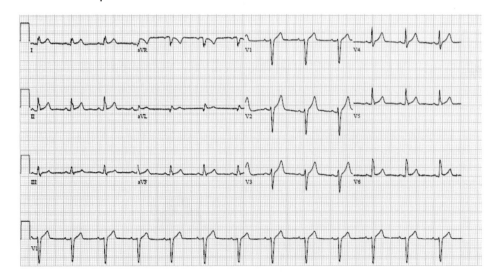

What is the most appropriate next step in management?

A. Emergent coronary angiography
B. Initiation of high-dose nonsteroidal anti-inflammatory drugs (NSAIDs)
C. Initiation of steroids
D. Pharmacologic stress testing with perfusion imaging

73. A 52-year-old man presents to your clinic for his annual physical. He is an active smoker with a history of chronic obstructive pulmonary disease and gastroesophageal reflux disease. His vital signs are notable for a HR of 65 beats/min and BP of 135/85 mmHg. Looking through his history, you note that his BP has ranged from 130/80 to 140/85 mmHg for the last 2 years. The patient asks you whether he should be on medications for his BP.

In addition to counseling him on diet and smoking cessation, which of the following do you recommend?

A. Calculating his atherosclerotic cardiovascular disease risk score and, if >10%, starting an antihypertensive agent now
B. Monitoring BP every 6 months and starting antihypertensives when BP >140/90 mmHg
C. Monitoring BP every 12 months and starting antihypertensives when BP >150/90 mmHg
D. Starting an antihypertensive medication now

74. A 50-year-old woman presents to your clinic to reestablish longitudinal care after not seeing a physician in 10 years. Her vital signs are notable for a BP of 148/92 mmHg. Her physical examination is otherwise unremarkable. Laboratory evaluation is notable for hemoglobin A_{1c} of 8.4% and creatinine of 1.2 mg/dL. You have her return for a repeat BP check and urine sample. Repeat BP is 150/94 mmHg and urine microalbumin/creatinine ratio is 45 mg/g.

Which of the following antihypertensives would you recommend?

A. Amlodipine
B. Carvedilol
C. Hydrochlorothiazide
D. Lisinopril

75. A 65-year-old man presents to the ED with a complaint of tearing chest pain radiating to the back. He has a history of poorly controlled HTN, hyperlipidemia, and CAD requiring CABG surgery 5 years ago. Initial vital signs reveal a HR of 110 beats/min, BP of 190/110 mmHg, and oxygen saturation of 94% on room air. The remainder of his physical examination is unremarkable. Workup includes CTA that shows a large aortic dissection distal to the takeoff of the left subclavian artery.

Which of the following agents should be given first to control his BP?

A. Intravenous hydralazine
B. Intravenous labetalol
C. Intravenous nitroprusside
D. Oral labetalol

76. A 32-year-old obese woman presents to your clinic for an annual visit. She has a history of HTN that is well controlled on lisinopril. She tells you that she is trying to conceive.

In addition to prescribing her a prenatal multivitamin, which change would you make to her antihypertensive regimen?

A. Stop lisinopril and monitor BPs as you would expect her BP to decrease during pregnancy
B. Substitute hydrochlorothiazide for lisinopril
C. Substitute labetalol for lisinopril
D. Substitute spironolactone for lisinopril

77. A 48-year-old man presents as a new patient to your clinic. He reports always having high BP. His BP today is 150/90 mmHg. His current medication regimen is amlodipine 10 mg daily, lisinopril 40 mg daily, and carvedilol 25 mg BID.

Which of the following medications should be added to his regimen?

A. Chlorthalidone
B. Clonidine patch
C. Doxazosin
D. Hydralazine

78. A 38-year-old black man with no prior medical history presents for a yearly appointment. He currently takes no medications. His body mass index (BMI) is 24. His initial BP taken by the medical assistant was 157/97 mmHg. A repeat BP was obtained by his physician and remained elevated at 152/91 mmHg. There are no clear provoking factors for his HTN. The patient is hesitant to start any medications, so he plans to buy a home BP cuff and monitor his BP at home. Two weeks later, he sends you a log of his home BPs, which range from 150 to 170/80 to 90 mmHg. He is now amenable to starting an antihypertensive agent.

Which is the best choice for an initial antihypertensive medication in this patient?

A. Amlodipine
B. Losartan
C. Spironolactone
D. Carvedilol

79. A 29-year-old woman with HTN presents to your clinic for a follow-up visit. Over the last few months, her BP medication doses have been increased, with only mild improvement in her BP. Her BP today is 168/92 mmHg. On physical examination, you auscultate an abdominal bruit. She has a normal serum creatinine.

Which of the following is the next best diagnostic test to order?

A. MR angiography (MRA) of the renal arteries
B. Noncontrast CT of the thoracic and abdominal aorta
C. Serum metanephrines
D. Sleep apnea testing

80. A 63-year-old man with HTN, hyperlipidemia, and a smoking history is incidentally discovered to have a thoracic aortic aneurysm (TAA) measured at 4 cm by CT of the chest.

When should the next assessment of aneurysm size be performed?

A. 3 months
B. 6 months
C. 12 months
D. 24 months

81. A 45-year-old man with no past medical history undergoes a TTE for an incidentally heard murmur. A bicuspid aortic valve is identified with a TAA measured at 4.5 cm.

Which of the following recommendations would you offer the patient with regard to screening of family members?

A. All first-degree male relatives should be screened
B. All first-degree relatives should be screened
C. Family members previously informed of a murmur should be screened
D. No additional screening is required

82. A 64-year-old woman with HTN, hyperlipidemia, and coronary disease has an abdominal aortic aneurysm diameter measured at 4.9 cm that has increased in size by 0.6 cm in the preceding 6 months.

    Which feature of her history merits consideration for early surgical repair of her aortic aneurysm?
    A. Aneurysm size of 4.9 cm
    B. Female sex
    C. Rate of growth of >0.5 cm in 6 months
    D. Surgical repair is not indicated

83. A 78-year-old man with a history of HTN and hyperlipidemia presents with chest pain. The pain initially started suddenly, radiated to his back, and was rated a 10 on a scale of 1 to 10. His pain is now an 8/10. He is diaphoretic and appears in distress. Initial vital signs are notable for a HR of 112 beats/min, BP of 168/72 mmHg, and oxygen saturation of 92% on room air. He undergoes emergent CTA of the chest, which reveals a large ascending aortic dissection. The cardiothoracic surgical team is consulted.

    What is the first step in medication management?
    A. Esmolol drip
    B. Metoprolol IV push
    C. Nitroglycerin drip
    D. Nitroprusside drip

84. A 65-year-old man with a history of tobacco use disorder, HTN, and hyperlipidemia presents with sudden-onset ripping chest pain that radiates to his back. Pain was maximal at onset and has subsequently decreased to an 8/10. He is diaphoretic and in moderate distress on arrival. Vital signs are notable for sinus tachycardia at a rate of 110 beats/min, a BP of 172/94 mmHg, and an oxygen saturation of 98% on room air. A chest x-ray (CXR) is obtained and is shown below:

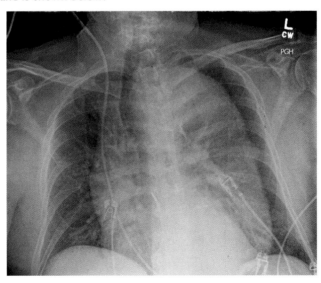

    The CXR is concerning for which of the following pathologies?
    A. Aortic dissection
    B. Pericardial effusion
    C. Pneumothorax
    D. Pulmonary edema

85. A 68-year-old man is admitted to the cardiac ICU following an inferior-posterior STEMI. He is currently supported by an intra-aortic balloon pump and norepinephrine. On reassessment 2 hours later, his left radial arterial line has lost its tracing and the radial and brachial pulse is difficult to palpate. Right radial and brachial artery pulses are intact and easily palpable. By PA catheter, cardiac output and CI are unchanged from prior.

    What is the most likely diagnosis?

    A. Aortic dissection
    B. Radial artery spasm
    C. Thromboembolism
    D. Worsening cardiogenic shock

86. A 38-year-old man presents with acute-onset 10/10 chest pain radiating to his back. Initial BP is 190/110 mmHg. ECG is without ischemic changes. Examination is notable for a tall, slender gentleman in moderate distress. Pectus excavatum is noted, and on cardiac examination he is noted to have a III/IV early diastolic murmur best heard at the right upper sternal border. Lungs are notable for bibasilar rales, with equal breath sounds bilaterally. A CTA chest is in process.

    Based on the above presentation, what will be the most likely definitive treatment?

    A. Coronary angiogram
    B. Medical management alone
    C. Needle decompression
    D. Surgery

87. A 74-year-old man with a history of tobacco use disorder, HTN, and hyperlipidemia is admitted to the ICU for hemodynamic monitoring for a type B aortic dissection extending from T4 to the diaphragmatic hiatus. His current medications include an esmolol drip and nitroprusside. The patient is noted to have diminishing urine output. The nitroprusside and esmolol doses have been reduced to maintain systolic BP of 100 to 120 mmHg and HR <60 beats/min. Repeat labs are obtained and are as follows:

    - Creatinine: 1.8 mg/dL (0.9 mg/dL previously)
    - Lactate: 4.2 mmol/L (1.8 mmol/L previously)
    - Arterial blood gas (ABG): pH: 7.25, P_{CO_2}: 28 mmHg, P_{O_2}: 98 mmHg, Fi_{O_2} 30%

    What is the most likely etiology of these hemodynamic changes?

    A. Cyanide toxicity
    B. Extension of the dissection below the diaphragmatic hiatus
    C. Extension of the dissection proximally into the ascending aortic arch
    D. Sedation effect

88. You evaluate a 22-year-old man who presents with intermittent fevers and light-headedness. Approximately 4 weeks earlier, he had been hiking in Massachusetts and shortly thereafter noted a rash on his left thigh that resolved on its own. Vital signs reveal a temperature of 38.5°C (101.3°F), HR of 25 beats/min, and BP of 80/55 mmHg. Cardiac examination is notable only for bradycardia. The remainder of the examination is unremarkable. ECG reveals CHB with a slow junctional escape rhythm at 25 beats/min. He receives appropriate IV fluid resuscitation; however, his BP remains 80/55 mmHg.

    What is the most appropriate acute management of this arrhythmia?

    A. IV ceftriaxone
    B. Oral doxycycline
    C. Permanent pacemaker implantation
    D. Transvenous temporary pacemaker

89. You are asked to evaluate a 68-year-old man for an abnormal ECG. He has a history of chronic obstructive pulmonary disease with reasonable symptom control on inhaled corticosteroids and long-acting β-agonists. Vital signs reveal an irregular HR of 101 beats/min and BP of 122/70 mmHg. Cardiopulmonary examination is otherwise unremarkable. ECG reveals an irregular rhythm with three distinct P-wave morphologies.

What is the most likely mechanism of this arrhythmia?

A. Chaotic atrial activation originating from the pulmonary veins
B. Increased automaticity at multiple sites in the atria
C. Reentry through dual pathways in the atrioventricular node
D. Reentry through the atrioventricular node and an accessory pathway

90. You are asked to evaluate a 44-year-old man with a known history of ventricular preexcitation (Wolff-Parkinson-White [WPW]) in the ED for palpitations that abruptly started an hour prior to presentation. Vital signs reveal an irregular HR of 120 beats/min and BP of 120/65 mmHg. ECG reveals AF with preexcitation.

What is the appropriate initial therapy for management of this arrhythmia?

A. Adenosine
B. Digoxin
C. Emergent direct current cardioversion
D. Procainamide

91. You are called emergently to the bedside after a 54-year-old healthy woman developed unstable polymorphic VT. She was admitted to the hospital 3 days earlier for treatment of a right lower lobe pneumonia and had been improving on levofloxacin. Prior to this hospitalization, she had been healthy and performed moderate- to high-intensity aerobic exercise for at least 40 minutes a day. After emergent defibrillation, she regains spontaneous circulation. An ECG is obtained.

Which of the following is most likely to be present on the ECG?

A. LBBB
B. Long QT interval
C. Pseudo-RBBB with ST-segment elevation in V_1 to V_3
D. T-wave inversion in V_1 to V_3

92. A 54-year-old woman is admitted with unstable monomorphic VT prompting defibrillation from her ICD. She has a history of ischemic cardiomyopathy (LVEF 20%) and three hospitalizations for monomorphic VT prompting ICD discharge in the past 2 months. Her most recent coronary angiogram last month demonstrates nonobstructive disease. Current medications include aspirin, atorvastatin, metoprolol, amiodarone, mexiletine, and furosemide. Vital signs reveal temperature of 37°C (98.6°F), HR of 75 beats/min, and BP of 110/60 mmHg. Cardiac examination reveals a laterally displaced apical impulse and normal heart sounds without murmurs. There is no JVD, lung sounds are clear, and there is no lower extremity edema.

What is the next most appropriate step in care?

A. Flecainide
B. Intra-aortic balloon pump
C. IV magnesium
D. Radiofrequency ablation

93. A 65-year-old man with a history of recurrent urinary tract infections presents to the hospital with pyelonephritis. Overnight, you are called by his nurse because he is bradycardic with an HR of 50 beats/min. BP is 95/60 mmHg. The following ECG is obtained:

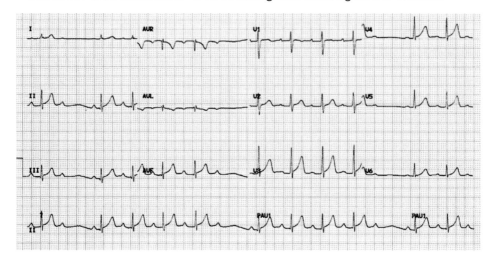

What is the next best step?

A. Adenosine
B. Atropine
C. Observation
D. Temporary pacemaker

94. A 21-year-old man with no medical history presents to the ED with palpitations. The following ECG is obtained:

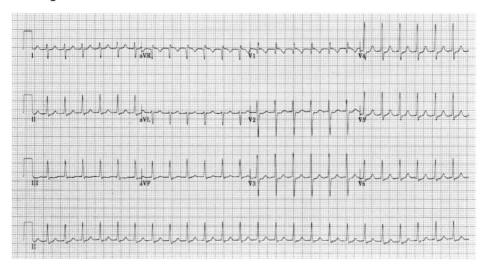

What is the most likely diagnosis?

A. AF
B. Atrial flutter with 2:1 block
C. Atrioventricular nodal reentrant tachycardia
D. Sinus tachycardia

95. You are asked to evaluate a 66-year-old woman with a history of HTN in the ED for palpitations during the past several days. Vital signs reveal a HR of 150 beats/min and BP of 100/60 mmHg. Cardiac examination is notable for a rapid irregular heart rhythm without murmurs or gallops. The remainder of the examination is unremarkable. ECG reveals new onset of AF with rapid ventricular response.

She is admitted to the hospital and her ventricular response rates are controlled to a range of 110 to 130 beats/min after atrioventricular nodal blockade, but her low BP limits further titration. TTE reveals mild left atrial dilation and LVEF of 40%. After thorough investigation, the etiology of her systolic dysfunction is determined to be tachycardia-induced cardiomyopathy.

What is the appropriate management of this arrhythmia?

A. Continue rate control with current regimen
B. Perform cardioversion without TEE
C. Perform TEE; if no left atrial thrombus, perform cardioversion
D. Refer for ablation

96. You are asked to evaluate a 69-year-old woman with a history of an ischemic cardiomyopathy in the cardiac ICU. Vital signs reveal a HR of 125 beats/min, BP of 95/65 mmHg, and oxygen saturation of 92% on 3 L of supplemental oxygen. The jugular venous pulsations are elevated. Cardiac examination is notable for a rapid, irregular heart rhythm with an S_3 gallop. Pulmonary examination reveals diffuse crackles. ECG reveals new onset of AF with rapid ventricular response. Her medications include aspirin, atorvastatin, metoprolol, lisinopril, and torsemide.

She is admitted to the hospital and started on unfractionated heparin and intravenous furosemide. Her respiratory symptoms improve by day 3 of hospitalization. TTE reveals left atrial dilation and LVEF of 30%. After consultation from the cardiology team, a rhythm control strategy is recommended for long-term management of her AF. The team would like to initiate drug therapy prior to consideration of cardioversion to help maintain long-term sinus rhythm.

What is the most appropriate medical therapy?

A. Amiodarone
B. Diltiazem
C. Flecainide
D. Propafenone

97. A 69-year-old woman with a history of HTN, diabetes, AF, and HFrEF presents to your outpatient clinic. Her current medication regimen includes aspirin, atorvastatin, empagliflozin, metformin, sacubitril-valsartan, and spironolactone. She has had difficult-to-control AF with multiple prior cardioversions, ablations, and significant side effects to β-blockers and other antiarrhythmics (dofetilide), so the plan is to initiate her on long-term amiodarone.

Which of the following tests is NOT recommended as a baseline screening test prior to initiation of amiodarone?

A. Liver function testing
B. Pulmonary function testing (PFT)
C. Serum creatinine
D. Ophthalmic exam

98. A 52-year-old woman presents to your clinic for a yearly physical examination. She has a history of hypothyroidism and rheumatic mitral stenosis. She reports that she has felt well, but over the recent months she notes intermittent episodes of palpitations. Medications include levothyroxine. Vital signs reveal a HR of 90 beats/min and BP of 105/55 mmHg. You perform an ECG in the office, which reveals new onset of AF. Her echocardiogram demonstrates moderate rheumatic mitral stenosis with a preserved LVEF.

Which of the following is the best choice regarding a decision about anticoagulation?

A. Do not start anticoagulation
B. Start aspirin
C. Start rivaroxaban
D. Start warfarin

99. You are asked to evaluate a 77-year-old woman in the ED after a fall. She has a history of CAD, HTN, and AF. She reports that she was vacuuming her home when she tripped on the edge of her rug and fell, landing on her outstretched arms and hitting her head against the coffee table. Medications include aspirin, metoprolol, furosemide, lisinopril, apixaban, and a multivitamin. Vital signs reveal a regular HR of 90 beats/min and BP of 105/55 mmHg. Cardiac and neurologic examinations are unremarkable. CT of the head is performed that reveals a large subdural hemorrhage. She is evaluated by neurosurgery and is planned to go to the operating room for surgical evacuation.

What is the next most appropriate pharmacologic therapy?

A. Andexanet alfa
B. Fresh frozen plasma
C. Idarucizumab
D. Vitamin K

100. A 43-year-old woman with a history of rheumatic mitral stenosis and AF returns to your office for routine follow-up. Her current medications include metoprolol and warfarin. She reports having seen an advertisement on television for apixaban and would like to learn more.

Which of the following statements about direct-acting oral anticoagulants is true?

A. Direct-acting oral anticoagulants are indicated for long-term antithrombotic therapy for patients with mechanical heart valves
B. Direct-acting oral anticoagulants are not indicated for patients with AF with rheumatic mitral stenosis
C. Direct-acting oral anticoagulants carry a higher risk of intracranial hemorrhage compared to warfarin
D. There are no reversal agents available for direct-acting oral anticoagulants in case of life-threatening bleeding

101. A 70-year-old woman has a history of long-standing, permanent AF. She also has amyloid angiopathy and is now admitted with a large intracerebral hemorrhage.

What option should be considered to reduce her risk of stroke or systemic embolism?

A. Amiodarone
B. Aspirin alone
C. Half-dose apixaban
D. Percutaneous left atrial appendage occlusion

102. A 64-year-old female with symptomatic paroxysmal AF and HF with an LVEF of 30% presents to clinic for evaluation. She has remained symptomatic despite nodal blockade, and had QTc prolongation with dofetilide. Her current medications include metoprolol, lisinopril, eplerenone, and empagliflozin. Her baseline lab work is notable for normal renal function and normal thyroid function, and she has mildly elevated hepatic enzymes.

What is the next best step in management of her symptomatic AF?

A. Propranolol
B. Amiodarone
C. Catheter ablation
D. Sotalol

103. A 63-year-old man with permanent AF on metoprolol, diltiazem, and digoxin presents to the ED following a syncopal episode. He reports that his syncopal episode was preceded by a very short period of light-headedness and a sensation of his heart racing. He has experienced one similar episode in the past approximately 1 week prior to presentation. He is monitored on 48 hours of telemetry without notable arrhythmic events. A decision is made to discharge the patient with an ambulatory ECG monitoring device.

Which type of monitor might best capture his arrhythmia?

A. 48-Hour Holter monitor
B. Event recorder
C. Implantable loop recorder
D. Long-term external cardiac event monitoring device

104. A 29-year-old female with muscular dystrophy and prior cardiac transplant presents to the hospital with 3 days of chest palpations and weakness. You get called the room as the patient reports acute-onset light-headedness and see the following rhythm on telemetry monitoring:

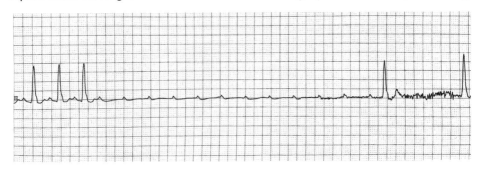

What should you do next?

A. Administer atropine for symptomatic bradycardia
B. Start an amiodarone infusion
C. Place a transvenous pacing wire
D. Perform a right heart catheterization and endomyocardial biopsy

105. A 72-year-old man with known moderate aortic stenosis and HTN presents with an episode of syncope while climbing a flight of stairs. He denies a prodromal syndrome.

Which one of the following may offer the highest yield for elucidating an etiology of his syncopal episode?

A. A TTE
B. An ECG
C. Carotid artery Doppler ultrasound examination
D. History and physical

106. A 74-year-old woman with no past medical history presents with syncope that occurred during micturition. The event was witnessed by her daughter, who notes that there was no evidence of seizure. Orthostatic vital signs on arrival demonstrate a 5 mmHg drop in systolic BP from supine to standing with a 20 beats/min increase in HR. Her physical examination is otherwise unremarkable. Her ECG is unrevealing. The patient presently has no complaints.

    What is the most likely etiology for her syncope?

    A. Arrhythmogenic
    B. Neurocardiogenic
    C. Neurologic
    D. Orthostatic hypotension

107. You are asked to evaluate an 83-year-old man who was admitted to the cardiology service who underwent implantation of a dual-chamber pacemaker earlier in the day for sick sinus syndrome and sinus pauses resulting in syncope. Your evaluation reveals a HR of 110 beats/min and BP of 70/55 mmHg. Heart sounds are normal and pulmonary examination reveals clear breath sounds. His neck veins are elevated to 15 cm H_2O with a blunted Y descent. There are no cannon A waves. ECG reveals sinus tachycardia and narrow QRS complex.

    What is the most likely etiology of his presentation?

    A. Flash pulmonary edema
    B. Lead perforation leading to cardiac tamponade
    C. Pacemaker-mediated tachycardia
    D. Pacemaker syndrome

108. You evaluate a 60-year-old man with a history of ischemic cardiomyopathy following an anterior MI in 2009. He reports New York Heart Association class III symptoms, including dyspnea on mild exertion and rare orthopnea. Vital signs reveal a HR of 60 beats/min and BP of 90/60 mmHg. Examination reveals no JVD, normal heart sounds, clear breath sounds on pulmonary auscultation, and no lower extremity edema. Medications include aspirin, atorvastatin, furosemide, metoprolol, lisinopril, and spironolactone. ECG reveals normal sinus rhythm with a LBBB (QRS = 152 ms). His last TTE reveals an LVEF of 25%.

    Which of the following will reduce his mortality risk?

    A. Cardiac resynchronization therapy
    B. Dual-chamber pacemaker
    C. ICD
    D. Both A and C

109. You are asked to evaluate a 65-year-old man with a history of sick sinus syndrome requiring pacemaker implantation 5 months ago. He has no complaints today; however, his wife has noted intermittent fevers over the past few days. Vital signs revealed a temperature of 39.4°C (103°F), HR of 70 beats/min, and BP of 90/60 mmHg. Examination reveals normal heart sounds with erythema and tenderness over his left pectoral pacemaker implantation site. The remainder of his examination is unrevealing. He is admitted and started on intravenous antibiotics. Blood cultures grew methicillin-sensitive *Staphylococcus aureus* (MSSA). TEE reveals no vegetations on cardiac valves or implanted hardware. By hospital day 3, he is afebrile and feels well.

    What is the next best step in care?

    A. Convert to oral antibiotics to complete a 6-week course and discharge
    B. Discharge and continue intravenous antibiotics to complete a 6-week course
    C. Plan for pacemaker system removal
    D. Refer for tricuspid valve replacement

110. A 55-year-old woman is admitted to the hospital for elective open sigmoid colectomy for recurrent diverticulitis (last episode 3 months ago). She has a history of diabetes mellitus, HTN, hyperlipidemia, and an inferior MI 3 years ago requiring PCI. Vital signs reveal temperature of 37°C (98.6°F), HR of 75 beats/min, and BP of 110/60 mmHg. Physical examination is unremarkable. Medications include aspirin, metoprolol, atorvastatin, and a multivitamin. She denies any recent angina or dyspnea on exertion since her MI. She continues to go to the gym weekly and runs 5 miles on the treadmill at least five times per week.

What is the next appropriate step in care?

A. Discontinue aspirin perioperatively
B. Perform stress testing
C. Proceed to surgery
D. Start clopidogrel to decrease risk of perioperative MI

111. You evaluate a 75-year-old woman in clinic for preoperative evaluation 1 week prior to an elective cholecystectomy for cholelithiasis. She also has a history of severe symptomatic aortic stenosis and will be undergoing a valve replacement in 1 month. Vital signs reveal temperature of 37°C (98.6°F), HR of 75 beats/min, and BP of 110/60 mmHg. Cardiac examination reveals a harsh III/VI late-peaking systolic ejection murmur. There is no JVD, lung sounds are clear, and there is no lower extremity edema. Medications include aspirin and a multivitamin. She reports mild dyspnea on exertion that has progressed over the past year.

What is the next appropriate step in care?

A. Initiate furosemide
B. Perform stress testing
C. Postpone cholecystectomy until valve intervention is completed
D. Proceed to cholecystectomy as scheduled

112. A 75-year-old man is seen in the emergency room with chest pain and anterior ST-segment elevations on ECG. He is referred for coronary angiography and was found to have an occluded LAD coronary artery and undergoes placement of a drug-eluting stent. He is started on aspirin, clopidogrel, metoprolol, and atorvastatin. Near the time of discharge, you learn that he is scheduled for elective knee surgery in 2 weeks and the surgeons would need to stop his clopidogrel.

What is the next appropriate step in care?

A. Postpone knee replacement for 1 month
B. Postpone knee replacement for 3 months
C. Postpone knee replacement for 6 to 12 months
D. Proceed to knee replacement as scheduled in 2 weeks

113. A 68-year-old man with a history of nonobstructive CAD and stage 4 chronic kidney disease presents with a nonhealing ulcer on the lateral aspect of his left foot. The ulcer has been present for 3 months and has no purulence or erythema. On further history, he describes muscle fatigue and cramping in his legs that has limited his exercise tolerance.

What is the best initial diagnostic test of choice?

A. Ankle-brachial index
B. Arterial lower extremity angiogram in the cardiac catheterization lab
C. CTA of the lower extremities
D. MRA of the lower extremities

114. A 59-year-old man with a history of CAD, stage 4 chronic kidney disease, and who is nonadherent with medications presents with acute-onset pain in the left leg. On examination, his leg is cool to the touch. He describes numbness and tingling in his foot. Neither posterior tibial nor dorsalis pedis pulses are palpable. His foot is white and cold, with pain on palpation.

    While you are obtaining confirmatory imaging, what is the next best step?
    A. Initiate low-molecular-weight heparin
    B. Obtain arterial Doppler ultrasound examination in the morning
    C. Obtain urgent vascular surgery or vascular medicine consultation
    D. Place warm blankets on foot

115. A 69-year-old man with a history of advanced chronic kidney disease, HTN, and hyperlipidemia presents with painful leg cramps while ambulating. He does not have pain at rest. You suspect he may have peripheral arterial disease (PAD). You order ankle-brachial index. The right leg ankle-brachial index is 1.0 and the left leg ankle-brachial index is 0.95.

    What would be the next best diagnostic test of choice?
    A. Angiography in catheterization lab
    B. CTA of the lower extremities
    C. Exercise ABI
    D. Venous ultrasonography of the lower extremities

ANSWERS

1. **The correct answer is: B. Inferior STEMI.** The patient has ST elevations $\geq$1 mm in two contiguous leads (III, aVF), meeting criteria for STEMI. The presence of ST depressions in leads I and aVL reflects reciprocal changes, whereas the presence of ST depressions in leads V_2 and V_3 may indicate posterior myocardial ischemia. In addition, there are T-wave inversions in V_4 to V_6. The patient meets STEMI criteria and requires urgent revascularization. The absence of anterior (V_3-V_4) elevations makes anterior involvement unlikely, and the territorial nature of the ECG changes argues against pericarditis.

2. **The correct answer is: C. Pericarditis.** The patient has diffuse concave upward ST elevations across multiple vascular territories, making pericarditis the most likely diagnosis. In addition, lead aVR has an ST depression with elevation of the PR segment. In sum, this ECG is most suggestive of pericardial inflammation. Given the viral prodrome, this patient most likely has viral pericarditis.

    Anterior STEMIs present with elevations in the anterior precordial leads (V_3 and V_4) and represent occlusion of the LAD artery or its branches. Inferior STEMIs present with ST elevations in leads II, III, and aVF and represent occlusion of the RCA (or its branches) in 85% of patients and the left circumflex artery (or its branches) in 15% of patients (in whom the posterior descending artery arises from the left circumflex artery).

3. **The correct answer is: C. AF with RBBB and left anterior fascicular block.** The irregular ventricular rate with lack of visible P waves makes AF the most likely underlying atrial rhythm. The patient has a RBBB manifesting with classic morphology in V_1 to V_3. A RBBB is defined by a QRS $\geq$120 ms (110-119 = intraventricular conduction delay or "incomplete"), rSR′ in R precordial leads (V_1, V_2), and wide S wave in I and V_6. Sometimes, ST depressions or T-wave inversions are seen in the right precordial leads. In addition, this patient has a left axis deviation, which does not normally occur with a RBBB, suggesting a left anterior fascicular block is also present. The presence of a RBBB with a left anterior fascicular block is called a bifascicular block.

    CHB requires evidence of atrial and ventricular dissociation with an atrial rate that is regular and exceeds the ventricular rate, and a regular ventricular rate. The width and rate of the ventricular depolarizations are determined by where in the His-Purkinje system the ventricular beats are originating from. Higher junctional escape beats have narrower complexes and faster rates than those originating from the Purkinje system.

    The patient does not have a LBBB. LBBBs are defined by a QRS $\geq$120 ms with a broad, slurred, monophasic R in I, aVL, and V_5 to V_6. RS may be present in V_5 to V_6 if the patient has cardiomegaly. In addition, there is an absence of Q waves in I, V_5, and V_6. The patient does not meet these criteria and therefore does not have a LBBB.

4. **The correct answer is: B. Hyperkalemia.** Hyperkalemia is characterized by ECG changes that may include hyperacute or peaked T waves. This can progress to a shortening of the QT interval, PR prolongation, atrioventricular block and, at extreme elevations, widened QRS and ST elevation. Hypercalcemia results in shortening of the QT interval with flattened T waves, P waves, and J point elevation. Hypokalemia manifests with flattening of the T waves on ECG, presence of U waves, and prolongation of the QT interval. Although ischemia can also present with hyperacute T waves, the lack of chest pain or anginal equivalents makes this diagnosis less likely.

5. **The correct answer is: C. Initiating β-blocker therapy.** The ECG shows QTc prolongation. The QT segment is measured from the beginning of the QRS complex to the end of the T wave. The QTc is corrected for the HR using Bazett's formula: $QTc = \frac{QT}{\sqrt{RR}}$ interval (RR is measured in seconds). Bazett's formula may overcorrect at high HRs and undercorrect at a low HR. The normal QTc for men is <440 ms and for women <460 ms. Once the QTc is >500 ms, the risk of torsades de pointes increases. Slower HRs, potentially induced by nodal agents such as β-blockers, increase the risk of torsades de pointes in the presence of QTc prolongation. Therefore, when initiating any QT-prolonging medications, ECG monitoring for QTc prolongation is prudent.

    The differential for QT prolongation is broad but includes certain antiarrhythmics (such as class Ic, III), antipsychotics (ie, chlorpromazine, haloperidol, ziprasidone, quetiapine), antimicrobials (ie, fluoroquinolones, macrolides, azoles), antiemetics (ie, ondansetron, droperidol), pain medications including methadone, and electrolyte disturbances (ie, hypocalcemia, hypokalemia). For this patient, the combination of methadone and new initiation of a fluoroquinolone may have contributed to this QTc prolongation.

    For patients in whom QT prolongation is seen, serial ECG monitoring, correction of PR electrolytes, and discontinuation of nonessential QT-prolonging medications are advised. No guidelines exist for discontinuation of QT-prolonging medications, and clinical judgment should be used.

6. **The correct answer is: D. Pulmonary embolism.** The ECG shows sinus tachycardia at a rate of approximately 100 beats/min. In addition, there is evidence of right heart strain manifested by the prominent S wave in lead I, T-wave inversion and Q wave in lead III as well as a RBBB. Additional findings of right heart strain (not seen on this ECG) include ST elevations in precordial leads. Given the patient's risk factor (tobacco use), physical examination findings (including hypoxemia with clear lungs and left greater than right lower extremity edema), and ECG findings, pulmonary embolism is the most likely diagnosis.

    Inferior STEMI presents with chest pain or other chest pain equivalent as well as >1 mm ST elevations in the inferior leads (II, III, aVF). Pericarditis manifests early with diffuse ST elevations with PR depressions (except aVR, which has PR elevation and ST depression). Non-ST-elevation MI (NSTEMI) may or may not have ECG findings, including ST depressions and T-wave inversions with positive troponin, but typically would not manifest with new RBBB.

7. **The correct answer is: A. Check posterior leads.** Posterior leads (V_7-V_9) should be checked in patients with a history consistent with an acute coronary syndrome when the initial standard 12-lead ECG reveals ST depressions in V_1 to V_3 (corresponding to posterior ST-segment elevations), R wave > S wave in V_1 (corresponding to a posterior Q wave), or no ST-segment changes. If posterior leads reveal ST-segment elevations, it would mandate urgent revascularization as this would be consistent with an acute STEMI. Although pulmonary embolism could cause chest pain, it is more commonly pleuritic. ECG changes in pulmonary embolism include evidence of right ventricular strain such as S wave in lead I, Q wave in lead III, T-wave inversion in lead III, RBBB, right axis deviation, and ST-segment elevations in the anterior precordial leads. Although pericarditis can cause chest pain, it is typically a sharp pain worse with inspiration and decreased with sitting forward. On physical examination, a pericardial friction rub may be present and the ECG may show diffuse ST elevation with PR depressions. Although colchicine is the first-line treatment, the history and examinations are not consistent with pericarditis. Gastroesophageal reflux disease can cause a burning chest pain. It often occurs following eating, may be associated with an acidic taste in mouth, and worsens postprandially and with recumbency. The chest pain history in this vignette is more concerning for an acute coronary syndrome.

8. **The correct answer is: A. Activate the cardiac catheterization lab for urgent revascularization.** The ECG is concerning for an acute inferoposterior STEMI, and the patient should go for urgent coronary angiography. ST-segment elevation in the right-sided leads (most typically V_4R) suggests right ventricle involvement. In these cases, the right ventricle is preload dependent and administration of a vasodilator such as nitroglycerin will decrease preload, which could lead to hypotension. A TTE may be utilized to evaluate for wall motion abnormalities to support a diagnosis of ischemia, but in this instance, the history and ECG are diagnostic, and an echocardiogram may contribute to delays in primary PCI. Posterior leads are not expected to be useful in this case as STEMI has already been diagnosed and will therefore not change management.

9. **The correct answer is: A. Acute pericarditis.** The vignette is most consistent with acute pericarditis. The description of a sharp, pleuritic pain that is improved by leaning forward and worsened by lying back is most consistent with pericarditis. This may have been precipitated by a recent viral illness. Classic ECG findings include PR depressions with a diffuse pattern of ST elevations that do not correlate to a unique coronary vascular distribution. An aortic dissection may also present with acute onset of sharp chest pain, although the pain is typically not positional and often radiates to the back. There are often no ECG findings in aortic dissection, although it may include low voltages if there is a pericardial effusion or ST elevations if the dissection extends into a coronary artery (typically the RCA). Acute coronary syndrome may have a variety of clinical presentations, including chest pain, pressure, shortness of breath, neck or jaw pain, arm pain, and arm numbness or tingling. Pain may even be epigastric or abdominal and include nausea or vomiting. Although ST elevations always raise concern for an acute coronary syndrome, the presence of upsloping ST elevations across multiple vascular territories is suggestive of a diffuse process such as pericarditis. Acute pulmonary embolism may also present with sudden-onset pleuritic chest pain. Hemodynamic markers include hypoxemia, tachycardia, and hypotension, depending on the size of the pulmonary embolism. ECG findings may range from sinus tachycardia to evidence of right ventricle strain. ST elevations in multiple vascular territories would be atypical.

10. **The correct answer is: A. Cardiac magnetic resonance imaging (MRI).** Despite a clinical presentation suggestive of NSTEMI, women are less likely than men to have obstructive coronary disease at catheterization. This entity is known as MI with no obstructive CAD. Individuals with MI with no obstructive CAD remain at increased risk for major adverse cardiac events, and alternate etiologies for the patient's presentation should be investigated. Coronary films should be reviewed for missed dissection, plaque erosion/disruption, emboli, or spasm. An LV functional assessment should be pursued. In this patient with depressed LV function and elevated troponin, a diagnosis of myocarditis should be considered, which can be confirmed with a cardiac MRI.

11. **The correct answer is: D. Pharmacologic stress test with perfusion imaging.** Given the patient has a LBBB at baseline, he cannot undergo an ECG exercise tolerance test as the ECG alone will not be diagnostic for ischemia. In addition, his recent knee replacement and poor exercise tolerance at baseline would make him a poor candidate for exercise stress testing. Exercise stress tests require achievement of at least 85% of a maximum predicted HR to maximize diagnostic yield. If a patient is unable to exercise long enough to reach this end point, the test will not be interpretable. For patients with underlying LBBB, a vasodilator stress is typically recommended, preferentially before either an exercise or chronotropic evaluation because there is a higher risk of a false positive at higher HRs (as dobutamine would cause) as a result of ventricular dyssynchrony.

12. **The correct answer is: C. Coronary CT angiography (CTA).** The patient has a somewhat atypical chest pain history, but does have risk factors including family history of early CAD, HTN, and hyperlipidemia, giving him an intermediate probability of CAD. A coronary CTA will give information about the anatomy of the coronary arteries as well as any stenoses and is therefore a reasonable test to exclude coronary disease. Although it has a high negative predictive value, positive findings may need to be confirmed with a coronary angiogram. Cardiac MRI without stress testing can be employed to examine cardiac function and structure, but is not optimal in the emergency room setting because of the length of the test. An exercise stress test has the benefit of evaluating functional capacity and provocation of symptoms with exercise. However, the patient's chronic knee pain may limit his ability to reach 85% of the maximum predicted HR, thus limiting the test's diagnostic ability.

13. **The correct answer is: C. CABG.** Given the patient has multivessel CAD, diabetes and HFrEF, he would benefit from CABG. Treatment of HF symptoms alone is inadequate. A stress test is not an appropriate next step given that the patient has already been found to have multivessel disease. Percutaneous revascularization can be considered if the patient is deemed not be a surgical candidate, but this would not be the first choice given diabetes and low EF.

14. **The correct answer is: B. Coronary angiography.** The patient has a high-risk stress test for several reasons. He achieved only four METs before stopping because of angina. Additionally, his BP did not augment with exercise, raising concern for left main or multivessel CAD. The ECG at 7 minutes into recovery has >2 mm ST depressions diffusely and an ST elevation in aVR. High-risk ECG findings are ST depressions ≥2 mm or ≥1 mm in stage 1 of an exercise stress test, depressions occurring in ≥5 leads or ≥5 minutes into recovery. In sum, the findings in the vignette are highly concerning for significant CAD requiring definition of his coronary anatomy and consideration of revascularization.

    Other high-risk features on stress tests include a Duke treadmill score <-11, a drop in EF during stress (if imaging is obtained), ≥1 large or 2 moderate perfusion defects, transient LV dilation, or increased lung uptake of radionuclide tracer (if perfusion imaging is obtained).

15. **The correct answer is: A. Initiate β-blocker and statin.** The patient presents with a syndrome consistent with stable angina. Exercise stress testing confirms the diagnosis of CAD with demonstrable ischemia in a single territory. The next best step in management would be the institution of optimal medical therapy that includes low-dose aspirin, β-blocker, and statin therapy (and possibly other lipid-lowering therapy). Coronary angiography should be considered in those patients with refractory symptoms despite optimal medical therapy and in those patients with high-risk stress test findings (low EF, transient ischemic dilation [suggestive of three-vessel disease], hypotensive response to exercise, ≥2 territories of moderate ischemia or >1 territory of severe ischemia, exercise-induced arrhythmias). In the absence of left main disease on coronary CTA, it is reasonable to first consider a trial of optimized medical therapy before considering coronary revascularization in patients with moderate-to-severe ischemia (ISCHEMIA trial). TTE would help identify structural heart abnormalities, which would be unlikely to explain the patient's symptoms.

16. **The correct answer is: D. Manual compression of the access site.** Access site bleeding should be suspected in postprocedural patients with hypotension, lower abdominal or back pain, or rapidly expanding hematoma. The first step in managing active

hemorrhage requires primary bleeding control with manual compression of the common femoral artery. Thereafter, consideration can be given to whether blood products should be administered empirically to facilitate hemodynamic stabilization. CT of the abdomen can be utilized when the diagnosis is uncertain and hemodynamic parameters have stabilized. Although most bleeding stops with manual pressure, surgical or percutaneous intervention can be considered following failure of manual compression. Aspirin and P2Y12 inhibitor therapy does not reverse quickly and thus stopping would not help in the acute setting. Any decisions about altering antiplatelet therapy long term (which would be unlikely) should be done in consultation with the cardiologist.

17. **The correct answer is: B. Clopidogrel can be held to permit a knee replacement.** In this clinical scenario, clopidogrel can be held to permit the patient to undergo a knee replacement. The initial decision on dual antiplatelet therapy duration depends on the indication for stent placement. Patients who undergo stent placement for management of an acute coronary syndrome are considered to be at higher risk for stent thrombosis and recurrent MI; therefore, dual antiplatelet therapy is ideally recommended for a minimum of 12 months, regardless of stent type. Some lower-risk patients may be eligible for shorter durations of dual antiplatelet therapy or possibly antiplatelet monotherapy. The intravenous P2Y12 inhibitor cangrelor does not have a role for elective procedures but can be considered as an off-label IV bridge for semi-urgent procedures for patients in whom the risk of stent thrombosis off of dual antiplatelet therapy is considered high. There is no role for stress testing to guide the duration of dual antiplatelet therapy.

18. **The correct answer is: A. A conservative strategy of aspirin, β-blocker, and nitrates as needed, followed by noninvasive risk stratification (stress testing) to help determine if coronary angiography is appropriate, provided the patient remains asymptomatic.** All patients presenting with unstable angina or NSTEMI should undergo risk assessment, which can be performed with two commonly used scores: Thrombolysis in Myocardial Infarction (TIMI) or Global Registry of Acute Coronary Events risk scores. Urgent/immediate diagnostic angiography with the intent to revascularize should be pursued in patients with NSTEMI who have refractory angina or hemodynamic/electrical instability. Early (within 24 hours) diagnostic angiography with the intent to revascularize is indicated in stabilized patients with NSTEMI who are at high risk of clinical events. In patients, such as this example, at low risk (TIMI score 0-2 or Global Registry of Acute Coronary Events score ≤108), a conservative strategy of optimal medical therapy with coronary angiography pursued in those with persistent or recurrent symptoms or high-risk stress test findings can be considered.

19. **The Correct answer is: A. Cardiac MRI.** This patient presented with signs and symptoms of MI and was found to have MINOCA or MI with nonobstructive CAD. MINOCA is defined as signs and symptoms of acute myocardial injury with rise and fall in cardiac biomarkers in the absence of obstructive epicardial CAD (stenosis ≥50%). Patients with MINOCA are often younger and more likely to be female. Studies suggest that an alternate etiology for the chest pain can be identified in a substantial proportion of patients. Cardiac MRI is able to identify areas of infarction as well as rule out alternative diagnoses such as myocarditis. In some patients, intracoronary imaging (such as optical coherence tomography [OCT] or intravascular ultrasound [IVUS]) may be appropriate to help identify less evident coronary etiologies such as plaque erosion or dissection. A TEE would not be helpful in this situation. A CCTA is not necessary as the patient has already had a coronary angiogram to evaluate her coronary arteries.

20. **The correct answer is: C. Metoprolol.** In this patient presenting with STEMI with plans for primary PCI, the clinical examination suggests features of evolving cardiac pump failure (elevated JVP, basilar rales, and an S_3) with suggestion of hypoperfusion (cool lower extremities) and marginal hemodynamics (tachycardia, hypotension with narrow pulse pressure). β-Blocker therapy is recommended within the first 24 hours in patients with STEMI but should be deferred in patients with HF, a low-output state, or at risk of developing cardiogenic shock as it may block the compensatory sympathetic response.

21. **The correct answer is: D. Urgent TTE.** Rapid reperfusion therapy has decreased the incidence of mechanical complications of MI. Nonetheless, a high index of suspicion is required. Patients with late presentations of larger territory MI, especially of the anterior wall, are at highest risk of developing a ventricular septal defect. The harsh holosystolic murmur at the lower sternal border, especially in the presence of a palpable systolic thrill, is pathognomonic for a ventricular septal defect. The diagnosis is typically made by TTE, although an increase of venous oxygen saturation between the right atrium and the PA by right heart catheterization can be suggestive. Definitive management necessitates surgical repair. Afterload reducing agents (ie, nitroprusside) and interventions (ie, intra-aortic balloon pump) can help decrease left to right shunting through the ventricular septal defect as a bridge to surgery.

22. **The correct answer is: B. Administer alteplase within 30 minutes of hospital arrival and proceed with urgent transfer to PCI-capable facility.** In patients with STEMI who are candidates for reperfusion presenting to a non-PCI-capable hospital, transfer to a PCI-capable hospital should be pursued if the anticipated time from first medical contact to device therapy is <120 minutes. When the anticipated transfer time is >120 minutes, fibrinolytic therapy should be administered within 30 minutes of hospital arrival. Patients with cardiogenic shock or severe HF should be transferred to a PCI-capable hospital as soon as possible, irrespective of the time delay since MI. In the absence of cardiogenic shock or HF, transfer can be pursued urgently if there is evidence of failed pharmacologic reperfusion (ongoing symptoms) or within 24 hours for those patients in whom an invasive strategy is being pursued.

23. **The correct answer is: A. Activate cardiac catheterization lab for coronary angiography.** This patient is presenting with symptoms of acute coronary syndrome and an ECG that meets STEMI criteria. The ECG above shows ST elevations in leads V_1, V_2, and I and aVL. There are also reciprocal ST depressions in II, III, aVF, V_4 to V_6. The overall clinical situation is most concerning for spontaneous coronary artery dissection (SCAD) given the age of the patient, lack of traditional cardiac risk factors, and peripartum period. SCAD is the most common cause of MI in the peripartum period, and is called pregnancy-associated SCAD. The majority of these cases occur within 1 week of delivery. Pregnancy-associated SCAD is more likely to involve the left main, LAD, or multiple vessels. A TTE would be helpful for patients with signs and symptoms of acute coronary syndrome, without ECG changes to look for wall motion abnormalities, however; given the ST elevations on the ECG and symptoms, this is not a necessary step prior to coronary angiography. An elective stress test would not be appropriate in this situation. A TEE is not the next best step given that it would delay cardiac catheterization. The ECG does not have classic findings of hyperkalemia, which include peaked T waves and widened QRS complex.

24. **The correct answer is: B. History of ischemic stroke <3 months prior to admission.** Absolute contraindications for fibrinolytic therapy include: prior history of intracranial hemorrhage, intracranial neoplasm, aneurysm, arteriovenous malformation, ischemic stroke or closed head trauma within the last 3 months, head or spinal surgery within the last 2 months, active internal bleeding or known bleeding diathesis, suspected aortic dissection, severe uncontrollable HTN, and previous treatment with streptokinase within the last 6 months. In the current case, the patient has a recent history of ischemic stroke 1 month prior to admission, which would be an absolute contraindication for fibrinolytic therapy. The patient should be considered for immediate transfer to a PCI-capable hospital even though the delay might be longer than typically recommended.

25. **The correct answer is: A. Make arrangements to stent the LAD in the next 45 days.** Randomized trials, including the COMPLETE trial, showed a lower risk of recurrent major adverse cardiovascular events when nonculprit lesions are stented in addition to the culprit lesion in patients with STEMI. This can be pursued either during the index hospitalization or within the first 45 days. Fractional flow reserve would be reasonable for a moderate stenosis (50%-69% stenosis) but is not required for more severe stenoses. The stenting of nonculprit lesions should not be pursued for patients with signs or symptoms of cardiogenic shock.

26. **The correct answer is: C. 5-fluorouracil (5-FU).** This patient's clinical presentation is consistent with coronary vasospasm. Vasospastic angina often manifests as substernal chest pressure at rest, which typically improves with short-acting nitrates. ECG changes such as ST-segment elevation or depression may be seen during an acute episode of chest discomfort; however, the changes are usually transient and return to baseline rapidly upon resolution of symptoms. 5-FU is commonly administered in the treatment of solid malignancies and can induce coronary vasospasm after initiation of treatment. 5-FU is the second most common cause of cardiotoxicity because of chemotherapy, after anthracyclines. Leucovorin and oxaliplatin are not commonly associated with cardiotoxicity. Stress cardiomyopathy is less likely given the normal echocardiogram.

27. **The correct answer is: C. Add ezetimibe.** All acute coronary syndrome patients should be prescribed a high-intensity statin, regardless of the baseline LDL-C. Data from the IMPROVE-IT trial suggest additive benefit for ezetimibe on a background of moderate-intensity statin and is recommended for patients in whom LDL-C is still not at goal.

28. **The correct answer is: E. A and C.** Even in the absence of stenting, patients with acute coronary syndrome should be considered for dual antiplatelet therapy for approximately 12 months. Some studies support longer durations of therapy. Prasugrel has not been shown to benefit patients with non–ST-elevation acute coronary syndrome who are conservatively managed. A dose reduction may also need to be considered with prasugrel for patients over the age of 75. In contrast, ticagrelor has been shown to reduce the risk of major adverse cardiovascular events on a background of aspirin, regardless of whether patients undergo coronary stenting. More recent data may suggest that aspirin may be safely stopped with continued P2Y12 inhibitor monotherapy 1 to 3 months post-PCI (TWILIGHT). Nonetheless, the initial treatment strategy should include dual antiplatelet therapy.

29. **The correct answer is: C. Invasive coronary angiography.** The patient is experiencing NSTEMI, and per the American College of Cardiology and American Heart Association (ACC/AHA) guidelines, an invasive strategy is recommended in these higher-risk patients to reduce the risk of recurrent spontaneous MI.

30. **The correct answer is: B. Within 24 hours.** For high-risk patients with elevated troponin, ST-segment changes, or high Global Registry of Acute Coronary Events score (>140), early angiography within 24 hours is recommended. Lower-risk patients (eg, those without the above features, but with diabetes, chronic kidney disease, PCI in the past 6 months, prior CABG, or LVEF <40%) can undergo angiography within 72 hours. Patients with refractory or recurrent angina or hemodynamic or electrical instability should undergo angiography immediately.

31. **The correct answer is: C. Diltiazem.** Vasospastic or Prinzmetal angina is a clinical syndrome of rest angina with transient ST-segment elevation, nitrate-responsive angina, or angiographically apparent coronary spasm. Obstructive coronary disease may be the cause of vasospasm and thus should be excluded by invasive or noninvasive means. Calcium channel blockers (CCBs) are first-line therapy for vasospastic angina as they prevent vasoconstriction and promote vasodilation. Long-acting nitrates can also be effective, but nitrate tolerance makes them less desirable. β-Blockers, particularly nonselective β-blockers, should be avoided as they can precipitate vasospasm. Aspirin should be used with caution as it is a prostacyclin inhibitor at high doses and may also precipitate vasospasm.

32. **The correct answer is: B. Posterior leads (leads V_7-V_9).** In a patient with cardiovascular risk factors and a clinical history consistent with acute coronary syndrome, a high index of suspicion should be maintained. If the presenting ECG is nondiagnostic, posterior leads should be checked to assess the distal left circumflex and RCA territory that may supply the posterior wall of the left ventricle. Posterior ST elevations can help diagnose a posterior STEMI that may not be electrically apparent on a standard 12-lead ECG. Right-sided precordial leads are useful in patients presenting with an inferior MI to help detect right ventricle involvement and would not be useful in this case. Serial troponin measurements would be appropriate following completion of the posterior lead ECG. In this patient with rest symptoms highly suggestive of acute coronary syndrome, pulmonary embolus CT would not be the next best step (but could be pursued after acute coronary syndrome was definitely ruled out).

33. **The correct answer is: B. Myocarditis.** This patient is presenting with a chest pain syndrome and was found to have very high cardiac biomarkers, indicating myocardial injury. Appropriately, she was initially evaluated for acute coronary syndrome, which is the most life-threatening etiology for this syndrome. Her coronary catheterization showed nonobstructive disease that rules out coronary thrombosis as a cause. This condition is now commonly referred to as MINOCA (MI with no obstructive CAD). There is a growing understanding that further workup should still be pursued for individuals with MINOCA to exclude alternate etiologies. The overall clinical picture of elevated serum troponin, nonobstructive coronary arteries, echocardiogram with reduced EF, regional wall motion abnormalities not in a vascular territory, and effusion point toward a diagnosis of myocarditis. These echo features are less consistent with a stress cardiomyopathy and there is no clear stressor. Patients are considered to have microvascular CAD when they have anginal symptoms, absence of obstructive CAD, and some evidence of ischemia on functional testing; the troponin elevations in this syndrome are typically modest.

34. **The correct answer is: D. Take clopidogrel for at least 1 year.** Current ACC/AHA guidelines support continued use of dual antiplatelet therapy for at least 12 months for patients after acute coronary syndrome. At 12 months, consideration can be given to continuing the P2Y12 inhibitor for a longer duration if the patient is believed to be at low bleeding risk and high ischemic risk. For patients who undergo elective PCI for stable CAD, shorter courses of dual antiplatelet therapy may be possible. Of note, emerging evidence suggests that monotherapy with a P2Y12 inhibitor can be considered with discontinuation of aspirin 1 to 3 months post-PCI.

35. **The correct answer is: B. Distributive shock.** This patient's normal cardiac output points toward distributive shock because with all the other etiologies one would expect a diminished cardiac output. For patients who are hospitalized, distributive shock should always remain on the differential given the high frequency of sepsis from a nosocomial infection. Patients with distributive shock typically have high cardiac output, low SVR, and low/normal filling pressures. In cardiogenic shock, we expect low cardiac output and high

filling pressures. In hypovolemic shock, we expect both low cardiac output and low filling pressures. The cardiac output is low in obstructive shock and filling pressures vary based on etiology of the obstructive shock.

36. **The correct answer is: D. Left atrial—same; LVEDP—lower.** The PA wedge pressure is an estimate of the LVEDP under ideal no-flow conditions, and assuming the left atrial and LV pressures are equal (ie, there is no transmitral gradient). The mean PA wedge pressure is often used to estimate LVEDP. Mitral regurgitation is one of several conditions in which mean PA pressure can significantly overestimate LVEDP because of chronic regurgitant flow returning to the left atrium during each cardiac systole. In mitral regurgitation, mean left atrial pressure is higher than the LVEDP. The mean left atrial pressure transmits to the wedge pressure. Therefore, in this scenario, wedge pressure = left atrial pressure > LVEDP.

37. **The correct answer is: C. Increase dobutamine.** This patient has a low CI, high SVR, and high filling pressures consistent with ongoing cardiogenic shock. Increasing the dobutamine will increase contractility, allowing for increased forward flow and diuresis. Increasing the diuretic dose without increasing contractility will have minimal benefit. Adding norepinephrine and vasopressin will increase the afterload on the heart and therefore will not be as beneficial as an inodilator like dobutamine.

38. **The correct answer is: A. Mixed—cardiogenic and distributive.** Her hypotension is suggestive of a mixed picture of both cardiogenic (with reduced cardiac output despite inotropic support because of diminished LV function) and distributive (low end of normal SVR but on a vasopressor) shock. In pure cardiogenic shock and in tamponade, we would expect high filling pressures. In pure distributive shock in a patient with sepsis, we would expect a normal/high cardiac output.

39. **The correct answer is: D. Emergent TTE.** The sudden change in hemodynamics in a post-MI patient is worrisome for a mechanical complication of MI. The rise in MVO_2 does not fit with her clinical picture of worsening cardiogenic shock and likely reflects development of a ventricular septal defect. Urgent echocardiography is needed to confirm the diagnosis, the treatment for which is typically urgent surgery. On physical examination, one might expect to hear a new, harsh holosystolic murmur with a thrill and see a step-up (>7%) in oxygen saturation from central venous (pre–left-to-right shunt) to mixed venous (post–left-to-right shunt).

40. **The correct answer is: B. Furosemide.** Diuretics have been shown in multiple trials to reduce symptoms related to congestion; however, they have never been proven to reduce mortality. The agents that have been shown to reduce mortality in patients with symptomatic HF with reduced EF include ACE inhibitors, angiotensin receptor blockers (ARBs; if ACE inhibitors are not tolerated), ARNIs (ARB+ neprilysin inhibitors), β-blockers (specifically carvedilol, metoprolol, and bisoprolol), mineralocorticoid receptor antagonists (MRAs; spironolactone and eplerenone), and sodium-glucose cotransporter 2 inhibitors (SGLT2i). Of note, ARNIs have been demonstrated to be superior to ACE inhibitors in patients with symptomatic HF and reduced LV function, but the two should never be used in combination.

41. **The correct answer is: B. Administer intravenous furosemide.** In this patient with suggestive evidence of a HF exacerbation, her AKI is likely explained by cardiorenal syndrome that is believed to be driven by a variety of factors, including venous congestion. The initial treatment of choice is diuresis, which should improve her symptoms of congestion and likely will improve her creatinine. She is mentating well with normal perfusion (warm extremities) and normal pulse pressure. Intravenous crystalloid likely would worsen

her HF exacerbation. Given her limited response to oral diuretics, she may be experiencing poor gut absorption from bowel edema. Therefore, the most appropriate step is to administer intravenous furosemide or another intravenous diuretic.

42. **The correct answer is: A. Decreased aortic regurgitation.** The benefits of an intra-aortic balloon pump are 2-fold: (a) inflation during diastole results in augmentation of coronary perfusion and (b) deflation during systole decreases afterload and improves cardiac output, which may further decrease myocardial oxygen demand. One of the major risks of the intra-aortic balloon pump is that inflation during diastole will increase preexisting aortic regurgitation. Aortic aneurysms and aortic regurgitation are relative contraindications to balloon pump placement.

43. **The correct answer is: C. Diuresis alone.** When patients present with acute decompensated HF, it is important to assess their degree of congestion (wet vs. dry) and adequacy of perfusion (warm vs. cold). This patient's elevated JVP, crackles on lung examination, and lower extremity edema are suggestive of volume overload (wet). His normal lactate, LFTs, creatinine, warm extremities, and reasonable urine output suggest adequate end-organ perfusion or forward flow (warm). In a patient who is "warm and wet," the initial step in therapy is diuresis alone. If inadequate perfusion is demonstrated, then the patient may also benefit from the addition of inotropes.

44. **The correct answer is: A. Dapagliflozin.** GDMT for patients with HFrEF includes medical therapy with β-blockers, renin-angiotensin-aldosterone system (RAAS) inhibitors, MRAs, and SGLT2i. This patient has HFrEF with excellent functional capacity and is already medically managed with metoprolol (β-blocker), sacubitril-valsartan (RAAS inhibitor), and spironolactone (MRA), and thus will benefit from the addition of dapagliflozin (SGLT2i). SGTL2i have mortality benefit in patients with HFrEF regardless of the presence of diabetes.

45. **The correct answer is: A. Nitroprusside.** This patient with known advanced HF is presenting in cardiogenic shock after an episode of sustained VT. On examination, he is found to be cold and dry as evidenced by lack of peripheral edema, JVD, and lung crackles. This is further supported by invasive data you receive from a PA catheter, which shows a low CI and a PCWP of 12 mmHg. The overarching goal in cardiogenic shock is to provide interventions that will improve cardiac output while maintaining systemic perfusion. As the patient's PCWP is at goal, furosemide would not be helpful and may lower the CI by dropping preload. The patient has a high SVR, which is a physiologic response to the low cardiac output in an attempt to preserve BP. Increased SVR, which functions as afterload, also increases myocardial demand and worsens cardiac output. Nitroprusside in this context can improve cardiac output by promoting arterial vasodilation. If the patient's BP drops to unacceptable levels with nitroprusside, then further sources of support may be required in the form of inotropes or mechanical devices. In this case, inotropes such as dobutamine also carry a risk of precipitating VT. Although amiodarone is indicated to suppress VT, it will not directly improve cardiac output. Metoprolol is contraindicated in cardiogenic shock as it has a negative inotropic effect.

46. **The correct answer is: D. Empagliflozin.** Many clinical trials have failed to demonstrate the benefit of pharmacotherapy to reduce mortality among patients with HF with preserved EF. In a clinical trial, spironolactone did not reduce mortality, but was shown to decrease the risk of rehospitalization for HF (*NEJM.* 2014;370:1383). Most recently, two trials in patients with HF with preserved EF patients have shown improved cardiovascular outcomes with an SGLT2i (EMPEROR-Preserved & DELIVER).

47. The correct answer is: C. No reduction in diuretic dosing after starting sacubitril/valsartan. This patient is presenting with signs and symptoms of hypovolemia including dizziness/light-headedness, tachycardia, hypotension, and low JVP. Laboratory studies demonstrate AKI. Sacubitril/valsartan is a combination neprilysin inhibitor and ARB. Neprilysin is an enzyme that degrades natriuretic peptides. Therefore, sacubitril prevents the degradation of natriuretic peptides and results in a diuretic effect. Patients being started on this medication should be monitored for over-diuresis and may require diuretic dosing adjustments. Patients with HF should be educated about adherence to fluid restriction, but here the clinical picture is most consistent with over-diuresis, not volume overload.

48. The correct answer is: C. Insert a percutaneous LV assist device (eg, Impella or TandemHeart). This patient is in cardiogenic shock because of profound acute decompensated HF. Increasing the pressor dose would not address his cardiogenic shock. Increasing the dobutamine is unlikely to be sufficient and could risk further end-organ damage. An intra-aortic balloon pump is also unlikely to offer adequate support. A percutaneous LV assist device can provide up to 5.5 L/min cardiac output and would be the next best step. It should be noted, however, that randomized trials supporting the use of assist devices are currently lacking.

49. The correct answer is: B. Initiation of venoarterial extracorporeal membrane oxygen. The patient has evidence of biventricular HF from a presumed influenza myocarditis. With supportive care, myocardial recovery is expected, and thus with escalation of pharmacologic support, mechanical circulatory support should also be considered. Given the patient's biventricular failure, a pure LV support device would be insufficient. Thus, the patient should be considered for venoarterial extracorporeal membrane oxygen. It should be noted that large, randomized trials supporting this approach are lacking.

50. The correct answer is: B. Initiation of angiotensin-converting enzyme (ACE) inhibitor and β-blocker; repeat TTE in 3 months. In this case, the patient presents with a dilated cardiomyopathy and is found to have influenza infection. Although this may be the etiology of his systolic HF, the cardiac MRI did not support a diagnosis of acute myocarditis. He also has a history of significant toxin exposure including alcohol and cocaine, which may lead to systolic dysfunction. He should pursue abstinence and immediately start appropriate GDMT to promote positive LV remodeling and possibly improve his EF. TTE can be repeated in 3 months to assess for recovery of function; 1 month may be too soon to expect any significant improvement. If he has persistent significant LV dysfunction, an ICD can then be considered at this time. A primary prevention ICD should not be placed if there is a reasonable expectation for recovery in LV function. Myocardial biopsy is not indicated in this case, as it is typically pursued in cases of hemodynamic or electrical instability when pathology is expected to change management.

51. The correct answer is: B. Discontinue norepinephrine and initiate phenylephrine. The patient has a history of HOCM, which indicates septal hypertrophy with a narrow subaortic outflow tract. β-Agonists, such as norepinephrine, will increase chronotropy and inotropy, which can worsen outflow obstruction and can lead to worsening hypotension. In this case, the vasopressor of choice would be phenylephrine, which is a pure α-agonist, and therefore will increase SVR without increasing chronotropy or inotropy. Slower HRs may be advantageous by increasing LV filling time and therefore decreasing the outflow gradient. The addition of other inotropes, such as dobutamine or epinephrine, will likely worsen her shock. Volume depletion can also worsen the obstruction, but at this time, she appears to be euvolemic with a central venous pressure of 12 mmHg on her most recent tracing.

52. **The correct answer is: A. BP decrease of ≥20 mmHg with exercise.** Patients with hypertrophic cardiomyopathy who have had prior episodes of VT/ventricular fibrillation are candidates for consideration of ICD placement. Patients with ≥1 of the following risk factors may be considered for primary prevention ICD placement and should be referred to an electrophysiologist. Risk factors include family history of sudden cardiac death, unexplained syncope (especially if exertional), LV wall thickness ≥30 mm, LV aneurysm, or EF <50%. ICDs may also be considered if nonsustained VT is documented, failure of systolic BP to increase or fall from peak ≥20 mmHg with exercise, >15% late gadolinium enhancement (fibrosis) on cardiac MRI. Changes in BP with exercise can be assessed with an exercise treadmill test. Answers B and C do not meet the criteria outlined in the guidelines and are therefore incorrect.

53. **The correct answer is: A. Amyloidosis.** The discordance of low voltages on ECG, despite thick ventricular walls on TTE, is a classic ECG finding for cardiac amyloidosis for someone who is suspected to be at risk. Additional diagnostic tests include serum and urine protein electrophoresis, quantification of SFLC ratio, technetium pyrophosphate scan, and possible fat pad biopsy and cardiac MRI. Sarcoidosis is another type of infiltrative cardiomyopathy; however, his history (including multiple myeloma and renal failure) and ECG findings are more characteristic of amyloidosis. Patients with sarcoidosis do not classically have increased LV wall thickness, as involvement may be quite patchy. With long-standing HTN or hypertrophic cardiomyopathy, a TTE will commonly show LV wall thickening because of concentric hypertrophy; however, this is typically reflected by normal or high voltages on ECG.

54. **The correct answer is: B. LV wall thickness of 15 mm.** LV wall thickness ≥15 mm is one of the diagnostic criteria for hypertrophic cardiomyopathy. LV wall thickness ≥30 mm, as well as answer choices A, C, and D, are all high-risk features for sudden cardiac death. An ICD is recommended for all patients with hypertrophic cardiomyopathy and a history of cardiac arrest or sustained VT. Patients with hypertrophic cardiomyopathy should be evaluated for high-risk features and, if any exist, considered for ICD implantation.

55. **The correct answer is: D. Refer for surgical myomectomy.** This patient with known HOCM meets criteria for surgical myomectomy based on symptoms of HF despite maximal medical therapy, and an LVOT gradient >30 mmHg at rest or with provocation. Surgical myomectomy reduces symptoms of HF in the vast majority of patients with HOCM and is preferred over alcohol septal ablation when patients are considered good surgical candidates. Digoxin would increase contractility and worsen the outflow tract obstruction. Furosemide should be used with caution in HOCM, as diuretics further reduce preload, which can worsen outflow tract obstruction.

56. **The correct answer is: A. Technetium-99m pyrophosphate scan.** This patient is presenting with new-onset HF and peripheral neuropathy; his echocardiogram has features concerning for an infiltrative cardiomyopathy. The clinical syndrome is most concerning for systemic amyloidosis, which can be broadly broken down into AL amyloidosis, a disease of immunoglobulin light chain deposition in the setting of plasma cell dyscrasia, and transthyretin (TTR) amyloidosis, which involves deposition of misfolded TTR proteins. Given the normal SPEP/SFLC, senile TTR amyloid is the most likely etiology. Although endomyocardial biopsy and fat pad biopsy are possible diagnostic tools, a technetium-99 PYP scan is a noninvasive method of assessing for TTR amyloid. Immunoglobulin light chain will not bind the radiolabeled pyrophosphate and this modality can only be used to assess for TTR amyloid. Cardiac PET is often utilized to assess CAD but also has utility in assessing for certain cardiomyopathies such as cardiac sarcoidosis.

57. **The correct answer is: A. Coronary angiography.** The next best step is to obtain an urgent coronary angiogram to exclude obstructive CAD. Although the history and echocardiogram are suggestive of Takotsubo cardiomyopathy because of the recent stressor and evidence of apical ballooning, it is necessary to definitively rule out acute plaque rupture prior to diagnosing a stress-induced cardiomyopathy.

58. **The correct answer is: A. Absolute abstinence from alcohol.** Although the cause of his new cardiomyopathy could be from alternate etiologies, it may be due to alcohol use or alcohol may be contributing. The treatment in addition to GDMT for HFrEF and rate or rhythm control for AF is complete abstinence from alcohol.

59. **The correct answer is: A. Proceed to dobutamine stress echo.** This patient should be evaluated with a dobutamine stress echo prior to consideration of aortic valve replacement in order to better understand whether he exhibits low-flow, low-gradient, severe aortic stenosis. In patients with reduced EF and aortic valve area <1 cm^2, it may be challenging to distinguish if the estimated aortic valve area is low because of the reduced EF or because of true severe aortic stenosis. If the calculated aortic valve area increases substantially with administration of dobutamine, then this would suggest "pseudo-aortic stenosis", as the initial aortic valve area estimate was likely explained by poor forward flow. Similarly, it is important to know whether the mean gradient across the valve significantly increases in response to dobutamine. If the mean gradient increases substantially and the aortic valve area does not change, then the patient benefits from aortic valve replacement.

60. **The correct answer is: D. Repeat TTE every 1 to 2 years.** This patient was incidentally found to have a bicuspid aortic valve and echocardiographic evidence of moderate aortic stenosis while undergoing workup for her fevers. Aortic valve intervention is not indicated for moderate aortic stenosis; therefore, she needs routine periodic monitoring with repeat TTE yearly to every other year. Patients with bicuspid aortic valve are also at risk of developing TAAs. In these cases, aortic valve replacement may be indicated in patients with aortic stenosis or regurgitation at the time of surgical intervention on the ascending aorta.

61. **The correct answer is: A. Heart team approach to determine recommendation for surgical versus transcatheter aortic valve replacement.** This patient has symptomatic severe aortic stenosis; therefore, aortic valve replacement is indicated. The STS score is used to determine the risk of surgical mortality for many surgical procedures, including aortic valve replacement. Transcatheter aortic valve replacement has been shown to be noninferior to surgical aortic valve replacement for high STS score ($>8\%$) patients (PARTNER A trial), intermediate STS score (4%-8%) patients (PARTNER 2 trial), and, most recently, low STS score ($<4\%$) patients (PARTNER 3 trial, published in 2019). A transcatheter aortic valve replacement approach typically offers faster hospital recovery but has a higher incidence of permanent pacemaker placement. For this patient with a low STS score, either surgical or transcatheter aortic valve replacement may be appropriate, and the decision of which to recommend to the patient should be made by a multidisciplinary heart team.

62. **The correct answer is: B. Mechanical aortic valve replacement.** Given the patient has symptomatic severe aortic stenosis, he has a Class I indication for aortic valve replacement. Current guidelines recommend mechanical aortic valve replacement for patients <50 years old who do not have a contraindication for anticoagulation. These recommendations are in place as mechanical valves have on average a significantly longer lifespan than bioprosthetic valves. For patients 50 to 65 years old, shared decision-making is recommended in the choice between mechanical and bioprosthetic valves. And in patients

>65 years old, bioprosthetic valves are preferred. In the current case, given the patient is young and has no known history of bleeding complications, a mechanical valve would be preferred.

63. **The correct answer is: B. Mitral regurgitation.** This patient most likely had a missed inferior MI that occurred 3 days ago as suggested by his symptoms and the appearance of inferior Q waves on his ECG. Patients are at risk of mechanical complications, including papillary muscle rupture, ventricular septal rupture, and pericardial wall rupture, approximately 2 to 7 days following MI. This is particularly true in larger infarcts that are not revascularized. The posteromedial papillary muscle is typically supplied by the posterior descending artery off of the RCA. Because of its sole blood supply, it is more prone to rupture than the anterolateral papillary muscle. Papillary muscle rupture is typically manifested with acute onset of dyspnea, hypoxia, pulmonary edema, holosystolic murmur (low pitched and may be hard to appreciate), and hypotension. This requires immediate surgical repair and can be evaluated by echocardiogram. A ventricular septal defect is another complication after MI but typically exhibits a louder systolic murmur and is often accompanied by a thrill. Although LV dysfunction and a pulmonary embolus are possible, a mechanical complication should be first considered during this time frame after MI.

64. **The correct answer is: C. Stop coumadin now and bridge with unfractionated heparin.** Patients with a mechanical valve in the aortic position and additional stroke risk factors such as AF, prior thromboembolism, hypercoagulability, and EF <30% to 35% should be managed with a coumadin goal of 2.5 to 3.5. Patients with a mechanical mitral valve or a mechanical aortic valve with risk factors for stroke should be bridged with heparin when coumadin is discontinued. For patients with a mechanical aortic valve replacement without high-risk features, the decision to bridge with anticoagulation may depend on patient factors, the procedure being performed, and other medical comorbidities. The novel anticoagulants, including the direct thrombin inhibitor dabigatran and factor Xa inhibitors, are contraindicated in patients with a mechanical valve.

65. **The correct answer is: C. Referral for aortic valve replacement.** In patients with chronic severe aortic regurgitation, aortic valve replacement is recommended for symptomatic patients (Class I, Level of Evidence B), patients with LVEF 55% (Class I, Level of Evidence B), patients with indication for another cardiac surgery (Class I, Level of Evidence C), or patients with LVEF >55% and LVESD >50 mm or LVESD indexed to body surface area of >25 mm/m^2 (Class 2a, Level of Evidence B). In the current case, although the patient has remained asymptomatic, her LVEF is now <55%, which would be an indication for aortic valve replacement.

66. **The correct answer is: C. Refer for mitral valve surgery.** Patients with chronic severe primary mitral regurgitation because of mitral valve prolapse should be referred for mitral valve replacement if they have an EF between 30% and 60% or a LVESD >40 mm, regardless of symptom status. She has no evidence of congestion, so furosemide is not indicated. Because she has an indication for mitral valve intervention, additional testing with ambulatory ECG monitoring or repeat echocardiography is not indicated.

67. **The correct answer is: C. Hold the warfarin and monitor.** In the setting of a patient with a mechanical valve, the risks of bleeding need to be weighed against the risks of valve thrombosis in the setting of subtherapeutic INR levels. In a patient with no overt signs of bleeding and an INR of 5 to 10, the general recommendations are to hold the warfarin and monitor for any signs of bleeding. If the patient becomes unstable, or develops signs of significant bleeding, then warfarin reversal is warranted and can be achieved by vitamin K, fresh frozen plasma, or prothrombin complex concentrate.

68. **The correct answer is: D. Refer for percutaneous mitral balloon commissurotomy as anatomy allows.** Patients with rheumatic mitral stenosis may have prolonged asymptomatic phases; however, the additional volume load of pregnancy often results in overt symptoms of HF. She currently describes symptoms consistent with New York Heart Association class III HF. In the presence of moderate-to-severe symptoms and pregnancy, consideration needs to be given to possible mitral valve intervention if the pregnancy is to be continued. For patients in whom the anatomy is amenable, a percutaneous procedure is preferred. Women of child-bearing age with known mitral valve stenosis should be counseled about the possible risks of pregnancy.

69. **The correct answer is: D. High-dose aspirin and colchicine.** This patient is presenting with acute pericarditis as evidence by sharp chest pain with an ECG demonstrating diffuse ST-segment elevation with PR-segment depression. First-line therapy in acute pericarditis includes high-dose aspirin or NSAIDs and colchicine. Although the patient has risk factors for CAD, her normal cardiac enzymes and absence of ischemic changes on ECG or wall motion abnormalities on echocardiogram are reassuring, and thus stress testing and cardiac catheterization are not warranted. Pericardiocentesis is not indicated in this patient with a small pericardial effusion without clinical evidence of cardiac tamponade.

70. **The correct answer is: C. Give 500 mL fluid bolus.** The patient is presenting with Beck's triad (distant heart sounds, elevated jugular vein pulsation, and hypotension) concerning for tamponade. Upfront treatment of suspected tamponade relies on volume expansion while a diagnostic and therapeutic plan is formulated. An emergent TTE must be obtained to measure the size and location of the effusion. Effusions amenable to pericardiocentesis are anterior in location and at least 10 mm in size (measured during diastole). A pericardial window may be needed in posterior effusions not amenable to pericardiocentesis. The history and physical are most suggestive of a pericardial effusion, so a pulmonary embolism CT scan would not be the first step.

71. **The correct answer is: B. Constrictive pericarditis.** Constrictive pericarditis may occur in 1% to 2% of cases following pericarditis. In patients with tuberculosis, bacterial infections, neoplasm, or, as in this case, exposure to radiation therapy, the risk of developing constrictive pericarditis is higher. Constrictive pericarditis occurs when there is adhesion between the visceral and parietal pericardium, resulting in a rigid pericardium limiting diastolic filling and increasing venous pressures. The limitation of venous return occurs only after the rapid filling stage following opening of the tricuspid valve. These patients often have Kussmaul sign present, which manifests as a jugular venous pulsation that does not decrease with inspiration. Sometimes, a pericardial knock may be present. ECG may show low voltages, but constrictive pericarditis does not cause conduction disease, which is more commonly seen with restrictive cardiomyopathy. Clinically, patients often have signs and symptoms of right-sided HF on examination and clear lungs. Diagnostically, TTE reveals respirophasic variation, where during inspiration there is increased flow seen across the tricuspid valve and decreased flow across the mitral valve. Other findings include expiratory hepatic vein flow reversal. On simultaneous left and right heart catheterization, there is equalization of the ventricular end-diastolic pressures between the right and left ventricles and discordance of the right ventricular and LV pressure peaks during the respiratory cycle.

72. **The correct answer is: B. Initiation of high-dose nonsteroidal anti-inflammatory drugs (NSAIDs).** Pericarditis may manifest with ECG changes, including ST elevations diffusely (often crossing multiple vascular territories such as leads I and II). The ST-elevation morphology is classically concave upward. PR depression may be seen as well.

The exception to these changes is in lead aVR where there may be ST depression and PR elevation as seen here. The ECG may ultimately reveal T-wave inversions.

High-dose NSAIDs remain the backbone of acute pericarditis treatment. In patients with a recent MI, aspirin can be used. Colchicine should be added for a period of 3 months to decrease the risk of refractory or recurrent pericarditis. Steroids should only be utilized in those patients with contraindications to NSAIDs or refractory pericarditis, as steroids have been shown to increase the risk of recurrence.

73. **The correct answer is: A. Calculating his atherosclerotic cardiovascular disease risk score and, if >10%, starting an antihypertensive agent now.** Per the most recent 2017 ACC/AHA BP guidelines, a confirmed BP between 130 and 139/80 and 89 mmHg is considered to be stage 1 HTN. For this patient population, the recommendation is to initiate an antihypertensive if clinical cardiovascular disease is present (ie, ischemic heart disease, HF, stroke) or their calculated atherosclerotic cardiovascular disease risk is >10%.

74. **The correct answer is: D. Lisinopril.** First-line antihypertensives include ACE inhibitors, CCBs, and diuretics. The choice of which antihypertensive to begin with is guided by the presence of comorbidities. Patients with diabetes mellitus with microalbuminuria should be treated first line with an ACE inhibitor, in the absence of contraindications.

75. **The correct answer is: B. Intravenous labetalol.** In this patient with hypertensive emergency complicated by aortic dissection, intravenous agents are needed initially to achieve rapid HR and BP control. The use of a pure vasodilator can lead to reflex tachycardia, thereby increasing LV contractile force and potentially propagating the aortic dissection. As such, the first choice of intravenous agent should limit HR response such as a β-blocker. A vasodilator can then be added to achieve BP control.

76. **The correct answer is: C. Substitute labetalol for lisinopril.** ACE inhibitors should be discontinued in women planning to conceive, given the risk of fetus malformation during the first trimester and renal failure in the second/third trimesters. The preferred agents for HTN during pregnancy are methyldopa, labetalol, and nifedipine. HTN can worsen during pregnancy and cause significant harm to the fetus. Therefore, it is not recommended to stop antihypertensive medications during pregnancy in women with an indication for their continued use.

77. **The correct answer is: A. Chlorthalidone.** Occult volume overload often underlies difficult-to-control HTN. Therefore, all patients with concern for resistant HTN should be on a diuretic. The definition of resistant HTN includes ≥3 drugs with at least one agent being a diuretic.

78. **The correct answer is: A. Amlodipine.** Current guidelines recommend either a CCB or a thiazide diuretic (eg, hydrochlorothiazide, chlorthalidone) in the initial treatment of black adults with HTN and no history of HF or chronic kidney disease. These agents lead to better BP control as monotherapy or as initial agents in multidrug regimens compared to other antihypertensive medications. The first-line therapy recommended for non-black patients includes thiazides, CCBs, ACE inhibitors, or ARBs.

79. **The correct answer is: A. MR angiography (MRA) of the renal arteries.** In this young patient with severe HTN and an abdominal bruit, renal artery stenosis secondary to fibromuscular dysplasia should be strongly suspected. An MRA of the renal arteries would be a reasonable first step in her diagnostic evaluation. Although a duplex ultrasound can be considered, it cannot definitively exclude fibromuscular dysplasia. A noncontrast CT scan

will not visualize the vasculature adequately. In some instances, direct visualization with renal angiography may be required if clinical suspicion remains high, but a diagnosis cannot be made noninvasively. For patients with confirmed fibromuscular dysplasia in whom BP cannot be controlled, percutaneous transluminal renal angioplasty should be considered.

80. **The correct answer is: B. 6 months.** All patients who have a newly discovered aortic aneurysm should undergo repeat assessment at 6 months to ensure aneurysm stability and rate of growth. Thereafter, TAAs can be monitored yearly if stable.

81. **The correct answer is: B. All first-degree relatives should be screened.** Screening for TAAs is recommended in all patients with a bicuspid aortic valve. First-degree relatives of patients with a TAA, bicuspid aortic valve, or connective tissue disorder should undergo screening for TAAs.

82. **The correct answer is: C. Rate of growth of 0.5 cm in 6 months.** Surgical repair of abdominal aortic aneurysms should be performed in patients with aneurysms ≥5.5 cm in size or those associated with symptoms. Surgical repair should be considered in females with aneurysms ≥5 cm and in those patients in whom the rate of growth is >0.5 cm/year.

83. **The correct answer is: A. Esmolol drip.** The patient has a type A aortic dissection and should have prompt surgical evaluation. In the interval, the key to upfront medical management is to decrease the impulse (dP/dt) with each heartbeat, targeting a HR <60 beats/min and systolic BP <120 mmHg. BP should be titrated off the highest BP reading, as dissection involving the subclavian artery can result in falsely low readings. The optimal first agent would be an esmolol drip—a β-blocker that provides predictable pharmacokinetics that is easier to titrate. Starting with either nitroprusside or nitroglycerin would cause reflex tachycardia and can propagate the dissection. Either of these may be started following β-blocker initiation. Nitroprusside should be avoided with renal dysfunction, as it can precipitate cyanide toxicity. A continuous IV β-blocker drip would likely offer better control and opportunities for titration than a single metoprolol IV push.

84. **The correct answer is: A. Aortic dissection.** The patient's mediastinal silhouette is enlarged, raising concern for aortic pathology such as dissection. An abnormal CXR is seen in 60% to 90% of patients with aortic dissection. A normal CXR, however, does not rule out aortic dissection or pathology. Given the clinical history of a tearing back pain that was maximal at onset and remains severe, with HTN, hyperlipidemia, and tobacco use history, the patient in the clinical vignette is most likely experiencing an acute aortic dissection and a CTA of the chest should be pursued.

    There are lung markings extending to the periphery of the lung fields, making pneumothorax incorrect. Although the trachea appears to be displaced to the right, it may be the result of the tortuous aorta and does not represent a tension pneumothorax, as both lungs appear fully inflated in the CXR. Although there may be subtly increased vascular markings in the lung fields, pulmonary edema is not the predominant finding. A pericardial effusion that results in an increased cardiac silhouette is more likely to be associated with tamponade (hypotension, tachycardia, JVD) than HTN.

85. **The correct answer is: A. Aortic dissection.** Intra-aortic balloon pumps are used to increase coronary perfusion pressure and augment cardiac output. One of the complications of intra-aortic balloon pumps includes aortic dissection. Propagation of the dissection into a subclavian, femoral, or carotid artery may cause pulse deficits. In the clinical vignette, the balloon caused dissection, which propagated to involve the left subclavian artery leading to loss of radial arterial line tracing. Although worsening cardiac output can cause distal

pulses to be more difficult to palpate (in the setting of increased SVR), the cardiac output and CI are unchanged in the vignette. In addition, the asymmetry of the examination makes a global process, such as worsening cardiogenic shock unlikely. Radial artery spasm can occur, particularly if the artery is catheterized, but it should not affect the brachial artery. Thromboembolism can occur with large anterior MIs in the setting of LV akinesis. This patient, however, experienced an inferior-posterior STEMI that is less likely to lead to LV thrombus compared to anterior MIs.

86. **The correct answer is: D. Surgery.** The patient has a body habitus that may be consistent with Marfan syndrome, and his diastolic murmur may be suggestive of a proximal dissection. Acute aortic regurgitation is present in approximately 44% of patients with a proximal aortic dissection. The patient also has new signs of HF (bilateral pulmonary rales), which may be a sign of proximal dissection leading to aortic regurgitation.

    The treatment for a proximal aortic dissection (type A) is typically urgent surgery. Distal dissections (type B) may be managed medically by decreasing dP/dt and targeting HR <60 beats/min and central systolic BP <120 mmHg. Although patients with Marfan syndrome are at increased risk for pneumothorax, this patient has a diastolic murmur, HTN, and back pain, which is therefore concerning for a proximal dissection.

87. **The correct answer is: B. Extension of the dissection below the diaphragmatic hiatus.** Acute renal failure, decreased urine output, and lactic acidosis are concerning for impaired blood flow into the renal arteries and visceral blood supply. This could be due to direct extension of the dissection into additional arteries or because of decreased blood flow as a result of obstruction by a false lumen in the dissection flap. Although proximal dissection can cause hypotension, the mechanism is typically through acute aortic regurgitation, tamponade, or cardiogenic shock. This patient has signs of malperfusion below the diaphragm, making this the more likely etiology. Cyanide toxicity is a complication of patients being treated with nitroprusside. Risk factors for cyanide toxicity include hypoalbuminemia and high doses of nitroprusside. However, the patient has no evidence of cellular hypoxia, making this diagnosis less likely. Alternative medications for afterload reduction should be considered given the acute renal failure. Sedation effect should not cause renal failure or lactic acidosis.

88. **The correct answer is: D. Transvenous temporary pacemaker.** This patient has a clinical syndrome concerning for early disseminated Lyme disease, including intermittent fevers, recent history of a target-shaped rash, and travel to an endemic area. In this setting, his ECG findings of CHB with a slow escape rhythm are likely secondary to acute Lyme carditis. His CHB may resolve following a course of antibiotics; therefore, a permanent pacemaker is not immediately indicated. However, a temporary pacemaker should be placed in this scenario as he remains hemodynamically unstable.

89. **The correct answer is: B. Increased automaticity at multiple sites in the atria.** The ECG reveals an irregular rhythm with three distinct P-wave morphologies, which is consistent with multifocal atrial tachycardia (MAT). The mechanism of this arrhythmia is believed to be through increased automaticity at multiple sites in the atria (each site responsible for a distinct P wave). MAT is not common but is sometimes seen in patients with chronic lung disease. Chaotic atrial activation originating from the pulmonary veins is often the presumptive mechanism of AF (no P waves seen on ECG). Reentry through dual pathways in the atrioventricular node is the mechanism of atrioventricular nodal reentrant tachycardia. Reentry through the atrioventricular node and an accessory pathway is the mechanism of atrioventricular reentrant tachycardia. Atrioventricular nodal reentrant rhythms may exhibit a retrograde P wave on ECG.

90. **The correct answer is: D. Procainamide.** For patients with WPW, a rapid supraventricular tachycardia may conduct through both the atrioventricular node and accessory pathway. If a drug is administered that purely blocks the atrioventricular node, then there is a risk that the rhythm might travel exclusively down the accessory pathway and degenerate to ventricular fibrillation. For this reason, procainamide is the drug of choice as it will stabilize the atrial rhythm. Digoxin and adenosine will primarily target the atrioventricular node and are therefore contraindicated. Direct current cardioversion may eventually be required but is not emergent at this time if the patient is stable.

91. **The correct answer is: B. Long QT interval.** This clinical vignette presents an otherwise healthy 54-year-old woman who is admitted with pneumonia and is undergoing treatment with antibiotics. Her recent exposure to levofloxacin and a polymorphic VT arrest raise concern for an acquired long QT syndrome. A new LBBB can suggest an acute infarct, which is a cause of polymorphic VT; however, she is a relatively young woman with no cardiovascular symptoms or risk factors and excellent cardiovascular fitness. In this case, the most likely cause of her polymorphic VT is an acquired long QT interval. Any QT-prolonging therapies should be immediately discontinued. A pseudo-RBBB with ST-segment elevation in V_1 to V_3 is a classic ECG pattern seen in Brugada syndrome (a rare, congenital channelopathy associated with sudden cardiac death). T-wave inversion in V_1 to V_3 can be seen in arrhythmogenic right ventricular change as well as other right ventricle cardiomyopathies; however, these are typically associated with monomorphic VT and are rare.

92. **The correct answer is: D. Radiofrequency ablation.** The patient presents with a fourth episode of monomorphic VT over the past 2 months. This has been occurring despite adequate medical therapy (β-blockers, mexiletine, amiodarone). Her most recent coronary angiogram would suggest that her VT is not driven by ischemia. For recurrent VT or VT storm, radiofrequency ablation can be an effective therapy and is the next most appropriate step in care.

93. **The correct answer is: C. Observation.** The ECG tracing reveals second-degree atrioventricular block type 1 (also called Mobitz I or Wenckebach). This arrhythmia is often asymptomatic and usually can be monitored without intervention. Symptomatic patients with second-degree atrioventricular block type 2 (also called Mobitz II) or third-degree heart block may require a pacemaker. Atropine is indicated for symptomatic bradycardia.

94. **The correct answer is: C. Atrioventricular nodal reentrant tachycardia.** The patient presents with a narrow complex tachycardia at 150 beats/min. ECG reveals a regular rate. A retrograde P wave can be seen immediately following the QRS complex in leads V_1 and V_2, suggesting this rhythm is atrioventricular nodal reentrant tachycardia. ECGs of atrial flutter often show flutter waves at a typical circuit of 300 beats/min that are best visualized in leads II, III, and aVF. AF is an irregular rhythm. Atrioventricular nodal reentrant tachycardia can typically be terminated with IV adenosine, as it disrupts the reentrant path involving the atrioventricular node.

95. **The correct answer is: C. Perform TEE; if no left atrial thrombus, perform cardioversion.** The patient presents with new AF complicated by a tachycardia-induced cardiomyopathy. She has inadequate rate control on her current regimen and her BP has limited further titration. Therefore, restoration of sinus rhythm is likely to provide her the best opportunity to recover LV function. As the duration of her AF is unknown, she should undergo TEE to evaluate for left atrial thrombus prior to any attempts at cardioversion. All patients after electrical cardioversion should receive several weeks of anticoagulation. This is independent from the decision of long-term anticoagulation. Typically, an ablation for AF is only pursued after several recurrences.

96. **The correct answer is: A. Amiodarone.** The patient has new-onset AF and a history of an ischemic cardiomyopathy. Both flecainide and propafenone are class Ic antiarrhythmic drugs and can be useful for the management of AF. However, class Ic drugs are contraindicated in patients with ischemia or structural heart disease. Although amiodarone has potential side effects, it can be used to maintain sinus rhythm in patients with structural heart disease. A non-dihydropyridine CCB such as diltiazem may be helpful for rate control but is contraindicated in HF.

97. **The correct answer is: C. Serum creatinine.** Long-term amiodarone use has been known to lead to toxicity of multiple organ systems (eg, thyroid, skin, liver, lungs, eyes). Current recommendations advocate a baseline ECG, PFT, CXR, thyroid function tests (TFTs), LFTs, and ophthalmic examination. Amiodarone is not known to lead to renal dysfunction, so monitoring for renal function is not routinely indicated.

98. **The correct answer is: D. Start warfarin.** This patient presents with valvular AF secondary to rheumatic mitral stenosis. The CHA_2DS_2-VASc score should be used to help assess a patient's risk of embolic stroke or systemic embolic events in patients with nonvalvular AF. However, anticoagulation is always indicated for patients with moderate or severe rheumatic mitral stenosis in the presence of AF. Patients with moderate or severe rheumatic mitral stenosis were excluded from trials of the novel or direct-acting oral anticoagulants, including rivaroxaban, and therefore are not indicated for use. Clinical practice guidelines recommend use of vitamin K antagonists, such as warfarin, to reduce the risk of stroke in these patients.

99. **The correct answer is: A. Andexanet alfa.** This patient presents with a life-threatening traumatic intracranial hemorrhage following a mechanical fall. She currently takes both aspirin and apixaban, which increases her risk of bleeding. In the acute setting, reversal of the effect of both agents would be indicated with both platelet transfusion and andexanet alfa. Andexanet alfa is a recombinant factor Xa protein that reverses the effect of factor Xa inhibitors, including apixaban. Idarucizumab is a monoclonal antibody that reverses the effect of the direct thrombin inhibitor dabigatran. Fresh frozen plasma contains all factors in the soluble coagulation system and can be utilized to restore factor deficiencies in patients who are bleeding or are planned to undergo procedures. Vitamin K will reverse the effects of warfarin but not a factor Xa inhibitor.

100. **The correct answer is: B. Direct-acting oral anticoagulants are not indicated for patients with AF with rheumatic mitral stenosis.** Direct-acting oral anticoagulants are not indicated for patients with AF with rheumatic mitral stenosis as these patients are at very high risk of stroke and were excluded from trials assessing efficacy of direct-acting oral anticoagulants in the prevention of stroke in AF. Warfarin is the only oral anticoagulant that should be used for patients with a mechanical heart valve because of a trial that indicated that dabigatran is inferior to warfarin in that setting. Reversal agents are now available for all the approved direct-acting oral anticoagulants. In head-to-head clinical trials, the direct-acting oral anticoagulants have been shown to have a lower risk of intracranial hemorrhage when compared to warfarin in patients with AF.

101. **The correct answer is: D. Percutaneous left atrial appendage occlusion.** Percutaneous left atrial appendage occlusion offers an alternative to long-term anticoagulation for reduction of stroke and systemic embolism. However, patients will still need to take some form of anticoagulation for a period of weeks surrounding the time of procedure. The efficacy of half-dose apixaban to prevent stroke has not been established and may still increase her risk of further intracranial hemorrhage. Aspirin alone is not believed to

significantly attenuate risk of stroke or systemic embolic event in a patient with AF and will still increase the risk of bleeding. Antiarrhythmic therapy such as amiodarone does not sufficiently lower the risk of stroke in a patient with AF to preclude anticoagulation.

102. **The correct answer is: C. Catheter ablation.** Catheter ablation should be considered for patients with symptomatic AF and HF. Specifically, in patients with symptomatic AF and LVEF <35%, catheter ablation reduces the risk of all-cause mortality and HF hospitalization when compared with medical therapy with antiarrhythmic therapy. Propranolol should not be initiated in this patient who is already on nodal blockade with metoprolol, and who has been symptomatic despite attempts at rate control in the past. Antiarrhythmic therapies such as amiodarone and sotalol may be considered in patients in whom antiarrhythmic therapies have not yet been attempted, or in patients who may not tolerate a catheter ablation procedure. Antiarrhythmic therapy has already been attempted in this patient and thus the next step in management should be a referral for catheter ablation. Furthermore, amiodarone should not be initiated in this patient with elevated liver enzymes.

103. **The correct answer is: D. Long-term external cardiac event monitoring device.** The salient features of this case include a syncope presentation with the frequency of symptoms occurring on a weekly basis. Thus, a 48-hour Holter monitor may not offer a sufficiently durable time interval to capture the event. Event recorders rely on activation by the patient, which may be impractical in patients experiencing syncope with limited prodrome. Implantable loop recorders can record up to 3 years and are generally considered in patients with a suspicion of arrhythmogenic syncope too infrequent to be captured by alternative means. A long-term external cardiac event monitoring device provides continuous monitoring for up to 14 days, a sufficient period of time to identify a potential cause in this case and does not rely on patient activation for recording.

104. **The correct answer is: C. Place a transvenous pacing wire.** This rhythm strip demonstrates CHB. There is an atrial rhythm present that is not conducting and there is no junctional or ventricular escape. A temporary transvenous pacing wire is required to provide a means of ventricular pacing until a more definitive pacing device can be installed. Atropine, an anti-muscarinic agent, is not helpful in bradyarrhythmias originating below the atrioventricular node, that is, Mobitz II and CHB, and may paradoxically cause CHB in heart transplant patients. Although it is important to get an endomyocardial biopsy to evaluate for rejection as a cause of arrhythmia, the more pressing concern is to provide a means of back-up pacing.

105. **The correct answer is: D. History and physical.** Evaluation of syncopal presentations is challenging and an etiology may not be determined in upward of 40% of cases. A history and physical with orthostatic vital signs have been shown to have the highest yield and cost-effectiveness in identifying a cause for syncope. ECG can demonstrate abnormalities in 50% of syncope cases but is only helpful in elucidating a cause for syncope in 10% of cases. A TTE can be considered to evaluate for structural heart disease, but even in the presence of structural heart disease, more than one potential cause may be contributing for which a history and physical remain most useful. Evaluation for evidence of severe carotid stenosis should be guided by clinical suspicion and examination.

106. **The correct answer is: B. Neurocardiogenic.** About 25% of syncopal episodes are deemed to be from a neurocardiogenic or vasovagal cause, often precipitated by increased vagal tone related to cough, defecation, carotid hypersensitivity, or micturition. This leads to an inappropriate decrease in HR and BP. Evaluation of orthostatic causes is

important. Orthostatic vital signs are considered positive if 15 seconds after moving from a supine to standing position there is a >20 mmHg drop in systolic BP, >10 mmHg drop in diastolic BP, or a >30 beats/min increase in HR. Arrhythmic cardiovascular causes are important to consider. In patients with no known cardiovascular disease at baseline, <5% of patients will have a cardiovascular explanation for their syncope. Neurologic causes explain about 10% of syncopal presentations. Given the presence of collateral information and the benign clinical examination with complete resolution of symptoms, a neurocardiogenic cause is more likely.

107. **The correct answer is: B. Lead perforation leading to cardiac tamponade.** This patient's hypotension and elevated neck veins are suggestive of cardiac tamponade secondary to lead perforation at the time of the procedure, resulting in a pericardial effusion. A blunted Y descent is typically observed in the jugular veins because there is impaired right ventricle filling during diastole. Pacemaker syndrome is typically described in patients who have a pacemaker that does not allow for synchrony between the atria and ventricles, thereby leading to a sensation of pulsations and fullness in the neck because of the right atrium contracting against a closed tricuspid valve. Pacemaker-mediated tachycardia is a wide complex tachycardia that occurs when retrograde P waves (because of the loss of atrioventricular synchrony) are sensed in an atrial tracking mode resulting in fast ventricular pacing. Flash pulmonary edema is not consistent with the history and the physical examination, which was notable for clear breath sounds.

108. **The correct answer is: D. Both A and C.** Patients with an irreversible ischemic cardiomyopathy and an LVEF <35% have been shown to have a mortality benefit from placement of a primary prevention ICD. Cardiac resynchronization therapy has also been shown to have a mortality benefit in patients with symptomatic HF and a reduced EF if they also have a wide QRS on ECG (>120 ms, ideally LBBB >150 ms). Patients should first be medically optimized before device placement is considered. Cardiac resynchronization is achieved by placement of an LV lead that allows the left ventricle to contract with greater synchrony. In addition to a mortality benefit, cardiac resynchronization may increase the EF and reduce HF symptoms. A dual-chamber pacemaker is typically indicated for atrioventricular block, sinus node dysfunction, and specific forms of syncope; however, right ventricle pacing may worsen HF by creating more dyssynchrony.

109. **The correct answer is: C. Plan for pacemaker system removal.** This patient presents with evidence of pacemaker infection as evidenced by fever, positive blood cultures growing *S. aureus*, and erythema around his device site. Despite a negative TEE, he has staphylococcal bacteremia and merits definitive therapy with system removal. Continuing oral or intravenous antibiotics without system removal would be inadequate therapy. He has no evidence of endocarditis and therefore does not merit valve surgery.

110. **The correct answer is: C. Proceed to surgery.** This patient presents for elective open colectomy. She denies active cardiac symptoms such as angina or HF and maintains >4 METs in physical activity. For this reason, she should proceed with planned surgical intervention without additional testing. Patients with surgical emergencies can also be brought to the OR without further testing. She should continue her aspirin and β-blocker perioperatively as she has an indication to continue taking both.

111. **The correct answer is: C. Postpone cholecystectomy until valve intervention is completed.** This patient presents for elective cholecystectomy; however, she also has severe symptomatic aortic stenosis requiring surgery. Given the risk for procedural com-

plications with untreated severe valvular disease, her elective abdominal surgery should be postponed until after her valve intervention. There is no clear indication for stress testing or initiation of furosemide in this patient.

112. **The correct answer is: C. Postpone knee replacement for 6 to 12 months.** The patient just had an MI and underwent placement of a drug-eluting stent. Ideally, he should be continued on dual antiplatelet therapy for at least 12 months after his acute coronary syndrome with stent. In patients with emergent indications for surgery, surgery can proceed and ideally the patient would be continued on dual antiplatelet therapy. Consideration can be given to stopping dual antiplatelet therapy earlier in certain lower-risk patients who require elective procedures.

113. **The correct answer is: A. Ankle-brachial index.** The ankle-brachial index is a measurement comparing the BP of a patient's arm with the BP in the ankle (posterior tibial and dorsalis pedis), utilizing a BP cuff and ultrasonography. A normal ankle-brachial index (BP in the ankle divided by BP in the arm) is between 1.0 and 1.4, borderline values are between 0.91 and 0.99. An abnormal ankle-brachial index is ≤0.9. Conversely, if the value is ≥1.40, the test is nondiagnostic as the vessel may be incompressible because of calcifications. If the ankle-brachial index is ≥1.40, the next best step would be to check pulse volume recording, which may help localize disease in calcified vessels. The other diagnostic tests listed are utilized to diagnose, quantify, and plan intervention on PAD. However, with stage 4 chronic kidney disease, contrast-sparing studies (such as ankle-brachial index) are the optimal first test.

114. **The correct answer is: C. Obtain urgent vascular surgery or vascular medicine consultation.** The patient is presenting with signs of acute limb ischemia. This is an emergent condition and requires immediate imaging and urgent consultation with either vascular surgery or vascular medicine. Anticoagulation may be utilized if there is concern for acute arterial thrombosis. With severe renal dysfunction, however, low-molecular-weight heparin is contraindicated and unfractionated heparin should be used preferentially. Arterial Doppler ultrasound examination is a diagnostic test for acute limb ischemia. However, delaying until the morning would not be appropriate given the threat to the limb. Placing warm blankets on the foot will not reverse the acute limb ischemia and could be dangerous in a patient with decreased sensation.

115. **The correct answer is: C. Exercise ABI.** Rest ABI are the preferred screening test, but if normal or borderline in a case in which the clinical suspicion is high, as it is in this case, exercise ABI should be performed. A venous ultrasound is useful for evaluation of deep venous thrombosis but does not have a role in the evaluation of PAD. Although angiography in the cardiac catheterization lab and CTA do offer delineation of vascular anatomy, modalities that do not require contrast should be initially favored in this patient with chronic kidney disease.

QUESTIONS

1. A 75-year-old man with a history of hypertension and peptic ulcer disease presents with dyspnea on exertion to the emergency department (ED). He notes black-colored stools for the past 2 weeks. His initial examination is notable for conjunctival pallor, clear lung fields without rales, wheezing, or rhonchi, as well as tachycardia with a regular rhythm, normal S_1 and S_2, and without murmurs, rubs, or gallops. Initial laboratory workup reveals a hemoglobin of 5.5 g/dL, reduced from a baseline of 12 g/dL on routine outpatient laboratory testing from 3 months prior. His basic metabolic panel, arterial blood gas (ABG), and lactate are all within normal limits. A chest x-ray (CXR) is normal.

    What is the mechanism of this man's dyspnea on exertion?

    A. Decreased cardiac output
    B. Decreased oxygen delivery
    C. Decreased systemic vascular resistance
    D. High-output heart failure
    E. Pulmonary edema

2. A 75-year-old woman with a 50-pack-year history of cigarette smoking presents to her primary care physician (PCP) with 10 years of progressive dyspnea on exertion. She notes episodic wheezing and experiences a "chest cold" about two times per year. Her examination reveals distant breath sounds to auscultation and hyperresonant chest to percussion, with otherwise unremarkable examination. A CXR demonstrates hyperinflation with flattening of the bilateral hemidiaphragms. Pulmonary function tests (PFTs) reveal a forced expiratory volume (FEV_1) of 50% predicted, forced vital capacity (FVC) of 70% predicted, and FEV_1/FVC of 0.50. There is no response to bronchodilator.

    What pattern best describes her PFT results?

    A. Cannot determine without more information
    B. Normal
    C. Obstructive
    D. Restrictive

3. A 65-year-old man with a 20-pack-year history of cigarette smoking is referred to pulmonary clinic with 6 months of progressive dyspnea on exertion. He has been prescribed an albuterol inhaler by his PCP without improvement. He reports an occasional dry cough, but otherwise denies chest pain, fevers, chills, weight loss, or other associated symptoms. His examination reveals fine inspiratory crackles at the bases of both lung fields, with a normal cardiovascular examination, absence of any lower extremity edema, absence of fingernail clubbing, and otherwise unremarkable examination. A CXR demonstrates scattered reticular opacities at the bilateral lung bases. PFTs reveal an FEV_1 of 50% predicted, FVC of 45% predicted, and FEV_1/FVC of 0.95. There is no response to bronchodilator.

What pattern best describes his PFT results?

A. Cannot determine without more information
B. Normal
C. Obstructive
D. Restrictive

4. A 40-year-old woman without past medical history presents for evaluation of 3 months of progressive dyspnea on exertion. She denies other associated symptoms such as cough, chest pain, or hemoptysis. She undergoes PFTs, which reveal a reduced diffusion capacity of 45% predicted. Her spirometry and total lung capacity are within normal limits.

Which of the following diseases could the PFT findings NOT support?

A. Early interstitial lung disease (ILD)
B. Neuromuscular disease
C. Pulmonary embolism
D. Pulmonary hypertension

5. A 75-year-old female with a history of diabetes, hypertension, and chronic low back pain is 2 days status post partial colectomy for a large bowel obstruction and is noted to be short of breath. Vital signs are as follows: temperature (T) 37°C, heart rate (HR) 85 beats/min, blood pressure (BP) 130/80 mmHg, respiratory rate (RR) 24 breaths/min, and SaO_2 97% on 2 L/min via nasal cannula. On examination, she is tachypneic and taking shallow breaths and has significant abdominal tenderness. CXR reveals low lung volumes and bibasilar atelectasis. The only medications she is receiving in the hospital are enoxaparin, metoprolol, and sliding scale insulin.

What is the most appropriate next step for management?

A. Pain management and incentive spirometry
B. Antibiotics
C. Anticoagulation
D. Observation

6. A 30-year-old woman with a history of asthma presents to her PCP complaining of occasional shortness of breath and wheezing despite her current asthma treatment. She currently takes a low-dose inhaled corticosteroid and is requiring her albuterol rescue inhaler daily.

Which of the following management options would NOT be appropriate at this time?

A. Addition of a leukotriene receptor antagonist to her current regimen
B. Addition of a long-acting β-agonist to her current regimen
C. Addition of prednisone 5 mg oral daily to her current regimen
D. Increasing the inhaled corticosteroid to medium dose

7. A 25-year-old man with a history of asthma, prescribed fluticasone/salmeterol twice daily and albuterol, as needed, presents to the ED with wheezing and severe shortness of breath for the past day. Additionally, he has had 2 days of rhinorrhea and dry cough. He states that his symptoms began after exposure to a sibling who is suffering from an upper respiratory infection (URI). His vital signs are as follows: T 37°C, HR 90 beats/min, BP 130/80 mmHg, RR 24 breaths/min, and SaO_2 97% on 2 L/min via nasal cannula. His examination is notable for decreased air movement throughout all lung fields with scattered wheezing. A CXR is unremarkable.

What is the next best step in his management?

A. Administer albuterol nebulizers and intravenous (IV) methylprednisolone
B. Administer epinephrine 1:1000 dilution, 0.3 mL intramuscularly (IM)
C. Administer magnesium 2 g IV
D. Apply noninvasive positive-pressure ventilation
E. Perform computed tomography (CT) scan of his chest

8. A 50-year-old woman with a history of asthma is referred to a pulmonary clinic for recent worsening of her symptoms with frequent intermittent wheezing. She has a 20-year history of asthma, which had been well-controlled with albuterol and a low-dose inhaled corticosteroid. She denies known exposure to cigarette smoke, vaping, or new allergens. She has lived in the same home for the past 5 years and has recently been renovating her basement. Basic laboratory evaluation is notable for a normal white blood cell (WBC) count with an absolute eosinophil count of 2000 cells/μL. PFTs reveal a worsening obstructive pattern.

Which of the following is the next most appropriate test?

A. Antinuclear antibody (ANA)
B. Flexible bronchoscopy
C. Methacholine challenge PFT
D. Total immunoglobulin (Ig)E and *Aspergillus*-specific IgE

9. A 40-year-old man has long-standing asthma that has been difficult to control with standard therapies. He requires rescue albuterol treatment multiple times daily despite treatment with a high-dose inhaled corticosteroid, a long-acting β-agonist, a leukotriene receptor antagonist, and oral corticosteroids. He has removed all allergens from his home, and evaluation with an allergist did not reveal any modifiable allergen exposures.

What is the next best step in his management?

A. Adding daily albuterol nebulizer treatments
B. Checking serum eosinophil count and IgE to consider immunologic therapy
C. Increasing the dose of oral corticosteroids
D. No change to management
E. Repeating allergy testing

10. A 20-year-old female with a history of asthma and seasonal allergies presents to her PCP for an annual examination. In her childhood years she had two asthma exacerbations in March requiring hospital admission. She has not had any asthma exacerbations for 1 year. Her current medications are a daily low-dose inhaled corticosteroid, daily long-acting β-agonist, and an as-needed albuterol inhaler. She requires the albuterol approximately once per week. Her cardiopulmonary examination is unremarkable.

What is the next step in management?

A. Continue current medication regimen
B. Increase to a medium-dose inhaled corticosteroid
C. Discontinue the long-acting bronchodilator
D. Stop all medications

11. A 36-year-old male with a long-standing history of asthma requiring multiple intensive care unit (ICU) admissions presents to the ED in respiratory distress. Treatment is initiated with supplemental oxygen, nebulized albuterol, and methylprednisolone. Despite these measures, he remains in respiratory distress. Vital signs are as follows: T 38°C, HR 110 beats/min, BP 147/83 mmHg, RR 32 breaths/min, and SaO_2 92% on 6 L/min NC. The ED makes the decision to proceed with intubation because of signs of respiratory fatigue.

Which of the following should NOT be part of the intubation and ventilator strategy?

A. Select a large endotracheal tube
B. Maximize the expiratory time
C. Aim for a plateau pressure <30 cm H_2O
D. Ensure RR is >22 breaths/min

12. The night after intubation, the patient in Question 11 has a ventilator alarm for high pressures (peak inspiratory pressure 50 mmHg, plateau pressure 35 mmHg). The ventilator tubing is assessed and working appropriately. He is already receiving the appropriate medications to treat his asthma exacerbation.

    What is the next best step in management?

    A. Disconnect the ventilator
    B. Decrease positive end-expiratory pressure (PEEP)
    C. Increase FiO_2
    D. Increase RR

13. A 45-year-old man with non-Hodgkin lymphoma experiences wheezing, dyspnea, and hypotension several minutes after the initiation of his second infusion of rituximab treatment. He was asymptomatic at the time of arrival to the infusion appointment. His vital signs are as follows: T 37.4°C, HR 115 beats/min, BP 100/60 mmHg, RR 28 breaths/min, and SaO_2 98% on room air. On examination, he is noted to be in acute distress with diffuse wheezing and urticaria on his abdomen and chest.

    What is the immediate first-line management?

    A. Administer 50 mg diphenhydramine IV
    B. Administer 0.5 mL of 1:1000 dilution epinephrine IM
    C. Administer 0.3 mL of 1:10 000 dilution epinephrine IV
    D. Perform emergent intubation

14. A 23-year-old man with a history of allergic reaction to peanuts presents to the ED with urticaria after an accidental exposure to peanuts at a restaurant. His vital signs are stable, and his examination is only notable for urticaria on the chest and upper back. He reports a history of similar reaction and denies any associated symptoms such as dyspnea, facial swelling, or throat tightness at this time.

    Which of the following statements about management of allergic reactions is FALSE?

    A. A biphasic reaction with recurrence of anaphylaxis may occur anywhere from 8 to 72 hours after an initial episode of anaphylaxis
    B. All patients should be admitted to an inpatient ward for management
    C. Observation for 6 to 12 hours is appropriate for reactions limited to urticaria
    D. Patients who are observed with resolution of symptoms should be prescribed epinephrine autoinjector pens at the time of discharge

15. A 52-year-old man with a history of chronic obstructive pulmonary disease (COPD) presents to his PCP's office for a routine visit. He is on albuterol four times a day as needed. He reports that overall, he has had an increase in symptoms in the last 6 months. He reports that he was treated for a COPD flare with steroids about 5 months ago. He has had no further flares requiring him to go to the hospital, but he has had worsening shortness of breath and increased sputum production recently. His PFTs are notable for an FEV_1 of 71%.

What medication should be added to his medication regimen?

A. Increase frequency of albuterol to six times a day

B. Start daily azithromycin

C. Start tiotropium

D. Start triple therapy (an inhaled corticosteroid/a long-acting muscarinic antagonist/a long-acting β-agonist)

16. Two months later, the patient in Question 15 presents to the ED with shortness of breath and wheezing in the setting of a recent viral URI. He is found to be hypoxemic to 86% on room air. He is started on nasal cannula oxygen and his SpO_2 improves to 99%. He is later found to be somnolent by his nurse.

What is the next best step in his management?

A. Decrease oxygen for goal SpO_2 88% to 92%

B. Give stacked ipratropium nebs

C. Initiate noninvasive positive-pressure ventilation

D. Start methylprednisolone 125 mg IV q6h

17. A 72-year-old female with a 50-pack-year smoking history and known COPD presents to her PCP's office for a posthospital discharge follow-up appointment. She was admitted for 5 days with a COPD exacerbation. She was treated with antibiotics and a short course of prednisone. While in the hospital, she required up to 4 L/min oxygen via nasal cannula and was discharged on 2 L/min of oxygen. Her medications include a long-acting muscarinic antagonist, long-acting β-agonist, as-needed albuterol nebulizer, lisinopril, loratadine, and omeprazole. This is the third hospitalization this year for a COPD exacerbation, and she has been requiring her nebulizer more frequently, up to three times per day.

What is the next most appropriate step in management?

A. Add a daily ipratropium nebulizer

B. Change inhaler to triple therapy with a LAMA-LABA-ICS

C. Start prednisone 5 mg daily

D. Continue current medication regimen

18. A 50-year-old male former smoker with COPD presents to his PCP for routine follow-up. He has no acute concerns today. He takes a long-acting muscarinic antagonist daily. He denies shortness of breath, cough, and sputum production and has no recent hospital admissions for COPD exacerbations. He has been vaccinated against the flu and COVID-19. He appears well and has a normal cardiopulmonary examination. He is saturating 98% on room air.

What is the next most appropriate step in management?

A. Refer to a pulmonologist

B. Obtain a sputum sample

C. Administer 20-valent pneumococcal conjugate vaccine (PCV20)

D. Obtain ambulatory oxygen saturations

19. An 80-year-old woman with a history of severe COPD presents to her PCP's office for increased dyspnea over the past 9 months. PFTs demonstrate a progressive worsening in her obstructive deficit over the past 5 years—currently, her FEV_1 is 18% of predicted. She takes a combination of a long-acting β-agonist, a long-acting muscarinic antagonist, and an inhaled corticosteroid daily. She uses albuterol two times per day. Her oxygen saturation is noted to be 87% at rest, which has declined from 90% at the last visit.

Which of the following statements about oxygen therapy in COPD is true?

A. Eliminates the need for an inhaled corticosteroid
B. Prolongs survival in patients with oxygen saturation of 88% or less at rest
C. Reduces frequency of exacerbations
D. Reduces hospitalizations for COPD

20. A 75-year-old woman with a history of hypertension and frequent pulmonary infections for the past 5 years presents to her PCP's office with chronic cough, shortness of breath, and copious sputum production. Examination is notable for inspiratory squeaks but is otherwise unremarkable. CXR demonstrates tram-tracking in the lower lung fields.

Which of the following tests is most likely to determine the etiology of this patient's symptoms?

A. ANA
B. Chest CT and sputum cultures (including mycobacterial and fungal cultures)
C. IgA, IgG, IgM, and IgG subclasses
D. Sweat testing

21. Two weeks later, the patient in Question 20 presents to the ED with severe hemoptysis. She has expectorated approximately 600 mL of blood in the past 24 hours and she continues to have episodes of hemoptysis. Her HR is 89 beats/min, BP is 129/89 mmHg, and O_2 saturation is 93% on 2 L/min by nasal cannula. CXR shows a patchy opacification in the right mid-lung field.

What is the next best step in her management?

A. Give cough suppressant
B. Obtain stat chest CT
C. Place the patient R-side down
D. Transfuse 1 U packed red blood cells

22. A 22-year-old man with cystic fibrosis is discharged from the hospital following an acute exacerbation. He completes 4 weeks of antibiotic treatment targeting *Pseudomonas aeruginosa* from his sputum culture. He continues to take lumacaftor as prescribed.

Which additional steps are essential to maintaining lung function and avoiding future exacerbation?

A. 0.9% NaCl nebulizer at least twice daily
B. Airway clearance at least twice daily with a high-frequency oscillation vest
C. Monthly bronchoscopy
D. Weekly monitoring of pulmonary function

23. Which laboratory test is it most important to monitor closely during treatment with cystic fibrosis transmembrane conductance regulator (CFTR) modulators?

A. Basic metabolic panel
B. Liver function tests
C. Complete blood counts
D. Urine microalbumin:creatinine

24. A 70-year-old man with a history of hypertension, coronary artery disease, and without past tobacco use presents to an outpatient pulmonary clinic for evaluation of a solitary pulmonary nodule. The nodule was found incidentally on a chest CT performed 3 weeks earlier in an ED for chest pain. He denies cough, dyspnea, hemoptysis, weight loss, anorexia, or other associated symptoms. Review of his chest CT reveals a 5-mm solid nodule with smooth borders in the right upper lobe, without other associated abnormalities noted.

Which of the following statements is INCORRECT regarding solitary pulmonary nodules in general?

A. A 9-mm high-risk pulmonary nodule should be followed with CT chest every 12 months
B. A history of smoking and cancer are risk factors for malignant nodules
C. Positron emission tomography (PET)-CT is a sensitive study for ruling out malignancy of nodules >8 mm
D. The majority of solitary pulmonary nodules are benign

25. What is the next best step in management of the patient in Question 24?
A. Bronchoscopy with biopsy
B. No further workup necessary
C. Serial CT imaging to follow nodule at 12-month intervals
D. Surgical lung biopsy

26. A 35-year-old woman presents to her PCP's office with cough and shortness of breath. She denies joint pain or swelling, rashes, fevers, or night sweats. She does recall a tender red rash on her R shin about 2 months prior, which self-resolved. The patient works as a secretary and does not have any pets. She has never smoked. Examination is notable for fine crackles throughout the lung fields, but no skin or joint findings. CT scan is performed, which shows enlarged hilar lymph nodes and fibrotic changes. PFTs are notable for a mixed obstructive and restrictive pattern.

What is the most likely diagnosis?
A. Hypersensitivity pneumonitis
B. Idiopathic interstitial pneumonia
C. Sarcoidosis
D. Scleroderma

27. For the patient in Question 26, angiotensin-converting enzyme (ACE) level, ANA, rheumatoid factor, antineutrophilic cytoplasmic antibody (ANCA), cyclic citrullinated peptide (CCP), SSA/SSB, and Scl-70 are all within normal limits.

What is the most appropriate diagnostic step?
A. Bronchoscopy with bronchoalveolar lavage (BAL)
B. Endobronchial ultrasound (EBUS)-guided lymph node biopsy
C. Myositis antibody panel
D. Video-assisted thoracoscopic surgery (VATS) lung biopsy

28. A 50-year-old male with a 30-pack-year smoking history presents to his PCP's office to follow up on a 7-mm solitary solid pulmonary nodule that was identified incidentally on a CT scan obtained for a fever and cough. His symptoms have completely resolved and he feels well today, denying shortness of breath, cough, fatigue, and weight loss. The patient has a family history of lung cancer.

What is the next most appropriate step in management?
A. CT scan in 6 months
B. CT scan in 18 months
C. PET-CT now
D. Transbronchial biopsy now

29. A 72-year-old female with bronchiectasis is admitted for a productive cough and shortness of breath, consistent with an exacerbation of her disease. She is treated with supplemental oxygen and empiric antibiotics. Her vital signs are as follows: T 37°C, HR 82 beats/min, BP 136/83 mmHg, RR 20 breaths/min, and SaO_2 92% on 2 L/min NC. On examination, she is breathing comfortably without accessory muscle use and on auscultation has diffuse crackles and inspiratory squeaks.

What additional intervention should be offered?

A. Airway clearance techniques
B. Noninvasive positive-pressure ventilation
C. Bronchoscopy
D. Diuresis

30. A 65-year-old farmer presents to your primary care clinic with progressively worsening shortness of breath and a dry cough over a four-month period. He denies fevers, chills, weight loss, and malaise. His vital signs are as follows: T 37°C, HR 65 beats/min, BP 142/80 mmHg, RR 16 breaths/min, and SaO_2 94% on room air. On examination, he has diffuse crackles and does not have clubbing. CXR reveals upper lobe–predominant reticular opacities.

What finding on CT would be most consistent with hypersensitivity pneumonitis?

A. Ground glass opacities in bilateral upper lobes
B. Bibasilar consolidative opacities
C. Isolated 5-mm left middle lobe nodules
D. Peripheral tree-in-bud nodules

31. A 65-year-old man with a 25-pack-year smoking history presents to the pulmonary clinic for continued management of idiopathic pulmonary fibrosis. After a recent exacerbation of idiopathic pulmonary fibrosis, he underwent a CT scan of his chest to reassess the extent of his disease.

Which of the following is NOT a CT feature of idiopathic pulmonary fibrosis?

A. Apical cystic changes
B. Bibasilar honeycombing
C. Subpleural reticular opacities
D. Traction bronchiectasis

32. A 60-year-old male with a history of hypertension and atrial fibrillation is referred to pulmonology for shortness of breath. His current medications include lisinopril, metoprolol, and amiodarone. His PFTs reveal a mild restrictive pattern and a CT scan reveals a combination of ground glass and reticular opacities. A comprehensive serologic workup to screen for an underlying autoimmune process or occult connective tissue disease is unrevealing.

Which of the following is INCORRECT regarding amiodarone pulmonary toxicity?

A. Prognosis is generally favorable after discontinuation of amiodarone
B. In patients with moderate-to-severe respiratory symptoms, glucocorticoids are often used but their benefit is unclear
C. Interstitial pneumonitis is the predominant pathology
D. All patients on amiodarone should be screened with annual PFTs

33. A 55-year-old man undergoes a chest CT scan after presenting to the ED with blood-tinged cough and pleuritic chest pain. The CT scan shows bilateral nodular opacities and masses in the peripheral lung fields with some areas of cavitation. Pulmonary emboli are not present. In the past 6 months, he has also noted new hearing loss and intermittent epistaxis. Additional testing is notable for a urinalysis with many red blood cells present on microscopy.

Which of the following tests would support this man's diagnosis?

A. ANCA
B. CT scan with ILD protocol
C. D-dimer
D. Transthoracic echocardiogram

34. A 66-year-old female with a history of alcoholic cirrhosis decompensated by ascites and encephalopathy is admitted to the hospital for left lower extremity cellulitis and is found to have an acute kidney injury. She is started on antibiotics for the infection. Because of her encephalopathy, she cannot recall her home medications when asked by the admitting clinician. Over the next several days, her infection improves, and the kidney injury resolves. On hospital day 3, she develops shortness of breath. A CXR reveals a moderate right-sided pleural effusion. She is given 2 L/min oxygen via nasal cannula. Her vital signs are as follows: T 37°C, HR 82 beats/min, BP 136/83 mmHg, RR 20 breaths/min, and SaO$_2$ 93% on 2 L/min NC. She appears to be breathing comfortably without accessory muscle use and has decreased breath sounds over the right lung base.

    What is the next step in management?

    A. Tube thoracostomy
    B. Thoracentesis
    C. Start oral diuretics
    D. Close monitoring

35. A 72-year-old male with hypertension, hyperlipidemia, and ischemic cardiomyopathy complicated by heart failure with reduced ejection fraction (EF) presents to the emergency room with shortness of breath and lower extremity edema. His N-terminal pro B-type natriuretic peptide (NT-proBNP) is elevated significantly above his baseline. Troponins are negative. His WBC count is normal. His vital signs are as follows: T 37°C, HR 92 beats/min, BP 146/83 mmHg, RR 22 breaths/min, and SaO$_2$ 93% on 4 L/min NC. CXR reveals bilateral moderate pleural effusions. After 3 days of IV diuretics, he appears euvolemic and is off supplemental oxygen. A repeat CXR reveals a moderate right-sided pleural effusion.

    What is the next appropriate step in management?

    A. Continue IV diuresis
    B. Thoracentesis
    C. Tube thoracostomy
    D. Repeat CXR in outpatient setting

36. A 46-year-old woman with a history of diabetes, ischemic cardiomyopathy (EF 45%), and current smoking presents to the ED with shortness of breath and productive cough. Vital signs are as follows: T 37.6°C, HR 96 beats/min, BP 112/68 mmHg, RR 28 breaths/min, and SpO$_2$ 91% on room air. CXR is performed that shows a right-sided pleural effusion. Thoracentesis is performed; 500 mL of fluid is removed. Fluid studies are notable for lactate dehydrogenase (LDH) of 202 units/L, protein 4.1 g/dL, cholesterol 52 mg/dL, glucose 49 mg/dL, and pH 7.1. Serum protein is 6.8 g/dL and serum LDH is 243 units/L. There is a predominance of polymorphonuclear neutrophils (PMNs) on cell count.

    This effusion is most likely because of which of the following underlying conditions?

    A. Congestive heart failure exacerbation
    B. Infection
    C. Malignancy
    D. Rheumatoid arthritis

37. What is the next best therapeutic step for the patient in Question 36?

   A. Indwelling pleural catheter
   B. No intervention
   C. Serial thoracentesis
   D. Tube thoracostomy

38. A 72-year-old man with a history of heart failure (EF of 38%), type 2 diabetes, and a remote history of stage 1 lung cancer status post resection presents to the ED with worsening dyspnea on exertion and orthopnea. Vital signs are as follows: T 35.9°C, HR 67 beats/min, BP 120/78 mmHg, RR 18 breaths/min, and SpO_2 91% breathing ambient air. Examination is notable for diminished breath sounds at the bases bilaterally and diffuse coarse crackles, elevated jugular venous pressure, and 2+ pitting edema in the lower extremities bilaterally. CXR is notable for bilateral pleural effusions and interstitial edema. The patient is admitted to the hospital for IV diuresis. On hospital day 4, the patient has lost 4 kg of weight and his lower extremity edema has improved significantly; however, he continues to complain of shortness of breath. Repeat CXR demonstrates persistence of the bilateral effusions but improved interstitial edema. The medical team proceeds with right-sided thoracentesis, and 700 mL of straw-colored fluid is removed. Pleural fluid studies are notable for LDH 77 units/L, protein 4.1 g/dL, cholesterol 35 mg/dL, glucose 100 mg/dL, and pH 7.4. There are no WBCs or red blood cells present. Cytology examination is unremarkable. Serum studies are notable for LDH 187 units/L, protein 7.2 g/dL, and glucose 110 mg/dL.

What is the most likely cause of this effusion?

   A. Congestive heart failure
   B. Pneumonia
   C. Pulmonary embolism
   D. Recurrence of lung cancer

39. A 77-year-old man with a history of diabetes, hypertension, and colon cancer is admitted for surgical resection.

Which of the following should be used for thromboprophylaxis?

   A. Apixaban
   B. Enoxaparin
   C. Fondaparinux
   D. Mechanical prophylaxis

40. The patient in Question 39 has a complicated postoperative course and a prolonged hospitalization. He is eventually discharged to a rehabilitation facility on his home medications. On his fifth day at the facility, he develops shortness of breath and tachycardia. His SpO_2 is 89% on room air. CXR is unremarkable and labs are pending.

What is the best diagnostic test to use in this patient?

   A. CT pulmonary angiogram
   B. D-dimer
   C. Echocardiogram
   D. V/Q scan

41. The patient in Questions 39 and 40 is found to have a pulmonary embolus in the right pulmonary artery. He is started on a heparin drip.

What agent should be used in this patient to treat his pulmonary embolus on discharge?

A. Apixaban
B. Argatroban
C. Fondaparinux
D. Warfarin

42. A 45-year-old woman with a history of type 2 diabetes presents to her PCP with pain and swelling in her left lower extremity. D-dimer was 1200 ng/mL. A lower extremity ultrasound demonstrates a deep vein thrombosis (DVT) in the left popliteal vein. She has no known risk factors or recent provoking factors that would explain this DVT. She undergoes thorough evaluation, including age-appropriate cancer screening, which is unremarkable.

Which of the following anticoagulation approaches is most appropriate?

A. Apixaban for 3 months, then reassessment with patient counseling regarding ongoing anticoagulation
B. Apixaban for 4 weeks
C. Lifelong apixaban
D. No anticoagulation; compression stockings only

43. The patient in Question 42 is worried about developing a pulmonary embolus and asks if there is anything she can do to prevent this.

What is the next best step in her management?

A. Continue apixaban
B. Continue apixaban and place inferior vena cava (IVC) filter
C. Discontinue apixaban and place IVC filter
D. Start half-dose apixaban and place IVC filter

44. A 42-year-old female with stage II breast cancer presents to the emergency room with acute-onset shortness of breath. Her home medications include tamoxifen and omeprazole. CT pulmonary angiogram reveals a pulmonary embolus in the right main pulmonary artery. Her vital signs are as follows: T 38°C, HR 122 beats/min, BP 80/50 mmHg, RR 32 breaths/min, and SaO$_2$ 93% on 4 L/min NC. She is started on norepinephrine and a heparin gtt.

What is an additional most appropriate next step in management?

A. Surgical thrombectomy
B. Administer systemic thrombolysis
C. Place an IVC filter
D. Admit to the ICU

45. A 52-year-old woman who has not seen a doctor in over 20 years comes to the ED for evaluation of dyspnea on exertion. She has an oxygen saturation of 92%. She is admitted to the internal medicine service for further workup. CXR is within normal limits and CT scan is without interstitial process. PFTs show mild restriction and no obstruction. Transthoracic echocardiogram shows an EF of 54%, normal valves, and right ventricular systolic pressure (RVSP) of 55 mmHg. She then undergoes right heart catheterization (RHC). Pulmonary capillary wedge pressure (PCWP) is 13 mmHg and mean pulmonary artery pressure is 35 mmHg.

What is the most likely cause of her dyspnea?

A. COPD
B. Heart failure
C. Idiopathic pulmonary arterial hypertension (PAH)
D. ILD

46. The patient in Question 45 follows up with a pulmonary hypertension specialist who decides to start her on a medication.

What is the first-line treatment for this patient?

A. Epoprostenol
B. Nifedipine
C. Riociguat
D. Sildenafil

47. A few months later, the patient in Questions 45 and 46 presents to the ED with an episode of presyncope when walking her dog. Vital signs on arrival are notable for T 37°C, HR 118 beats/min, BP 78/41 mmHg, RR 22 breaths/min, and SpO_2 82% on room air (that improves to 88% on 6 L/min via nasal cannula). Examination is notable for elevated jugular venous pressure and cool extremities. Lactic acid is elevated to 4.0 mmol/L. Bedside ultrasound shows a dilated and diffusely hypokinetic right ventricle.

What is the next best step in her management?

A. Give 1 L bolus of 0.9% NaCl solution
B. Increase sildenafil dose
C. Initiate inotropic and vasopressor support
D. Intubate

48. A 66-year-old male with a history of hypertension and hyperlipidemia is undergoing work-up for shortness of breath. PFTs do not reveal obstructive or restrictive deficits. Chest CT is unremarkable. Echocardiogram revealed normal biventricular function, absence of valvular disease, and an RVSP of 45 mmHg. He underwent a RHC, and the following pressures (mmHg) were obtained: right atrium 10, right ventricle 40/11, pulmonary artery 40/23, and PCWP 10. There was no response to a vasodilator study.

What is the next most appropriate step in evaluation?

A. V/Q scan
B. Start sildenafil
C. Start oral diuretics
D. Cardiopulmonary exercise test

49. A 52-year-old female with a long-standing history of idiopathic pulmonary fibrosis on pirfenidone is seen in follow-up for 4 months of progressively worsening dyspnea. Her CT scan appears similar to her scan 6 months prior. Her PFTs reveal a FEV_1 of 1.32 L (69% predicted), which is also similar to 6 months prior. She is sent for a RHC and the following hemodynamics are obtained: RA 5, RV 45/10, PA 45/21, and PCWP 8.

What is the next most appropriate step in management?

A. Start tadalafil
B. Start inhaled treprostinil
C. Increase the dose of pirfenidone
D. Monitor symptoms and repeat CT scan, PFTs, and RHC in 6 months

50. A 72-year-old male is recently diagnosed with chronic thromboembolic pulmonary hypertension (CTEPH).

Which of the following is CORRECT regarding this diagnosis?

A. Pulmonary thromboendarterectomy is potentially curative
B. Riociguat is first-line therapy
C. Balloon pulmonary angioplasty is recommended as the first-line intervention in all patients
D. All patients have a history of pulmonary embolus and/or DVT

51. A 100-kg, 77-year-old man is admitted to the medical ICU for multifocal pneumonia and intubated for hypoxemia. Following intubation, his SpO_2 is 87% on volume control with the following settings: V_T 500 mL, RR 15 breaths/min, PEEP 5 cm H_2O, and FiO_2 70%.

How should the ventilator be adjusted?

A. Increase FiO_2
B. Increase PEEP
C. Increase RR
D. Increase V_T

52. On hospital day 2, the patient in Question 51 has an acute desaturation event and the ventilator alarms for high pressures (peak inspiratory pressure 46 cm H_2O, previously 27 cm H_2O). Plateau pressure is unchanged at 22 cm H_2O.

What is the most likely etiology of this change?

A. Auto-PEEP
B. Excessive secretions
C. Pneumothorax
D. Vent asynchrony

53. The patient in Questions 51 and 52 shows steady improvement, and the team plans to work toward extubation and decreases the pressure support from 10/5 cm H_2O with FiO_2 30% to 5/5 cm H_2O with FiO_2 30%.

Which of the following would suggest that the patient is not ready for extubation?

A. Decrease in mean arterial pressure (MAP) from 75 to 65 mmHg
B. Decrease in RR from 20 to 12 breaths/min; decrease in tidal volumes from 380 to 340 mL
C. Fall in SpO_2 from 96% to 90%
D. Increase in RR from 20 to 30 breaths/min; decrease in tidal volumes from 380 to 280 mL

54. A 26-year-old man with a history of asthma develops fevers to 38.8°C, chills, sore throat, and myalgias. He presents to his PCP's office where he is found to be influenza A positive. He is started on oseltamivir. Two days later, he develops severe shortness of breath. His roommate becomes concerned and brings him to the ED.

Vital signs on arrival to the ED are as follows: T 40°C, HR 119 beats/min, BP 96/54 mmHg, RR 28 breaths/min, and SpO_2 83% on room air. He is placed on high-flow nasal cannula with improvement in his SpO_2 to 93%. During the ED course, he is given 2 L lactated Ringer (LR) for ongoing hypotension as well as broad-spectrum antibiotics. On arrival to the ICU, he is noted to be hypoxemic to 79% despite high-flow nasal cannula at maximal settings. He is subsequently intubated. Postintubation CXR is notable for diffuse bilateral infiltrates. Postintubation ABG is 7.3/30/80 on 100% FiO_2.

Which of the following should NOT be part of the ventilator strategy?

A. Keeping FiO_2 as low as possible to maintain $PaO_2 > 65$ mmHg
B. Low tidal volume ventilation with $V_T < 6$ mL/kg
C. Maintaining pH > 7.3
D. Titrating PEEP to prevent tidal alveolar collapse

55. Despite optimizing PEEP and initiating paralytics, the patient in Question 54 continues to have a P/F ratio < 100.

Which of the following interventions has been found to have a mortality benefit in acute respiratory distress syndrome of all types?

A. Early extracorporeal membrane oxygenation (ECMO)
B. Proning
C. Pulmonary vasodilators (inhaled nitric oxide, prostacyclins)
D. Steroids

56. A 66-kg, 75-year-old man with a history of hypertension, atrial fibrillation, COPD, diabetes, and chronic kidney disease on hemodialysis presents to the ED from his assisted living facility after his wife found him confused and unable to get off of the couch the evening after a dialysis session. On Emergency Medical Services (EMS) arrival, the patient was found to be hypotensive to 78/33 mmHg, so he was taken to the ED for further management. He received 1 L of normal saline en route to the hospital.

Vital signs on arrival to the ED are as follows: T 35.6°C, HR 82 beats/min, BP 92/52 mmHg, RR 28 breaths/min, and SpO_2 88% on room air. On examination, he is somnolent. Lungs are clear and abdomen is soft. Labs are notable for a WBC count of 11×10^9/L, creatinine 4.9 mg/dL, and lactate 3.7 mmol/L. Blood cultures are pending.

What is the next best step in his management?

A. Give an additional liter of normal saline for a total of 2 L
B. Start broad-spectrum antibiotics
C. Start hydrocortisone and fludrocortisone
D. Start norepinephrine

57. What antibiotic regimen is most appropriate in the patient from Question 56?

A. Ceftriaxone/azithromycin
B. Levofloxacin
C. Vancomycin/cefepime
D. Vancomycin/cefepime/metronidazole/micafungin

58. The BP of the patient in Questions 56 and 57 falls to 75/40 mmHg despite 2 L LR fluid resuscitation.

What is the initial pressor of choice in this patient?

A. Dopamine
B. Norepinephrine
C. Phenylephrine
D. Vasopressin

59. A 33-year-old male with a history of depression is found in his garage by family members and subsequently brought to the emergency room by EMS. He is alert, reporting that he has a headache and nausea. His vital signs are as follows: T 38°C, HR 95 beats/min, BP 116/80 mmHg, RR 22 breaths/min, and SaO_2 94% on room air. His physical examination is unrevealing.

What is the next most appropriate step in management?

A. Start 100% oxygen
B. Refer for hyperbaric oxygen
C. Obtain carboxyhemoglobin level
D. Toxicology screen

60. A 44-year-old woman with a history of depression, hypertension, and asthma is taken to the ED by EMS after being found down at home with a bottle of empty pills nearby. Vital signs on arrival to the ED are as follows: T 36.2°C, HR 88 beats/min, BP 80/40 mmHg, RR 20 breaths/min, and SpO_2 92% on room air. Examination is notable for a somnolent woman who is slow to respond to questions. Tongue lacerations are present. Neurologic examination is notable for confusion. Reflexes are normal. Electrocardiogram (ECG) is notable for a QRS of 140 ms and a QT interval of 560 ms.

Overdose of which medication is most likely responsible for her presenting symptoms?

A. Amitriptyline
B. Carvedilol
C. Diltiazem
D. Lithium

61. What is the next best step in the management of the patient from Question 60?

A. Flumazenil
B. Glucagon
C. IV sodium bicarbonate
D. Urgent dialysis

62. A 72-year-old male with a history of hypertension, hyperlipidemia, and uncontrolled insulin-dependent type II diabetes presents to the ED with altered mental status. His vital signs are as follows: T 38°C, HR 122 beats/min, BP 76/54 mmHg, RR 22 breaths/min, and SaO_2 92% on room air. Basic labs and blood cultures are obtained. He receives empiric broad-spectrum antibiotics and 30 cc/kg of normal saline. Subsequent vital signs are T 38°C, HR 105 beats/min, BP 82/56 mmHg, RR 22 breaths/min, and SaO_2 93% on room air. He is started on norepinephrine, which is slowly uptitrated to 10 μg/min given persistent hypotension. Despite this, his BP is 80/54 mmHg.

What is the next most appropriate step in management?

A. Administer an additional 1 L/min NS
B. Increase norepinephrine to 15 μg/min
C. Start vasopressin 0.04 units/min
D. No change in current management

63. A 45-year-old man with cystic fibrosis has had progressive decline over the past 2 years. His FEV_1 is now 28% and he requires 6 L/min nasal cannula at all times. He is referred to a lung transplant center, and 3 months later, he undergoes bilateral lung transplantation.

He initially does well; however, 2 months later he develops fever, cough, and shortness of breath, and when he checks his home pulse oximeter, he notes that he is hypoxemic to 88% on room air. He is seen by his pulmonologist who performs a CXR that is unremarkable.

What etiology of his new symptoms must be ruled out?

A. Acute rejection
B. Chronic rejection
C. Pneumonia
D. Primary graft dysfunction

64. What is the next best diagnostic step for the patient in Question 63?

    A. Antibody testing

    B. Chest CT

    C. Sputum culture

    D. Transbronchial biopsy

65. How should the condition of the patient in Questions 63 and 64 be treated?

    A. Azithromycin, montelukast, and change in immunosuppressant therapy

    B. Broad-spectrum antibiotics

    C. Increasing immunosuppression

    D. No intervention

66. Which of the following is NOT an absolute contraindication to lung transplant?

    A. Age >65

    B. Current smoking

    C. Active malignancy

    D. Chronic kidney disease requiring dialysis

ANSWERS

1. **The correct answer is: B. Decreased oxygen delivery.** This patient is likely suffering from an upper gastrointestinal (GI) bleed, as evidenced by melena, new anemia, and history of peptic ulcer disease. His presenting symptom of dyspnea on exertion is secondary to decreased oxygen delivery to tissues. Delivery of oxygen to tissues is dictated by cardiac output and the oxygen content of blood. The major determinant of oxygen-carrying capacity in blood is the hemoglobin concentration. His examination and testing do not support a diagnosis of heart failure or pulmonary edema. High-output heart failure may develop in the setting of chronic anemia; however, his known hemoglobin 3 months prior was normal.

2. **The correct answer is: C. Obstructive.** The patient's presentation is suggestive of COPD. Her PFTs demonstrate a reduced FEV_1/FVC, supportive of an obstructive ventilatory deficit.

3. **The correct answer is: D. Restrictive.** The patient's presentation is suggestive of ILD. Her PFTs demonstrate a reduced FEV_1 and FVC with a normal FEV_1/FVC ratio, supportive of a restrictive ventilatory deficit.

4. **The correct answer is: B. Neuromuscular disease.** A reduced diffusion capacity indicates a reduced surface area of lung participating in gas exchange and/or a disruption to diffusion at the interface of alveoli, interstitium, and capillaries. In the absence of other abnormalities on PFT, this may indicate pulmonary vascular disease or early ILD. Reduced diffusion capacity is routinely corrected for hemoglobin concentration to exclude anemia as a cause. Neuromuscular disease would not affect reduced diffusion capacity, but rather would result in progressive restriction and reduced forces generated during inspiration and expiration.

5. **The correct answer is: A. Pain management and incentive spirometry.** This patient is likely suffering from atelectasis in the setting of postoperative pain. This is evidenced by her postoperative state, tachypnea with shallow breaths, and CXR findings of basilar atelectasis. The most appropriate management strategy for postoperative atelectasis is pain management and incentive spirometry. Lack of fever and x-ray findings argue against a bacterial pneumonia that would require antibiotics. Receipt of thromboprophylaxis and lack of tachycardia make pulmonary embolism less likely. Empiric anticoagulation is therefore not indicated at this juncture.

6. **The correct answer is: C. Addition of prednisone 5 mg oral daily to her current regimen.** This patient presents with continued uncontrolled asthma symptoms despite her current regimen of low-dose inhaled corticosteroid. It would not be appropriate to add daily oral corticosteroids given that the patient has many other options for escalation in her asthma management. Appropriate changes at this time would include increasing the dose of her inhaled corticosteroid, or addition of another medication such as a long-acting β-agonist or a leukotriene receptor antagonist.

7. **The correct answer is: A. Administer albuterol nebulizers and IV methylprednisolone.** This patient with a history of asthma presents with evidence on history and physical examination of acutely worsened airflow obstruction in the setting of a likely viral exacerbation of asthma, without evidence of pneumonia. The mainstays of treatment in the acute setting include short-acting β-agonist therapy at frequent intervals, corticosteroids, and supportive care. There is no clear benefit to epinephrine over usual care in asthma,

and this patient does not have other signs to suggest anaphylaxis. Magnesium may be considered in patients who fail to respond to first-line therapies but is not the best initial step. Noninvasive positive-pressure ventilation is controversial in asthma as it cannot reverse the inflammatory lung process and may contribute to hyperinflation and complications such as pneumothorax and hemodynamic instability.

8. **The correct answer is: D. Total immunoglobulin (Ig)E and *Aspergillus*-specific IgE.** This patient presents with previously controlled asthma that has suddenly worsened. This warrants a search for exacerbating factors or asthma mimics. Given her recent exposure to a basement renovation and elevated serum eosinophil count, one consideration would be allergic bronchopulmonary aspergillosis (ABPA). This appears in patients with asthma or cystic fibrosis who have been exposed to *Aspergillus*—this may occur in areas such as damp basements, water-damaged homes, or wet organic matter such as from leaves, compost, and barns. Central bronchiectasis on chest imaging would support this diagnosis. The tests necessary to fulfill diagnostic criteria include elevated total IgE and *Aspergillus*-specific IgE. Additionally, *Aspergillus*-specific IgG and absolute eosinophilia support this diagnosis.

9. **The correct answer is: B. Checking serum eosinophil count and IgE to consider immunologic therapy.** This patient has poorly controlled asthma despite escalation of inhaled therapy and adjunctive treatments. Given a desire to avoid long-term oral corticosteroid treatment, continuation of the current regimen or an increased dose of corticosteroids is not a preferred option. Similarly, repeat allergy testing or albuterol nebulizers are not preferred, as the patient has failed to benefit from allergy testing and albuterol only serves as a rescue therapy. Obtaining serum, eosinophil, and IgE levels to evaluate candidacy for anti-IgE and anti-interleukin-5 therapies would be the next best step in management. Of note, tezepelumab can be prescribed for patients with severe uncontrolled asthma even if eosinophils and IgE are normal.

10. **The correct answer is: C. Discontinue the long-acting bronchodilator.** This patient suffered from childhood asthma requiring two admissions for exacerbations in March, presumably triggered by seasonal allergies. Given she has now remained free from exacerbation for 1 year and only requires albuterol once per week, it is appropriate to "step down" her therapy. It is important to always consider "stepping down" therapy in patients who have been well-controlled on their current regimen for at least 3 to 6 months to protect patients from the side effects of therapy. It is reasonable to start with discontinuation of the LABA given discontinuation of inhaled corticosteroids prematurely can lead to exacerbations. Based on the history provided, there is no indication to increase therapy. Although this is not listed as an answer choice, another option based on the GINA guidelines would be to continue ICS/LABA, but as a PRN only.

11. **The correct answer is: D. Ensure RR is >22 breaths/min.** This patient is suffering from a severe asthma exacerbation with persistent respiratory failure despite oxygen therapy, nebulized albuterol, and IV corticosteroids. Appropriately, the decision is made to proceed with intubation. The risk of mechanical ventilation in patients with severe asthma is dynamic hyperinflation (aka "auto-PEEP"), which is when the expiratory time is insufficient to allow for complete emptying of the lungs between inhalations. When this occurs, given retained air, the plateau pressure increases, which can lead to cardiac arrest, barotrauma, and pneumothorax. Thus, it is crucial to employ mechanical ventilation strategies to mitigate the risk of dynamic hyperinflation: selecting a large endotracheal tube; maximizing expiratory time; and continuing optimal medical therapy with the goal of a plateau pressure under 30 cm H_2O. Increasing the RR would increase the risk of dynamic hyperinflation and should be avoided.

12. **The correct answer is: A. Disconnect the ventilator.** This patient has developed dynamic hyperinflation, discussed earlier, as indicated by his high peak inspiratory pressure and plateau pressure. He is at risk for barotrauma, pneumothorax, and cardiac arrest. Disconnecting the ventilator is the next best option in the acute setting. This allows time for complete lung emptying (which may require assistance from those at the bedside by providing pressure to the precordium), resolving the hyperinflation. Decreasing the PEEP will not address the underlying issue that he is hyperinflated and has insufficient time to exhale with his current obstruction. Changing the FiO_2 will also not address his hyperinflation. Increasing the RR will likely worsen his hyperinflation because it will allow even less time to exhale between breaths.

13. **The correct answer is: B. Administer 0.5 mL of 1:1000 dilution epinephrine IM.** The patient is experiencing anaphylaxis secondary to a rituximab infusion. The first most appropriate and important step is to administer epinephrine IM. A dilution of 1:1000 refers to 1 mg/mL concentration. Therefore, to administer 0.5 mg, one administers 0.5 mL IM. IV epinephrine is reserved for refractory shock despite initial treatment and aggressive fluid administration, or cardiac arrest. Histamine antagonists, glucocorticoids, and inhaled β-2 agonists are adjunctive therapies for anaphylaxis but do not serve as first-line management.

14. **The correct answer is: B. All patients should be admitted to an inpatient ward for management.** Patients with urticaria or mild bronchospasm may be observed in an ED or observation unit for at least 6 hours, obviating the need for universal admission of allergic reactions.

15. **The correct answer is: C. Start tiotropium.** The patient has had increased symptoms over the past 6 months, but his FEV_1 is Global Initiative for Chronic Obstructive Lung Disease (GOLD) stage 2 and he has fewer than two exacerbations per year, so starting a long-acting muscarinic antagonist (tiotropium) alone at this time is reasonable. Increasing the albuterol frequency without adding another controller medication is not appropriate. Daily azithromycin was found to decrease exacerbations, but it is not routine to start daily azithromycin, particularly in this patient who does not have frequent exacerbations. Triple therapy is not necessary at this time, although it could be considered in the future if his COPD continues to worsen.

16. **The correct answer is: C. Initiate noninvasive positive-pressure ventilation.** The patient likely is altered in the setting of hypercarbia and noninvasive positive-pressure ventilation should be initiated. Targeting a lower O_2 goal may help prevent CO_2 retention by avoiding V/Q mismatch, maintaining respiratory drive, and preventing the Haldane effect (more oxygenated blood has less CO_2-carrying capacity); however, now that the patient is altered, he likely needs noninvasive positive-pressure ventilation to improve ventilation and breathe off the CO_2. Ipratropium nebulizers and steroids are also important in managing acute COPD exacerbations, but are unlikely to improve his CO_2 and his mental status now that he has already begun to retain.

17. **The correct answer is: B. Change inhaler to triple therapy with a LAMA-LABA-ICS.** This patient has GOLD Group D COPD as evidenced by ≥2 exacerbations per year and severe symptoms requiring chronic oxygen therapy. Given she had an exacerbation and remains symptomatic despite chronic therapy with a LAMA and LABA, the next step in treatment is "triple therapy" with a LAMA-LABA-ICS. Studies have shown a decreased rate of exacerbations in some patients receiving triple as opposed to dual therapies, and some have demonstrated an improvement in FEV_1 and decreased mortality.

18. **The correct answer is: C. Administer 20-valent pneumococcal conjugate vaccine (PCV20).** This patient has COPD that is stable on his current regimen. It is crucial to ensure that patients with chronic lung disease are up to date on all vaccines including pneumococcal, influenza, pertussis, and COVID-19. Recently in 2022, the Advisory Committee on Immunization Practices recommended receipt of PCV20 alone *or* PCV15 followed by PPSV23 for adults aged 19 to 64 years with chronic lung disease.

19. **The correct answer is: B. Prolongs survival in patients with oxygen saturation of 88% or less at rest.** This patient has severe COPD with a decline in lung function and worsening symptoms over time. She also has severe resting hypoxemia, with an oxygen saturation of 87% at rest. In patients with COPD and a resting oxygen saturation of 88% or less, long-term oxygen treatment has been shown to improve survival. However, routine treatment with inhaled therapies and adjunctive treatments remain necessary to reduce the frequency of exacerbations and hospitalizations.

20. **The correct answer is: B. Chest CT and sputum cultures (including mycobacterial and fungal cultures).** This patient is presenting with symptoms consistent with bronchiectasis, most likely secondary to recurrent pulmonary infection. Thus, chest CT and sputum cultures are the next most appropriate diagnostic steps. Cystic fibrosis generally does not present in late age, so sweat testing would not be a first-line diagnostic test in this patient. Immunodeficiency (diagnosed with IgA, IgG, IgM, and IgG subclasses) is also a cause of bronchiectasis, but is less likely in this patient given she lacks a history of frequent infections throughout her life. Autoimmune diseases such as systemic lupus erythematosus and rheumatoid arthritis are also possible, but she lacks examination findings to suggest either of these as probable etiologies.

21. **The correct answer is: C. Place the patient R-side down.** The patient is experiencing massive hemoptysis, defined as >500 mL of expectorated blood in 24 hours, likely in the setting of her bronchiectasis. The first step in managing this patient is stabilizing her and preventing asphyxiation. The patient should be placed with affected side down, and if she becomes unstable from a respiratory perspective, she should be intubated (selectively intubate the nonaffected lung) while she awaits definitive treatment. Cough suppressants may actually increase the risk of asphyxiation. Blood transfusion is not necessary at this time given that the patient is hemodynamically stable, and the patient is much more likely to die from asphyxiation than from exsanguination. Chest CT may be useful to better determine the location/source of the bleeding, but the first step is to stabilize the patient.

22. **The correct answer is: B. Airway clearance at least twice daily with a high-frequency oscillation vest.** Airway clearance is an essential component of the daily care of patients with cystic fibrosis. Techniques such as manual chest physical therapy or wearing a vest serve to mobilize thickened secretions, which would otherwise predispose patients to infections. These techniques are accompanied by the use of nebulized hypertonic saline and dornase alfa, which serve to thin secretions. When performed routinely, airway clearance techniques can help maintain lung function and decrease exacerbation of cystic fibrosis because of infection. A 0.9% or normal saline nebulizer would not be sufficient to thin the airway mucus of patients with cystic fibrosis. Although PFTs are performed intermittently, they are not done as frequently as weekly intervals. Finally, routinely scheduled bronchoscopy does not play a role in the treatment of cystic fibrosis.

23. **The correct answer is: B. Liver function tests.** Drug-induced liver injury is a risk with treatment of all CFTR modulators and thus liver function tests should be monitored regularly. Discontinuation of therapy may be indicated based on the results given liver failure secondary to CFTR modulator has been documented.

24. **The correct answer is: A. A 9-mm high-risk pulmonary nodule should be followed with CT chest every 12 months.** For patients with solid solitary pulmonary nodule, PET/CT or biopsy should be considered, and if deferred, then a CT scan should be performed at a 3-month interval. Following at 12 months would not be appropriate for a large nodule in a high-risk patient.

25. **The correct answer is: C. Serial CT imaging to follow nodule at 12-month intervals.** Serial imaging is appropriate for this patient without risk factors for lung cancer and with a solitary, solid 5-mm nodule without high-risk appearance.

26. **The correct answer is: C. Sarcoidosis.** Sarcoidosis is the most likely diagnosis. The patient's demographics are consistent (female in fourth decade of life). Other salient historical features are the patient's history of painful red rash on her shin (erythema nodosum), findings of hilar lymphadenopathy on CT scan, and PFTs with a mixed obstructive and restrictive pattern. She does not have any exposures to suggest hypersensitivity pneumonitis, and although she is the right demographic for collagen vascular disease, she does not have any skin, joint, or muscle involvement that would suggest scleroderma. Idiopathic interstitial pneumonia is considered when the cause of a patient's ILD is unknown.

27. **The correct answer is: B. Endobronchial ultrasound (EBUS)-guided lymph node biopsy.** ACE has only 60% sensitivity for sarcoidosis without symptoms (closer to 90% with symptoms). EBUS-guided lymph node biopsy is the best diagnostic test for evaluation of sarcoidosis. VATS is often used for diagnosis of the idiopathic interstitial pneumonia and might be used if lymph node biopsy does not yield a diagnosis. BAL can be used to diagnose infection, hemorrhage, and eosinophilic syndromes. Because the concern is highest for sarcoidosis, myositis panel would be a low-yield diagnostic test.

28. **The correct answer is: A. CT scan in 6 months.** Per the Fleischner guidelines, CT imaging at 6 to 12 months is recommended for a solitary solid pulmonary nodule between 6 and 8 mm.

29. **The correct answer is: A. Airway clearance techniques.** This patient is suffering from a bronchiectasis exacerbation and is undergoing appropriate treatment with supplemental oxygen and antibiotics. Airway clearance techniques are also a mainstay of treatment for bronchiectasis exacerbations to improve the cough and assist with expelling secretions.

30. **The correct answer is: A. Ground glass opacities in bilateral upper lobes.** As noted in the question, this patient's presentation is most consistent with hypersensitivity pneumonitis, an immunologic reaction to an inhaled agent that can cause ILD. Although there are many radiologic patterns associated with the condition, classic findings are upper- and middle lobe–predominant centrilobular nodules and ground glass opacities, though basilar-predominant inflammatory changes can be seen in the early, nonfibrotic stages of disease. Bibasilar consolidative opacities are more consistent with aspiration. Peripheral tree-in-bud nodules are most commonly seen in infective bronchiolitis.

31. **The correct answer is: A. Apical cystic changes.** The characteristic features of idiopathic pulmonary fibrosis include a subpleural, bibasilar distribution of reticular opacities, honeycombing, and traction bronchiectasis. Ground glass opacities are classically absent, although their presence does not exclude idiopathic pulmonary fibrosis. Apical cystic changes are not seen as part of idiopathic pulmonary fibrosis.

32. **The correct answer is: D. All patients on amiodarone should be screened with annual PFTs.** Amiodarone is associated with several pulmonary diseases including interstitial pneumonitis, eosinophilic pneumonia, and organizing pneumonia, among others.

The pathogenesis of how amiodarone causes these conditions is not well described. Patients should receive baseline PFTs and an annual CXR to monitor for pulmonary toxicity. However, annual PFTs are not helpful in detecting all types of amiodarone pulmonary toxicity, so should only be done if dyspnea or other pulmonary symptoms develop, and then compared to the baseline values. Should pulmonary toxicity develop, discontinuation of therapy is the mainstay of treatment given the majority regain lung function. In severe/refractory cases, it may be reasonable to trial glucocorticoids, although results are mixed.

33. **The correct answer is: A. ANCA.** This man presents with cavitating peripheral lung nodules and masses. The differential diagnosis for this includes cancer (eg, primary lung or metastasis), vasculitis (eg, ANCA associated), pulmonary embolism (when just nodules with cavitation are present), autoimmune disease (eg, rheumatoid arthritis), infection (eg, fungal pneumonia, tuberculosis), and congenital abnormalities. The presence of hearing loss, bloody nasal discharge, and hematuria raises concern for a systemic vasculitis, specifically the ANCA-associated vasculitis granulomatosis with polyangiitis. The pulmonary imaging manifestations of granulomatosis with polyangiitis include solid and ground glass nodules with or without cavitation, waxing-and-waning pulmonary opacities, and lymphadenopathy.

34. **The correct answer is: C. Start oral diuretics.** This patient is suffering from hepatic hydrothorax related to her known cirrhosis as evidenced by development of a right-sided pleural effusion while holding home diuretics. Thoracentesis of a hepatic hydrothorax is rarely indicated as the fluid will reaccumulate. Thus, diuretics are the mainstay of treatment.

35. **The correct answer is: B. Thoracentesis.** This patient is suffering from a heart failure exacerbation as evidenced by his clinical volume overload and elevated NT-proBNP in the setting of his known cardiac history. The bilateral pleural effusions are likely secondary to the same, and initial treatment with diuretics is appropriate. However, given persistence of a unilateral pleural effusion, a thoracentesis and pleural fluid studies are indicated to ensure there is not an additional process, that is, malignancy, at play prior to discharge.

36. **The correct answer is: B. Infection.** This is an exudative effusion with PMN predominance, most consistent with a parapneumonic effusion. Congestive heart failure effusions are generally transudative. Both malignancy and rheumatoid arthritis can cause exudative effusions but do not have a PMN predominance on cell count.

37. **The correct answer is: D. Tube thoracostomy.** Tube thoracostomy is indicated for complicated parapneumonic effusions given the concern for development of organization and potential need for decortication later on. Serial thoracentesis is not appropriate in this case as there is a need for continual source control. Indwelling pleural catheters are used in some patients with malignancy; one is not indicated in this case, as the effusion is not expected to be recurrent. Because this is a complicated parapneumonic effusion, it must be tapped as explained above; thus, answer B (no intervention) is not appropriate.

38. **The correct answer is: A. Congestive heart failure.** Despite meeting Light's criteria for an exudate by effusion protein/serum protein ratio >0.5, this effusion is most likely a "pseudo-exudate" (in this case, an effusion that is due to congestive heart failure but has elevated total protein following diuresis). He does not meet more specific criteria for exudate (in this case, with a low-effusion cholesterol). The other effusions listed here will have pleural fluid studies consistent with an exudate (including elevated cholesterol), and should demonstrate other findings such as elevated WBCs or abnormal cytology.

39. **The correct answer is: B. Enoxaparin.** Low-molecular-weight heparin (LMWH) (enoxaparin) is the most appropriate prophylaxis for this patient who is having surgery.

Mechanical prophylaxis is more appropriate for ambulatory patients having minor surgery. Direct-acting oral anticoagulants (DOACs) are increasingly being studied for prophylaxis but are not currently a standard practice. Fondaparinux would be appropriate if this patient had a contraindication to heparin products (such as history of heparin-induced thrombocytopenia).

40. **The correct answer is: A. CT pulmonary angiogram.** Because there is a high suspicion for pulmonary embolus and the patient does not have any obvious contraindications to CT scan, CT pulmonary angiogram is the most appropriate test. V/Q would be appropriate if the patient had contraindication to CT scan. D-dimer will almost certainly be positive in this patient and thus will not help narrow the differential diagnosis. Echocardiogram may be useful for risk stratification; however, it is not sensitive for pulmonary embolus.

41. **The correct answer is: A. Apixaban.** This patient has a malignancy-associated venous thromboembolism. Per the CHEST guidelines in 2021, whereas edoxaban and rivaroxaban are associated with a higher risk of GI major bleeding than LMWH in patients with cancer-associated thrombosis (CAT) and a luminal GI malignancy, apixaban is not. Apixaban or LMWH is thus the preferred option in patients with luminal GI malignancies. Argatroban is an IV direct thrombin inhibitor that is sometimes used in the inpatient setting in patients with a history of heparin-induced thrombocytopenia, and fondaparinux is a subcutaneous option for this population.

42. **The correct answer is: A. Apixaban for 3 months, then reassessment with patient counseling regarding ongoing anticoagulation.** For a first, unprovoked proximal DVT, anticoagulation should be continued for at least 3 months. There is likely benefit for prolonged anticoagulation, but the decision should be made considering the nature of the clot, the patient's bleeding risk, and patient preference. Compression stockings alone or 4 weeks of anticoagulation is an option for superficial venous thrombosis (depending on risk factors for development of DVT), but not for DVT.

43. **The correct answer is: A. Continue apixaban.** The next most important step is to continue full-dose apixaban. There is no proven benefit to adding an IVC filter in patients who are able to take anticoagulation (this patient has no contraindications). Historically, IVC filters have been used in patients who have a contraindication to anticoagulation, but they are falling out of favor because of numerous potential complications and a recent study raising the question of increased mortality in patients with contraindications to anticoagulation who had IVC filters placed.

44. **The correct answer is: B. Administer systemic thrombolysis**. This patient is suffering from a high-risk pulmonary embolus given her hypotension, and thus systemic thrombolysis is indicated. Admission to the ICU is appropriate but should not delay administration of thrombolysis. Surgical thrombectomy is reserved for patients with contraindication to systemic thrombolysis or in patients who remain hemodynamically unstable despite systemic thrombolysis. IVC filters are rarely indicated in acute pulmonary embolism unless there are absolute contraindications to anticoagulation.

45. **The correct answer is: C. Idiopathic pulmonary arterial hypertension (PAH).** The patient has a mean pulmonary artery pressure >25 mmHg, which is elevated, the PCWP is normal, and the transpulmonary gradient (mean pulmonary artery pressure-PCWP) is 22 mmHg (normal <12-15 mmHg), suggesting precapillary pulmonary hypertension (ruling out answer B). Given that the patient has no evidence of COPD on PFTs or ILD on CT, this is less likely a group 3 pulmonary hypertension, and overall consistent with idiopathic PAH.

46. **The correct answer is: D. Sildenafil.** The first-line agent in this patient should be sildenafil given the minimal side-effect profile. All of the other agents are also approved in PAH.

47. **The correct answer is: C. Initiate inotropic and vasopressor support.** This patient is presenting with decompensated right heart failure in the setting of her known PAH. The first step is to improve her systemic BP with the initiation of an agent such as norepinephrine or vasopressin. Once her MAP has improved, the addition of milrinone will be appropriate to increase contractility (and decrease vascular resistance). Additional inhaled pulmonary vasodilators may be appropriate once the patient has stabilized. Intubation in patients with decompensated right heart failure can cause hemodynamic collapse and should be avoided if not absolutely necessary. IV fluid administration is also contraindicated in this patient, as it would likely increase her right ventricular filling pressures that are already high as evidenced by the patient's elevated jugular venous pulse and result in worsening right heart failure.

48. **The correct answer is: A. V/Q scan.** Based on the hemodynamics obtained during RHC, this patient has precapillary pulmonary hypertension (elevated mean pulmonary artery pressure with a normal PCWP). Lack of response to vasodilator study suggests against WHO Group 1 pulmonary hypertension, and raises the suspicion of WHO Group 4 disease (ie, chronic thromboembolic pulmonary hypertension). A ventilation-perfusion scan is the appropriate next step in evaluation. Starting treatment at this juncture is not necessary given he is hemodynamically stable and awaiting a final etiology of precapillary pulmonary hypertension to better guide therapy. Among patients with known pulmonary hypertension, cardiopulmonary exercise testing can better elucidate the etiology of exercise limitation (pulmonary vascular limit to exercise vs left-sided heart disease) and document response to treatment initiation.

49. **The correct answer is: B. Start inhaled treprostinil.** Among patients with ILD-related pulmonary hypertension, treprostinil has been shown to increase exercise capacity as compared to placebo. Her stable CT scan and PFTs suggest that symptom worsening is not because of progression of ILD, but instead may be related to development of precapillary pulmonary hypertension. Monitoring symptoms alone is not appropriate given there is an efficacious therapy available.

50. **The correct answer is: A. Pulmonary thromboendarterectomy is potentially curative.** CTEPH is the only etiology of pulmonary hypertension that is potentially curative via pulmonary thromboendarterectomy and should be considered the first-line treatment in all patients. Riociguat and balloon pulmonary angioplasty are reserved for patients who are not surgical candidates or who decline surgery. Up to 30% of patients who develop CTEPH have no known history of venous thromboembolism.

51. **The correct answer is: B. Increase PEEP.** The patient's SpO_2 is below goal (goal 88%-92%). Because the patient is already on a high FiO_2 (>0.6), increasing the PEEP is the most appropriate next step. Increasing the RR and V_T improves ventilation and should be employed if there are problems with hypercapnia.

52. **The correct answer is: B. Excessive secretions.** Auto-PEEP, pneumothorax, and vent asynchrony all can lead to increased peak inspiratory pressures; however, they are also associated with increased plateau pressures. In this case, the peak inspiratory pressure is elevated, but the plateau is unchanged, indicating increased resistances. Bronchospasm, secretions, aspiration, and problems with ventilator tubing can all lead to increased resistance (elevated peak inspiratory pressure-Pplat).

53. **The correct answer is: D. Increase in RR from 20 to 30 breaths/min; decrease in tidal volumes from 380 to 280 mL.** A number of parameters must be considered when liberating patients from ventilator support. An increase in RR and decrease in tidal volume, and thus an elevated rapid shallow breathing index (RR/tidal volume [L]) >105, predicts failure and may indicate that the patient is not ready for extubation. Fall in MAP merits close monitoring but does not necessarily mean that the patient is not ready for extubation.

54. **The correct answer is: C. Maintaining pH >7.3.** The major goal in ventilating patients with acute respiratory distress syndrome is to avoid ventilator-induced lung injury. This is done in a number of ways, including low tidal volume ventilation (<6 mL/kg), titrating PEEP, and avoiding high FiO_2 to prevent worsened V/Q mismatch (as well as theoretical risk of O_2-induced lung injury). To allow for low tidal volume ventilation, permissive hypercapnia is common practice (but goal should be to maintain pH >7.15-7.20).

55. **The correct answer is: B. Proning.** Many interventions have been studied in acute respiratory distress syndrome. Both proning and lung-protective low tidal volume ventilation have been shown to decrease mortality. There has been no proven mortality benefit to pulmonary vasodilators. In one trial, although steroids were associated with increased number of vent-free days and shock-free days during the first 28 days, they were associated with increased mortality at both 60 and 180 days when started ≥14 days after the onset of acute respiratory distress syndrome; they are not recommended in acute respiratory distress syndrome. There is no proven mortality benefit for early ECMO in acute respiratory distress syndrome.

56. **The correct answer is: B. Start broad-spectrum antibiotics.** It is important to start empiric IV antibiotics as soon as sepsis/septic shock is identified (patient meets 3/3 quick Sequential Organ Failure Assessment criteria: RR >22 breaths/min, change in mental status, and systolic BP <100 mmHg). Every hour of delay in starting antibiotics is associated with increasing mortality. Resuscitation with fluid (~30 mL/kg) and pressors may also play a role to maintain MAP >65 mmHg; however, at this time the patient is maintaining his MAP and priority should be given to starting antibiotics. There are some data to support the use of hydrocortisone and fludrocortisone in refractory shock; however, this is not an initial intervention.

57. **The correct answer is: C. Vancomycin/cefepime.** Broad-spectrum antibiotics should be initiated for septic shock. Generally, if a patient is without risk factors for fungal infection, antifungals are not necessary. Treatment for community-acquired pneumonia with either ceftriaxone/azithromycin or levofloxacin is insufficient in this patient with septic shock (particularly given his additional risk factors for bacteremia because he is on dialysis).

58. **The correct answer is: B. Norepinephrine.** Norepinephrine is generally the first-line pressor of choice in septic shock. It was associated with fewer arrhythmias when compared with dopamine (*NEJM.* 2010;362:779). The action of norepinephrine on α-receptors counteracts the vasodilatory state of sepsis, and β-agonist provides increased cardiac output. There may be benefit to adding vasopressin to norepinephrine in less severe septic shock (patients on 5-14 μg/min of norepinephrine) (*NEJM.* 2008;358:877).

59. **The correct answer is: A. Start 100% oxygen.** This patient is likely suffering from carbon monoxide poisoning and prompt initiation of 100% should not be delayed while awaiting definitive diagnosis. Oxygen therapy reduces the half-life of carboxyhemoglobin, promoting to prompt symptom resolution.

60. The correct answer is: A. Amitriptyline. The patient is presenting with seizures, hypotension, and prolonged QRS and QTc, consistent with tricyclic antidepressant overdose. Calcium channel blockers and β-blockers are associated with bradycardia, atrioventricular block, and hypotension. Lithium is associated with not only seizure and long QT but also nausea/vomiting/diarrhea, hyperreflexia, clonus, atrioventricular block, and bradycardia.

61. The correct answer is: C. IV sodium bicarbonate. IV NS and IV sodium bicarbonate are used in tricyclic antidepressant overdose. Glucagon may be used in β-blocker toxicity. Flumazenil can be used for benzodiazepine overdose; however, it should be avoided as it can precipitate withdrawal/seizures. Dialysis may be needed in the case of certain ingestions such as lithium, digoxin, methanol, or ethylene glycol.

62. The correct answer is: C. Start vasopressin 0.04 units/min. Vasopressin is the second-line agent in distributive shock, most often added to norepinephrine. Addition of vasopressin has been shown to reduce the dose of norepinephrine required, protecting patients from catecholamine-associated adverse effects (ie, arrythmias) and may reduce the risk of renal failure. Addition of vasopressin has not been shown to have a mortality benefit.

63. The correct answer is: A. Acute rejection. Acute rejection must be ruled out in any posttransplant patient presenting with fever, cough, shortness of breath, or any decline in pulmonary function. Pneumonia is less likely given unremarkable CXR. Primary graft dysfunction generally occurs immediately in the posttransplant period. Chronic rejection generally manifests itself as worsening obstruction on PFTs and is less associated with acute symptoms.

64. The correct answer is: D. Transbronchial biopsy. Whenever there is concern for rejection, transbronchial biopsy must be obtained.

65. The correct answer is: C. Increasing immunosuppression. Increased immunosuppression is the treatment for acute rejection. Azithromycin, montelukast, and change in immunosuppressant therapy may be used in chronic rejection. The patient does not appear to have an infection, so broad-spectrum antibiotics are not warranted.

66. The correct answer is: A. Age >65 years. Current smoking, active malignancy, and chronic kidney disease requiring dialysis are absolute contraindications to lung disease. Although older age confers a higher risk for transplant, there is not an absolute cut-off across all transplant centers.

GASTROENTEROLOGY

1. A 65-year-old man with a history of diabetes mellitus, hypertension, chronic obstructive pulmonary disease (COPD), and coronary artery disease (CAD) presents to the emergency department (ED) with several days of foul-smelling breath, vomiting after meals, and epigastric pressure. He has a 50-pack-year smoking history and has not been evaluated by a physician in several years. Computed tomography (CT) of the chest reveals a patulous and dilated esophagus with food and gas within the esophagus lumen, narrowing at the gastroesophageal junction, and evidence of ground glass opacities in the lungs consistent with possible aspiration pneumonia.

   What is the most appropriate next step in management?

   A. Gastroenterology consultation for possible esophagogastroduodenoscopy (EGD)
   B. Initiation of a calcium channel blocker
   C. Surgery consultation for possible esophagectomy
   D. Antifungal therapy for empiric coverage of Candida

2. A 75-year-old woman with a history of diabetes mellitus, hypertension, hyperlipidemia, and peripheral artery disease presents with a chief complaint of cough while eating. On further history, she describes trouble initiating her swallow as well as recent dysarthria.

   Which of the following is the most likely cause of her symptoms?

   A. Achalasia
   B. Esophageal web
   C. Stroke
   D. Zenker diverticulum

3. A 55-year-old man with a history of diabetes mellitus, hypertension, obesity, tobacco smoking, and gastroesophageal reflux disease (GERD) presents to his primary care physician (PCP) with the new onset of trouble swallowing. He describes a sensation of solid food becoming stuck in his mid-chest. He has been taking omeprazole 20 mg daily for GERD for the past 3 years. He only occasionally misses a dose of this medication.

   Which of the following is the next best step in the management of this patient?

   A. Do a barium swallow
   B. Do an EGD
   C. Encourage the patient not to miss any doses of omeprazole
   D. Increase the dose of omeprazole to 40 mg daily

4. A 35-year-old man presents with epigastric pain. The pain is gnawing and burning in nature and worsens after eating. Since a recent shoulder injury, he has been taking ibuprofen "around the clock" for pain control. He denies recent weight loss, nausea and vomiting, dysphagia, melena, or hematochezia. He has no family history of gastrointestinal (GI) cancers. On examination, vital signs are normal, and the abdomen is benign.

Which of the following is the next most reasonable step in his management?

A. Begin a proton pump inhibitor
B. Do an EGD
C. Prescribe quadruple therapy for *Helicobacter pylori*
D. Provide reassurance

5. A 35-year-old man presents to your primary care office to establish care. He reports several months of epigastric pain that improves with food. He has no hematochezia or melena. He came from China to America with his family 10 years ago. He does not take any medications and abstains from alcohol intake. Based on your clinical history and examination, you are concerned that he may have peptic ulcer disease and prescribe omeprazole 20 mg daily. You also want to rule out *H. pylori* infection.

Which is the most appropriate next test to assess for *H. pylori* infection?

A. *H. pylori* serum antibody
B. EGD with gastric biopsies and immunohistochemical staining
C. Stool sample for *H. pylori* antigen test
D. Start omeprazole now and perform urea breath test in 2 weeks

6. The patient described in Question 5 undergoes workup for his symptoms and is found to be positive for *H. pylori* infection.

Which of the following is the most appropriate initial treatment regimen?

A. Metronidazole, tetracycline, bismuth, and omeprazole for 14 days
B. Metronidazole, tetracycline, bismuth, and omeprazole for 10 days
C. Amoxicillin, tetracycline, and bismuth for 14 days
D. Clarithromycin, tetracycline, bismuth, and omeprazole for 14 days

7. A 65-year-old man with a history of hypertension, diabetes mellitus, CAD, and gout is brought to the ED by his wife for hematochezia at home. Five days ago, he began taking prednisone and ibuprofen for a gout flare. His other medications include aspirin, clopidogrel, metformin, and hydrochlorothiazide. Yesterday, he reported gnawing epigastric pain that worsened with meals. This morning, he reported feeling dizzy and began passing large amounts of bright red blood per rectum. An ambulance was called, and on arrival to the ED, his vital signs were as follows: pulse 120/min, blood pressure (BP) 89/50 mmHg, temperature 37°C, and O_2 saturation 100% on room air. Two large-bore intravenous (IV) lines were placed in the field.

Which of the following is the most appropriate immediate next step?

A. Gastroenterology consultation for EGD
B. Pantoprazole 40 mg IV
C. Type and cross
D. Volume resuscitation with crystalloid fluids

8. A 56-year-old woman with a history of cirrhosis secondary to alcohol use and ongoing alcohol use disorder presents to the ED with two episodes of hematemesis at home. She has no history of bleeding. She underwent EGD screening 3 years ago and had no gastroesophageal varices at that time. She currently takes furosemide and spironolactone. Her initial vital signs are as follows: pulse 110/min, BP 90/56 mmHg, temperature 37°C, and O_2 saturation 98% on room air. Her physical examination is notable for dried blood around the lips, spider telangiectasias on the chest, palmar erythema, shifting dullness and splenomegaly, and 1+ lower extremity edema. Two large-bore IVs are placed, and she is given 2 L

of normal saline, with normalization of her BP. Since arrival to the ED, she has had no further hematemesis. She is started on IV pantoprazole, IV ceftriaxone, and an octreotide bolus followed by a continuous octreotide infusion.

Which of the following is the next most appropriate step in her management?

A. Gastroenterology consultation for EGD

B. Interventional radiology consultation for arteriography and embolization of likely gastric varices

C. Interventional radiology consultation for placement of a transjugular intrahepatic portosystemic shunt (TIPS)

D. Placement of a Sengstaken-Blakemore tube

9. A 75-year-old man with a history of obesity and hypertension presents to the ED with hematochezia. He was at home in his usual state of health when he began having bright red blood per rectum several hours ago. He estimates blood loss of approximately 700 mL at home. By the time he arrived at the ED, his bleeding had stopped. His vital signs are normal. He denies dizziness, light-headedness, or abdominal pain.

The presentation is most consistent with which of the following?

A. Bleeding from peptic ulcer

B. Diverticular bleeding

C. Ischemic colitis

D. Variceal bleeding

10. A 75-year-old woman with a history of diabetes mellitus and CAD is seen by her PCP for progressive dyspnea on exertion. She was recently seen by her cardiologist with similar complaints. Her examination and workup at that time were not suggestive of a cardiac cause of dyspnea, and a stress test was negative for cardiac ischemia. Lab work, however, did demonstrate a new anemia with a hemoglobin of 8.5 g/dL, a mean corpuscular volume (MCV) of 75 fL per cell (normal 80-100), and a red cell distribution width of 19% (normal 11.5-14.5). At her PCP's office, she reports that she has had regular, normal bowel movements without melena, hematochezia, or hematemesis. Physical examination reveals a non-toxic-appearing woman with a nonfocal abdominal examination. Digital rectal examination reveals no masses, fissures, or hemorrhoids but is notable for brown stool that is positive for occult blood. A colonoscopy followed by an EGD are both unrevealing for a source of blood loss.

Which of the following is the next best step in her management?

A. Reassurance

B. CT arteriography

C. Tagged white blood cell (WBC) scan

D. Video capsule endoscopy

11. An 18-year-old woman presents for evaluation of diarrhea. She has a several-year history of intermittent cramping, abdominal pain, and bloating, and for the past 4 to 6 months she has had worsening diarrhea. She reports that her stools are foul-smelling and float in the toilet water. The diarrhea is relieved by fasting. Workup reveals an elevated fecal fat, as well as iron deficiency anemia.

Which of the following best describes the nature of the diarrhea?

A. Acute inflammatory diarrhea

B. Acute noninflammatory diarrhea

C. Chronic malabsorptive diarrhea

D. Chronic secretory diarrhea

12. An 83-year-old woman presents to the ED with 3 days of persistent watery diarrhea, abdominal discomfort, and fever. She recently finished a course of antibiotics for a urinary tract infection (UTI) and has had no recent travel or sick contacts. Her vital signs are notable for a heart rate of 110/min, BP of 95/65 mmHg, respiratory rate of 25/min, and temperature of 39.3°C. Abdominal examination reveals a diffusely tender abdomen and absence of bowel sounds. Her lab results are significant for a WBC count of 23 000/mm^3, and a positive stool polymerase chain reaction (PCR) for *Clostridioides difficile*.

What is the most appropriate next step in her management?

A. Surgery consultation
B. Infectious disease consultation for consideration of bezlotoxumab therapy
C. CT of the abdomen and pelvis
D. Fidaxomicin 200 mg BID

13. A 65-year-old woman with osteoporosis is hospitalized for repair of a hip fracture. Preoperatively, she is given cephalexin to reduce the risk of postoperative wound infection. Postoperatively, she is placed on MiraLAX to prevent constipation while she remains on narcotics for pain control. On postoperative day 1, she reports four to six loose stools. Her vital signs are normal. Laboratory testing shows a WBC count of 10 000/mm^3. A stool *C. difficile* PCR is positive, and stool *C. difficile* enzyme-linked immunoassay (EIA; toxin A/B test) returns negative.

Which of the following is the next most appropriate step in her management?

A. Discontinue the MiraLAX
B. Order glutamate dehydrogenase
C. Prescribe PO (oral intake) vancomycin
D. Prescribe PO vancomycin and metronidazole

14. A 35-year-old woman develops fever, diarrhea, and abdominal cramping after consuming raw eggs. Stool culture reveals nontyphoidal *Salmonella* species. She has normal PO intake and appears nontoxic, with a reassuring abdominal examination, and conservative management is employed.

For which of the following groups should antibiotics be considered in the treatment of *Salmonella* infection?

A. Antibiotics should never be employed for nontyphoidal *Salmonella* infection
B. Immunocompromised patients
C. Persons <20 years old
D. Persons with a history of prior *Salmonella* infection

15. A 22-year-old man presents with acute-onset nonbloody, nonbilious vomiting occurring 10 times a day. He has had occasional episodes like this in the past, lasting days at a time, and notes that hot showers have improved his symptoms during prior episodes. Episodes occur two or three times a year and last up to a week. He has no abdominal pain, change in stool pattern, weight loss, or evidence of GI bleeding. In between episodes, he feels normal without GI symptoms. He takes no regular medications and has no other past medical history. The social history is notable for regular marijuana use (multiple times daily) and intermittent cigarette use. He is given IV fluids for hydration as well as antiemetics for his symptoms.

Which of the following would you also recommend?

A. Cessation of marijuana
B. EGD
C. Lorazepam long term
D. Ondansetron long term

16. A 26-year-old woman presents to the GI clinic for 1 month follow-up of constipation-predominant irritable bowel syndrome (IBS-C). Based on her prior history and examination, you believe she has mild disease with no "red flag" symptoms. During her last visit she was started on psyllium in increasing doses and a high-fiber diet. On follow-up she reports a slight improvement in her constipation, with bowel movements occurring every 4 days compared with every 5 days previously. She has read about several medical therapies now available to treat IBS-C and wonders what the best next step in her management should be.

What is the most appropriate treatment for her?

A. MiraLAX
B. Lubiprostone
C. Linaclotide
D. Alosetron

17. A 45-year-old woman with a history of alcohol use disorder is hospitalized in the intensive care unit (ICU) for severe pancreatitis with hypotension requiring vasopressors. She is given IV fluids and IV morphine for pain control. On hospital day 3, she is noted to have absent flatus and bowel movements, and physical examination reveals a distended abdomen with decreased bowel sounds in all four quadrants. Abdominal CT shows interstitial edematous pancreatitis without necrosis and new, diffuse colonic dilatation (cecal diameter of 11 cm) without evidence of obstruction. She is made NPO, a nasogastric tube is placed for decompression, and she is given methylnaltrexone, without effect.

Which of the following would be the next most appropriate step?

A. Administer neostigmine
B. Minimize narcotic administration
C. Place a rectal tube
D. All of the above

18. In the patient in Question 17, a rectal tube is placed for decompression, and narcotics are weaned to minimize bowel-slowing effect. On hospital day 5, she is noted to have spontaneous passage of both stool and flatus. She is weaned off vasopressors, and the rectal tube is able to be discontinued. The nurse notes that the patient has been NPO for several days and is receiving IV D5NS; she inquires about the next steps in the patient's nutrition plan.

Which of the following is most appropriate?

A. Begin enteral nutrition
B. Begin peripheral parenteral nutrition
C. Begin total parenteral nutrition
D. Continue IV D5NS

19. A 70-year-old man with a history of obesity and hypertension presents with 2 days of fever and left lower quadrant pain. He has noted loose stools in the past 48 hours but denies nausea, vomiting, diarrhea, or constipation. He reports a normal appetite and PO intake. In the ED, he is febrile to 38.2°C, and the remainder of his vital signs are normal. Abdominal examination demonstrates focal left lower quadrant tenderness to deep palpation without rebound tenderness or guarding. CT of the abdomen and pelvis with IV and oral contrast is performed and demonstrates focal diverticulitis of the sigmoid colon without evidence of abscess or fistula. He is given acetaminophen with adequate pain control.

Which of the following is the next most appropriate step in his management?

A. Hospitalization with IV piperacillin-tazobactam
B. Interventional radiology consultation for abdominal drain placement
C. Outpatient therapy with PO metronidazole and ciprofloxacin
D. Surgical consultation for sigmoid resection

20. The patient in Question 19 is treated successfully with outpatient antibiotic therapy and returns to his PCP for follow-up. He is worried about a recurrence of diverticulitis.

Which one of the following is TRUE about recurrence and prevention of diverticulitis?

A. Because his first episode was uncomplicated, he can be almost certain that a subsequent episode will also be uncomplicated

B. Surgical resection should only be considered after a fourth recurrence of diverticulitis

C. The combination of amoxicillin/clavulanic acid has proven to be efficacious for the prevention of recurrent diverticulitis

D. The risk of recurrence within 10 years is approximately 20%

21. A 45-year-old woman presents to her PCP to discuss colorectal cancer screening options. She would like to avoid colonoscopy if possible because of concerns about the invasiveness of the test and wonders what other screening modalities are available. She has no family history of colorectal cancer and follows an active and healthy lifestyle.

Which of the following screening approaches is currently recommended by the American Gastroenterological Association?

A. Fecal occult blood test (FOBT) every other year

B. Flexible sigmoidoscopy every 10 years

C. Fecal DNA testing every 3 years

D. CT colonography every 3 years

22. A 50-year-old woman with a history of hypertension, diabetes mellitus, CAD with a prior myocardial infarction (MI), and heart failure with reduced ejection fraction (40%) presents for her first screening colonoscopy. She is currently feeling at her baseline. She is a nonsmoker and does not drink alcohol. Her medications include aspirin, lisinopril, furosemide, and metoprolol. Her family history is notable for a mother with colorectal cancer diagnosed at age 59 years, a maternal cousin with ulcerative colitis, and an early MI in her father.

Which of the following elements of her history places her at increased risk of colorectal cancer compared with the baseline population?

A. Aspirin use

B. Family history of colorectal cancer in her mother

C. Family history of ulcerative colitis in a cousin

D. Personal history of hypertension

23. A 19-year-old man presents with worsening bloody diarrhea and abdominal pain. His symptoms began 6 days ago with low abdominal pain that was quickly followed by overtly bloody diarrhea accompanied by intense rectal urgency and tenesmus. Over the past several days, his stools have become more frequent, now occurring 8 to 10 times per day. He has had no recent travel, antibiotic use, or hospitalization. He denies fever, oral ulcers, ocular symptoms, or joint or dermatologic symptoms. Family history is positive for ulcerative colitis in his mother and a maternal cousin. You suspect that the patient may have ulcerative colitis.

Which of the following would you expect a colonoscopy to show?

A. Deep ulcerations in a cobblestone pattern with skip lesions throughout the colon

B. Grossly normal-appearing mucosa with biopsies showing active chronic colitis

C. Mucosal inflammation in the rectum and extending proximally

D. Pseudomembranes throughout the colon

24. The patient in Question 23 undergoes colonoscopy, which demonstrates continuous, circumferential ulceration beginning in the rectum and extending proximally to the splenic flexure. Stool culture and *C. difficile* testing return negative. Biopsies from his colonoscopy demonstrate severe, active, chronic colitis with crypt distortion and abscesses, most consistent with a diagnosis of ulcerative colitis. He asks what he can expect with this disease.

Which one of the following would you tell him?

A. Cigarette smoking increases the risk of ulcerative colitis
B. He has an increased risk of colorectal cancer compared with the baseline population
C. His overall life expectancy is decreased compared with that of the general population
D. Unlike Crohn disease, patients with ulcerative colitis are not at risk for stricturing disease

25. A 21-year-old woman with a known history of stricturing Crohn disease involving the ileum has undergone several ileal resections for bowel obstruction secondary to strictures.

With her history of ileal disease and resection, she is at increased risk for which of the following?

A. Gallstones
B. Kidney stones
C. Osteoporosis
D. All of the above

26. A previously healthy 27-year-old woman presents with 4 weeks of new-onset bloody diarrhea, accompanied by lower abdominal pain, rectal urgency, and tenesmus. On evaluation, she has normal vital signs and is nontoxic appearing. Examination reveals tenderness to deep palpation in the left lower quadrant without accompanying guarding or rebound. Digital rectal examination reveals red blood on the gloved finger with no fissures, fistulas, or masses. She undergoes a colonoscopy, which reveals circumferential ulceration, friability, and contact bleeding that extends contiguously from the rectum to the descending colon. Biopsies show severely active chronic colitis with few crypt abscesses, confirming a diagnosis of ulcerative colitis with severe disease activity. She is started on IV glucocorticoids with improvement.

Which of the following would be the most appropriate medication for long-term maintenance therapy?

A. Cyclosporine
B. Infliximab
C. Methotrexate
D. Prednisone

27. A 79-year-old nursing home resident with atrial fibrillation (AF; not on anticoagulation because of frequent falls), hypertension, prior stroke, diabetes mellitus, and dyslipidemia presents with sudden onset of severe abdominal pain, which he describes as "the worst of his life." He was reported to be hypotensive (70/40 mmHg) at the nursing home but now has a BP of 102/55 mmHg. On examination, the abdomen is mildly tender to palpation, and there is a small amount of bright red blood in the rectal vault. Labs are notable for a serum lactate level of 4.0 mmol/L, WBC of 18 000/mm^3, normal lipase, and normal bilirubin. The serum creatinine level is 0.7 mg/dL.

Which of the following would be the next most appropriate step?

A. CT angiography of the abdomen
B. Duplex ultrasonography of mesenteric vessels
C. Flexible sigmoidoscopy
D. Magnetic resonance imaging (MRI) abdomen with gadolinium

28. An 83-year-old woman with CAD, prior coronary artery bypass grafting (CABG), hypertension, chronic kidney disease (baseline creatinine 2.0 mg/dL), tobacco use, and diabetes mellitus is admitted to the hospital after presenting with 6 months of worsening abdominal pain associated with eating. She has lost 10 lb because of a reluctance to eat (eating triggers the pain). On examination, vital signs are within normal limits, and she is well appearing. Laboratory results, including chemistries, liver biochemical tests, complete blood count (CBC), and lactate, are normal. The abdomen is nontender to palpation and there is a soft systolic bruit in the mid-abdomen. She currently has no pain.

Which of the following is the most likely pathophysiologic cause of her symptoms?
A. Decreased blood flow to the gut because of mesenteric atherosclerosis
B. Decreased perfusion in the superior mesenteric artery territory because of arterial embolism
C. Increased venous congestion because of mesenteric vein thrombus
D. Ischemic colitis because of decreased blood flow to the colon

29. The patient described in Question 28 undergoes workup for her symptoms.

Which of the following is the next most appropriate step in her diagnosis?
A. CT angiography with venous phase contrast
B. Invasive angiography
C. Magnetic resonance angiography
D. Ultrasonography with Doppler ultrasound of the mesenteric vessels

30. A 45-year-old woman with long-standing alcohol use disorder, multiple prior episodes of pancreatitis, and depression presents to the ED with abdominal pain radiating to the back. She had 10 alcoholic drinks on the day of presentation. On examination, she has a pulse of 110/min, BP 90/65 mmHg, dry mucous membranes, and epigastric tenderness and is vomiting green liquid. The hemoglobin is 10 g/dL (baseline), creatinine is 1.4 mg/dL (baseline 0.5 mg/dL), lactate is 2.0 mmol/dL (normal <1), and lipase is 32 U/L (normal <40). Abdominal ultrasonography shows no cholelithiasis, and the pancreas is obscured by bowel gas.

Which of the following is the next most appropriate step in her management?
A. IV lactated Ringer's solution and pain management
B. IV lorazepam (for alcohol withdrawal)
C. IV pantoprazole
D. Oral fluids, with antiemetics, if needed

31. A 40-year-old woman presents to the ED with epigastric pain, vomiting, and malaise. Two weeks prior to her presentation, she developed intermittent right upper quadrant (RUQ) pain after meals that has progressively worsened. She drinks alcohol occasionally and has not taken any new medications recently. Her vital signs show a heart rate of 104/min, BP 100/80 mmHg, respiratory rate 20/min, and temperature 38.1°C. Physical examination is significant for dry mucus membranes, moderate epigastric abdominal tenderness, and vomiting. Her labs reveal a sodium of 130 mmol/L, potassium 3.0 mmol/L, creatinine 1.4 mg/dL (baseline 0.8 mg/dL), blood urea nitrogen (BUN) 40 mg/dL, WBC count 16 000/mm³, lipase 200 U/L, alkaline phosphatase 176 U/L, and serum bilirubin 2.3 mg/dL. CT of the abdomen and pelvis shows a 1-cm stone within the common bile duct with evidence of fat straining and inflammation around the pancreas consistent with acute pancreatitis.

Which of the following is the most appropriate next step in management?
A. Consult GI for endoscopic retrograde cholangiopancreatography (ERCP)
B. Consult surgery for cholecystectomy
C. An oral diet
D. Magnetic resonance cholangiopancreatography (MRCP)

32. A 42-year-old woman with a history of alcohol use disorder (at least four beers daily) is admitted with epigastric pain, nausea, and vomiting and found to have a serum lipase level of 3200 U/L. Ultrasonography of the abdomen reveals no cholelithiasis or bile ductal dilatation, and the patient is diagnosed with a first episode of alcohol-related acute pancreatitis. She is treated with IV lactated Ringer's solution and analgesia. Within 4 days of hospital admission, she develops worsening abdominal pain and hypotension. She has a fever of 38.8°C, pulse 120/min, and BP 76/40 mmHg. On examination, she has marked abdominal tenderness, particularly in the epigastrium. Urgent CT of the abdomen with IV contrast reveals a 7-cm nonenhancing region of low attenuation within a mildly enlarged pancreas. She is started on carbapenem and levofloxacin and is no better after 12 hours.

Which of the following would you recommend?

A. Endoscopic placement of a pancreatic duct stent
B. IV fluids and octreotide
C. Open surgical debridement (necrosectomy)
D. Percutaneous drainage

33. A 35-year-old man with no history of alcohol, drug, or tobacco use presents to the GI clinic with 6 months of nonspecific epigastric pain, nausea after eating, and greasy foul-smelling stools. Initial testing reveals a decreased fecal elastase level and the presence of fecal fat. The hemoglobin A_{1c} (HbA$_{1c}$) level is 9.0%. Blood testing reveals elevated serum alkaline phosphatase of 350 U/L and total bilirubin of 3.2 mg/dL, and normal alanine aminotransferase (ALT) and aspartate aminotransferase (AST) levels.

While awaiting imaging, which of the following would be the next most appropriate lab test or tests?

A. Antinuclear antibody and immunoglobulin (Ig)G subtypes
B. Blood and stool cultures
C. *H. pylori* serology and human immunodeficiency virus (HIV) testing
D. Serum alcohol level

34. A 74-year-old woman with diabetes mellitus, hypertension (on hydralazine), dyslipidemia, COPD (on azithromycin three times a week), osteoarthritis (on acetaminophen), recurrent UTIs (on suppressive nitrofurantoin), and depression is seen by her PCP for annual physical. Liver enzymes are drawn as part of routine blood work and reveal an elevated total bilirubin of 2.5 mg/dL (direct bilirubin 1.5 mg/dL), an elevated alkaline phosphatase of 650 U/L, ALT 15 U/L, AST 20 U/L, international normalized ratio (INR) 1.2, and albumin 3.5 g/dL.

Which of the following medications would be most likely to cause this pattern of abnormalities?

A. Acetaminophen
B. Azithromycin
C. Hydralazine
D. Nitrofurantoin

35. A 29-year-old man undergoes an annual physical examination for an immigration visa. His workup reveals an abnormal lab result. The total bilirubin level is elevated to 3.0 mg/dL with a direct bilirubin of 0.3 mg/dL. Serum AST and ALT levels are 20 and 18 U/L, respectively. The alkaline phosphatase is 70 mg/dL and the INR, CBC, blood smear, reticulocyte count, and albumin are within normal limits. He has no symptoms and denies alcohol use. He takes no regular medications.

Which of the following would be the next best step in his diagnosis?

A. Abdominal ultrasonography
B. γ-Glutamyl transpeptidase
C. Review prior lab results and ask about a current illness or stressor
D. Urine ethyl glucuronide for surreptitious alcohol use disorder

36. A 59-year-old woman with a history of osteomyelitis and depression presents to her PCP with itching for 2 months. She has no new exposures to potential allergens. She denies a rash or family history of autoimmune liver disease. She takes no medications. On examination, there is no conjunctival icterus and she is well appearing. The abdominal examination is unremarkable. Fasting laboratory tests are notable for a normal serum creatinine, BUN, and CBC. The total bilirubin is 0.9 mg/dL, AST 19 U/L, ALT 23 U/L, and alkaline phosphatase 198 U/L.

Which of the following would you recommend?

A. An oral antioxidant
B. Antimitochondrial antibodies
C. γ-Glutamyl transpeptidase
D. Ultrasound elastography of the liver

37. A 26-year-old man presents to the ED with new-onset RUQ abdominal pain, conjunctival icterus, nausea, and vomiting. He reports no recent travel but may have been exposed to sick contacts (young cousins with nausea, vomiting, and diarrhea) over the past month. On examination, he is jaundiced with tenderness to palpation over the RUQ. Mental status is normal. He denies IV drug use and has not taken any medications. He drinks two alcoholic drinks daily and has had no tattoos or blood transfusions. Labs are notable for a serum ALT level of 5430 U/L, AST 3598 U/L, alkaline phosphatase 234 U/L, bilirubin 7.8 mg/dL, and INR 1.2.

Which of the following is the test most likely to confirm the diagnosis?

A. Anti–hepatitis B core (HBc)
B. Hepatitis C virus (HCV) RNA
C. IgM anti–hepatitis A virus (HAV)
D. Serum ethanol

38. A 54-year-old man is admitted to the ICU after cardiac arrest. Emergency Medicine Services (EMS) discovered him on the floor in ventricular fibrillation and performed cardiopulmonary resuscitation (CPR) for 10 minutes prior to return of spontaneous circulation. His ED electrocardiogram (ECG) revealed ST elevations in the inferior leads, and he was urgently taken for coronary angiography during which a drug-eluting stent was placed in the right coronary artery. He is now hemodynamically stable on minimal vasopressor support. Admission labs reveal an ALT of 6000 U/L, AST 7000 U/L, alkaline phosphatase 260 U/L, total bilirubin 4 mg/dL, lactate dehydrogenase (LDH) 5000 U/L, and INR of 2.

What is the most likely etiology of the abnormal liver enzyme levels?

A. Alcohol intoxication
B. Ischemic hepatitis
C. Acute viral hepatitis
D. Acetaminophen toxicity

39. A 47-year-old man from China presents to a hepatology clinic to establish care after moving to the United States. He is asymptomatic but has been told that he has had hepatitis B virus (HBV) since childhood. Serologic testing reveals that he is hepatitis B surface antigen (HBsAg) positive, hepatitis B surface antibody (anti-HBs) negative, IgG anti-HBc positive, IgM anti-HBc negative, hepatitis B e-antigen (HBeAg) positive, and hepatitis B e-antibody (anti-HBe) negative. An HBV DNA level (viral load) is 120 000 IU/mL. The serum ALT level is 256 U/L, and the alkaline phosphatase and bilirubin levels are normal. A liver fibrosis test suggests no fibrosis.

Which of the following is the next most appropriate step in his management?

A. Begin lamivudine

B. Begin tenofovir

C. Repeat testing in 3 to 6 months

D. Vaccinate against HBV

40. A 37-year-old man with a history of alcohol use disorder, IV drug use, and multiple prior admissions for alcohol-associated hepatitis presents with abdominal pain, fever, ascites, and conjunctival icterus. He was recently discharged from the hospital after treatment for spontaneous bacterial peritonitis (SBP). On examination, he is tachycardic with dry mucous membranes and is tender in the RUQ. The serum bilirubin level is 11.3 mg/dL and INR is 2. A Maddrey discriminant function is 57. A repeat paracentesis shows 650 nucleated cells (80% polymorphonuclear leukocytes [PMNs]) and gram-negative rods on Gram stain.

Which of the following would be the most appropriate management?

A. IV ceftriaxone

B. Oral prednisolone

C. Oral prednisolone and pentoxifylline

D. Referral for urgent liver transplant

41. A 57-year-old woman with type 2 diabetes mellitus complicated by nephropathy (chronic kidney disease stage IV with a baseline estimated glomerular filtration rate [eGFR] of 25 mL/min) and retinopathy, hypertension, prior IV drug use, and HCV infection presents to residents' clinic to establish care. She was diagnosed with HCV infection approximately 5 years ago, after an antibody screening test returned positive and was confirmed on repeat testing. Her current medications are insulin, cinacalcet, lisinopril, cholecalciferol, furosemide, and doxazosin. Examination reveals no stigmata of liver disease.

Labs are notable for platelets of 205 000/mm^3, total bilirubin 0.6 mg/dL, albumin 4.1 g/dL, INR 1.1, AST 21 U/L, and ALT 18 U/L. The HCV genotype is 1b, and the HCV RNA level is 2 305 000 IU/mL. HBV serologies are consistent with immunity to HBV as a result of prior vaccination. HIV testing is also negative. Ultrasound of the abdomen shows a normal-sized liver with slightly increased echogenicity and no splenomegaly. Vibration-controlled transient elastography reveals a liver stiffness of 5.5 kPa (normal). She inquires about treatment for her HCV.

What would you recommend?

A. Defer treatment, because there is no evidence of liver fibrosis or cirrhosis and the aminotransferase levels are normal

B. Treatment with pegylated interferon and ribavirin

C. Perform a liver biopsy before offering treatment

D. Suggest treatment with glecaprevir-pibrentasvir (a direct-acting antiviral regimen)

42. A 65-year-old woman is following up with her gastroenterologist to discuss the results of her recent liver biopsy. She has a history of morbid obesity (body mass index [BMI] 45), diabetes mellitus, hypertension, obstructive sleep apnea, and hyperlipidemia. During a routine physical examination 5 months ago, she was found to have abnormal liver enzyme levels and underwent an extensive medical workup including RUQ ultrasound, viral studies, autoimmune serologies, celiac serology, and thyroid-stimulating hormone (TSH), all of which were within normal limits. She does not drink alcohol. A nonalcoholic fatty liver disease (NAFLD) fibrosis score was elevated, and she underwent a liver biopsy, which revealed stage F1 to F2 fibrosis and hepatic steatosis most suggestive of NAFLD.

What is the most appropriate initial step in the management of NAFLD?

A. 10% loss of the patient's total body weight through diet and exercise
B. Metformin
C. Referral for bariatric surgery
D. Vitamin E supplementation

43. The patient described in Question 42 undergoes repeat liver biopsy in 1 year that demonstrates progression to cirrhosis.

What workup do you advise at this time?

A. Screening EGD for esophageal varices, biannual RUQ ultrasound ± alpha fetoprotein (AFP) to screen for hepatocellular carcinoma (HCC), and hepatitis A and B vaccination
B. Screening EGD and colonoscopy and biannual RUQ ultrasound ± AFP
C. Biannual RUQ ultrasound ± AFP, and hepatitis A, B, and C vaccination
D. Hepatitis A and B vaccination and careful follow-up if new symptoms arise

44. A 21-year-old woman with a history of depression, anxiety, and prior suicide attempts is brought in by ambulance after taking an intentional overdose of 40 g of acetaminophen 20 hours prior to presentation. On arrival to the ED, she is arousable but lethargic with asterixis. The serum bilirubin level is 5.6 mg/dL and INR is 1.6. The acetaminophen level is pending.

In addition to supportive care in an ICU, checking arterial ammonia and lactate, and transfer to a liver transplant center, which of the following treatments should be initiated first?

A. Activated charcoal
B. *N*-acetylcysteine
C. Pentoxifylline
D. Hemodialysis

45. The patient described in Question 44 is transferred to a liver transplant center ICU. She becomes more obtunded and unable to protect her airway. She is then intubated, and intracranial pressure monitoring is initiated. The arterial ammonia is 200 μmol/L, and the intracranial pressure is elevated. The serum sodium is 135 mEq/L, and bilirubin continues to rise (now 21.4 mg/dL). INR is increased to 2.3. She has no evidence of bleeding.

What is the best therapeutic measure to perform next for the elevated intracranial pressure?

A. Hypothermia
B. IV barbiturate
C. IV mannitol
D. Lactulose

46. A 34-year-old pregnant woman with acute liver failure because of hepatitis E virus (HEV) is intubated in the ICU and listed for a liver transplantation. She is being covered with broad-spectrum antibiotics for fever. She has hypoglycemia and requires a continuous dextrose infusion. Her labs are notable for an INR of 1.5, platelet count of 21 000/mm^3, fibrinogen of 123 mg/dL, and BUN of 45 mg/dL. She needs to have central access placed in the ICU.

Which of the following is the most appropriate blood product to administer immediately prior to line insertion?

A. Cryoprecipitate
B. Fresh frozen plasma
C. Platelets
D. Vitamin K

47. A 57-year-old man with biopsy-proven cirrhosis because of HCV infection, MELD (Model for End-Stage Liver Disease) score of 20, and prior sustained virologic response with sofosbuvir/ledipasvir treatment presents with 3 days of abdominal pain and fever. He is hemodynamically stable without encephalopathy. He has no history of SBP but meets the criteria for SBP prophylaxis and is taking ciprofloxacin daily. A diagnostic paracentesis demonstrates 500 nucleated cells (75% neutrophils); fluid cultures are sent.

Which of the following is the best empiric antibiotic to start in this case?

A. IV ceftriaxone
B. IV ciprofloxacin
C. IV vancomycin and meropenem
D. PO trimethoprim-sulfamethoxazole

48. A 60-year-old woman with cirrhosis caused by NAFLD, a prior variceal bleed, refractory ascites (requiring a paracentesis every 2 weeks, on furosemide and spironolactone), and a baseline serum creatinine level of 0.6 mg/dL presents with confusion and coffee-ground emesis. EGD reveals a gastric ulcer with a visible vessel, which is cauterized. She has not been adequately fluid resuscitated, and the serum creatinine level is noted on admission to be 1.5 mg/dL; the urine sediment is bland, and mean arterial pressure (MAP) is around 60 mmHg (which is close to her baseline).

Which of the following is the best first step in her management?

A. Draw blood cultures and administer IV meropenem
B. Hold diuretics and give IV albumin 1 g/kg
C. Reduce the dose of β-blocker
D. Transfer her to the ICU for IV norepinephrine and octreotide

49. A 45-year-old woman with a history of alcohol-related Child-Pugh class C cirrhosis and on-going alcohol use presents with hematemesis. She has no history of esophageal varices. She is initially hypotensive with a BP of 75/45 mmHg and tachycardic with a pulse of 120/min. The hemoglobin is 6.6 g/dL (with a baseline of 10 g/dL). Medications prior to admission were furosemide, spironolactone, lactulose, rifaximin, and omeprazole. She is resuscitated with 2 units of packed red blood cells and admitted to the ICU for urgent EGD, which reveals grade 3 esophageal varices with positive red wale signs.

Which of the following would be the most appropriate management for this patient?

A. Endoscopic variceal ligation and nonselective β-blocker
B. Nonselective β-blocker
C. Sengstaken-Blakemore tube placement
D. TIPS

50. A 50-year-old male veteran with HCV-related cirrhosis (no prior EGD or HCC screening), hypertension, and diabetes mellitus presents with abdominal pain for 5 days. He is hemodynamically stable with no change in the serum bilirubin, INR, and creatinine from baseline. CT with IV contrast is performed and reveals a heterogeneous liver, moderate amount of ascites, no focal liver lesions, and acute thrombosis of the portal vein. He is feeling well and would like to be discharged home.

Which of the following is the most appropriate management plan for this patient?

A. Admission to the hospital for IV heparin
B. Admission to the hospital for monitoring of clot progression and pain
C. Discharge home with repeat CT of the abdomen in 1 month
D. EGD screening for varices and initiation of anticoagulation

51. A 75-year-old man with end-stage renal disease (on hemodialysis), type 2 diabetes mellitus, hypertension, Waldenström macroglobulinemia, dyslipidemia, and obesity presents to the ED with acute onset of RUQ pain and new onset of ascites. His wife notes that his eyes have been yellow, and he has been confused for the past day. He has no history of liver disease. On examination, he is nontoxic appearing with conjunctival icterus, large-volume ascites, and RUQ tenderness. Labs are notable for a serum bilirubin of 6.5 mg/dL, INR of 2.0, AST 350 U/L, ALT 235 U/L, and alkaline phosphatase 323 U/L.

Which of the following would be the next most appropriate diagnostic test?

A. Abdominal ultrasonography with Doppler ultrasound
B. Liver elastography
C. MRI with MR venography (MRV) of the liver
D. Noncontrast CT of the abdomen and pelvis

52. A 20-year-old man, 12 days after hematopoietic stem cell transplantation (HSCT) for acute myelogenous leukemia, develops hepatomegaly, RUQ pain, ascites, weight gain of 12 lb over 2 days, and lower extremity edema. He has no rash or diarrhea. Two days later, his serum bilirubin level rises to 6.5 mg/dL with mildly elevated AST and ALT levels. Ultrasonography demonstrates reversal of flow in the portal vein.

Which of the following is the most likely diagnosis?

A. Acute cytomegalovirus infection
B. Acute graft-versus-host disease
C. Drug toxicity from pre-HSCT conditioning chemotherapy
D. Sinusoidal obstruction syndrome

53. A 46-year-old woman from Puerto Rico presents to the ED with new ascites, malaise, weight loss, and conjunctival icterus. A diagnostic paracentesis reveals an ascitic protein concentration of 0.8 g/dL, ascitic albumin of 0.5 g/dL (serum albumin of 3.0 g/dL), and 145 nucleated cells (65% neutrophils).

Based on the ascitic fluid studies, which of the following is the most likely diagnosis?

A. Nephrotic syndrome
B. Peritoneal carcinomatosis
C. Portal hypertension
D. Tuberculous ascites

54. A 68-year-old man with a history of AF, type 2 diabetes mellitus, hypertension, dyslipidemia, CAD, and prior percutaneous coronary intervention presents to the ED with abdominal pain, fever, and chills 9 days after open laparotomy for bowel obstruction. He is tender to palpation in the left upper quadrant. Broad-spectrum antibiotics are started, and a diagnostic paracentesis reveals polymicrobial growth within 24 hours, fluid LDH of 697 mg/dL, and glucose of 16 mg/dL. The following day he becomes acutely hypotensive with increasing abdominal pain.

Which of the following is the next most appropriate diagnostic test?

A. CT of the abdomen and pelvis
B. EGD with mucosal biopsies of the stomach and duodenum
C. Repeat paracentesis
D. Ultrasonography of the abdomen with Doppler ultrasound

55. A 67-year-old woman with a history of type 1 diabetes mellitus, end-stage renal disease (on peritoneal dialysis), hypertension, hypercholesterolemia, and COPD presents with abdominal pain, fever, and nausea. She reports that her dialysate fluid looks cloudy. Diagnostic peritoneal fluid studies reveal 320 WBCs (96% polymorphonuclear neutrophils). Her pulse is 110/min, BP 95/40 mmHg, and temperature 39°C.

Initial empiric antibiotic therapy should be with which of the following?

A. IV cefepime
B. IV ciprofloxacin and metronidazole
C. IV meropenem
D. IV vancomycin and gentamicin

56. An 80-year-old white woman with a history of morbid obesity, hypertension, gout, and type 2 diabetes mellitus presents with 2 days of RUQ pain, confusion, fever of 40°C, chills, and lethargy in the nursing home where she resides. On arrival to the ED, she is toxic appearing, tachycardic to 110/min, and hypotensive to 86/46 mmHg and is noted to have conjunctival icterus in addition to severe RUQ tenderness. She is volume-resuscitated in the ED, empiric antibiotics are given, and blood cultures are drawn. Abdominal ultrasonography shows dilatation of the bile duct to 1.5 cm with dilated intrahepatic ducts and cholelithiasis without cholecystitis. The serum bilirubin level is 6.8 mg/dL, ALT 154 U/L, AST 125 U/L, alkaline phosphatase 609 U/L, and WBC 30 000/mm³. In the ED, the patient remains hypotensive despite adequate fluid resuscitation and is started on vasopressors with escalating requirements. Broad-spectrum antibiotics are begun.

Which of the following is the most appropriate next step in her management?

A. Endoscopic ultrasonography
B. Cholecystostomy tube
C. ERCP
D. Surgical consultation for cholecystectomy

57. A 41-year-old morbidly obese woman with a history of hypertension and type 2 diabetes mellitus and who is currently 12 weeks pregnant presents with new onset of belching, nausea, and RUQ pain after eating, particularly after eating fatty foods. The pain lasts approximately 1 to 2 hours and radiates toward her right scapula. She has a family history of peptic ulcer disease. On examination, she is clinically well appearing and afebrile with a normal heart rate and BP. She also has mild RUQ tenderness. Liver enzymes and CBC are within the normal range. She is concerned about the pain and asks what she should do next.

Which of the following is most appropriate?

A. EGD
B. Esophageal probe monitoring
C. Referral for cholecystectomy
D. Transabdominal ultrasonography

58. A 56-year-old man with idiopathic pulmonary fibrosis who is 2 weeks post-bilateral lung transplantation remains in the ICU with postoperative pneumonia and multiple failed extubations. He is on total parenteral nutrition because of an inability to tolerate tube feeds. He is persistently febrile with a pressor requirement despite broad-spectrum antibiotics. CT of the abdomen and pelvis reveals a thick gallbladder wall with intramural gas, pericholecystic fluid, and sludge in the gallbladder without gallstones.

Which of the following is the next most appropriate step in his management?

A. Cholecystectomy
B. Cholecystostomy drain
C. Discontinuation of total parenteral nutrition
D. ERCP

ANSWERS

1. **The correct answer is: A. Gastroenterology consultation for possible esophago-gastroduodenoscopy (EGD).** This man presents with classic symptoms of late-stage achalasia, typically a neuromuscular disorder that causes progressive difficulty with swallowing both solids and liquids. A barium swallow study would reveal evidence of a dilated esophagus and distal "bird beak" narrowing that can also be appreciated on endoscopy. As the lower esophageal sphincter loses its ability to relax, food and liquid become stuck in the distal esophagus over time. The buildup of food can cause pressure in the chest, a foul-smelling odor, and dysphagia. The differential diagnosis of achalasia includes Chagas disease and malignancy at the gastroesophageal junction, which should be ruled out with EGD. Most often, however, the cause is idiopathic achalasia. After EGD is performed and malignancy is excluded, further evaluation with esophageal manometry may be considered, and the clinical team can decide on the most appropriate management (eg, peroral endoscopic myotomy, pneumatic dilation). Aspiration pneumonia is a frequent complication of this disease, and speech and swallow specialists should be consulted while interventions are pending to determine the safest means of enteral nutrition.

2. **The correct answer is: C. Stroke.** The patient describes trouble initiating a swallow, which suggests that the origin is oropharyngeal rather than esophageal. The combination of dysphagia and dysarthria raises concern for a neuromuscular rather than strictly structural cause. In this patient with known vascular disease, this constellation of symptoms is consistent with a stroke.

3. **The correct answer is: B. Do an EGD.** The patient has long-standing GERD and risk factors for Barrett esophagus and esophageal adenocarcinoma. The development of dysphagia is an alarm symptom for potential malignancy. Alarm symptoms include dysphagia, excessive vomiting, weight loss, and anemia. Risk factors for Barrett esophagus include age >50 years, Caucasian race, hiatal hernia, central adiposity, smoking, and a family history of Barrett esophagus or esophageal adenocarcinoma. The next best step in the management of this patient is to refer him for EGD to exclude malignancy. Although other complications from GERD, such as esophagitis and strictures, may cause dysphagia, malignancy should be excluded first. EGD is more sensitive and specific for Barrett esophagus and malignancy than a barium swallow.

4. **The correct answer is: A. Begin a proton pump inhibitor.** This patient presents with symptoms that are typical for peptic ulcer disease, specifically a gastric ulcer, because his pain worsens with meals (the pain of a duodenal ulcer is typically relieved with food). His use of nonsteroidal anti-inflammatory drugs (NSAIDs) is the most likely etiology of the presumed peptic ulcer disease. With a history of NSAID use, an absence of alarm symptoms, and a reassuring physical examination, it is reasonable to treat empirically with acid-suppressive therapy while he remains on NSAIDs and monitor him closely for symptom resolution. If his pain continues after a week or two, he should be advised to switch to acetaminophen for an NSAID-free period. EGD is not needed at this point but should be considered if his symptoms prove refractory to proton pump inhibitor therapy. Empiric treatment for *H. pylori* without testing is not recommended. Reassurance alone would be inappropriate.

5. **The correct answer is: C. Stool sample for *H. pylori* antigen test.** This patient presents with findings consistent with a duodenal ulcer. His pain is relieved with food because of the release of bicarbonate into the duodenum after consumption of a meal, with brief relief of pain. *H. pylori* infection is associated with duodenal ulcer in patients who do not take NSAIDs, and the Chinese population has a high prevalence of *H. pylori* infection,

thus increasing the pretest probability of disease. In a patient who has not yet started an acid-suppressive therapy, urea breath test and stool antigen test are the best noninvasive means of confirming *H. pylori* infection. *H. pylori* serologic testing cannot delineate prior infection from active disease and is helpful primarily in excluding infection in lower prevalence areas. The gold standard test for confirmation of *H. pylori* infection is EGD with biopsy and immunostaining; however, EGD is typically only performed if a patient fails treatment or has another indication for EGD.

6. **The correct answer is: A. Metronidazole, tetracycline, bismuth, and omeprazole for 14 days.** Of the available treatment regimens listed, answer A, referred to as "quadruple" therapy, is the preferred first treatment regimen for *H. pylori* infection. Evidence suggests that a 14-day regimen has higher clearance rates and reduced resistance as compared to a 7-day regimen and is recommended over a 10-day regimen (*Gastroenterology* 2016;151:51). In patients with an allergy to tetracyclines, the combination of metronidazole, amoxicillin, clarithromycin, and omeprazole for 14 days can be prescribed. In areas with a >15% resistance rate to clarithromycin, however, these clarithromycin-based regimens are not recommended.

7. **The correct answer is: D. Volume resuscitation with crystalloid fluids.** The patient is presenting with several risk factors for peptic ulcer disease (ibuprofen and aspirin use in combination with prednisone use) as well as symptoms and signs of a rapid upper GI bleed (hypotension, tachycardia in combination with hematochezia). Although red blood cell transfusion, IV proton pump inhibitor, and EGD are all appropriate steps in the management of brisk upper GI bleeding, immediate volume resuscitation with crystalloid fluids is of utmost priority given his hypotension and the rapid availability of IV fluids in the emergency room. Tachycardia and supine hypotension suggest that he has lost approximately 30% of his effective arterial blood volume and he needs urgent volume resuscitation.

8. **The correct answer is: A. Gastroenterology consultation for EGD.** The patient has cirrhosis and presents with an upper GI bleed and signs of portal hypertension (ascites and splenomegaly), raising concern for a possible variceal source. She has been hemodynamically resuscitated, and appropriate medical management has been initiated. The next best step is to perform an EGD with endoscopic band ligation if varices are found. A Sengstaken-Blakemore tube is not necessary because the bleeding is not uncontrollable. A Sengstaken-Blakemore tube is typically used in patients with unstable, large-volume hematemesis to allow subsequent EGD or for refractory bleeding in spite of band ligation to allow subsequent TIPS. A TIPS is not an appropriate first management step without first attempting EGD. Although gastric varices are possible, they must first be confirmed by EGD.

9. **The correct answer is: B. Diverticular bleeding.** The patient has had overt hematochezia but has remained hemodynamically stable. Therefore, the bleeding is most likely localized to a lower GI bleed (as opposed to a brisk upper GI bleed). The presentation with painless bleeding, along with a sudden onset and abrupt cessation, is typical of a diverticular bleed. His age is a clear risk factor for diverticulosis; obesity is also thought to be a risk factor. Ischemic colitis is less likely and is typically accompanied by abdominal pain and bloody stool. An upper GI source is unlikely in a patient who is hemodynamically stable and usually presents with melena rather than hematochezia.

10. **The correct answer is: D. Video capsule endoscopy.** This patient has a new, symptomatic anemia, with labs suggestive of iron deficiency (low MCV, elevated red cell distribution width). Although she has no overt symptoms of bleeding, her positive FOBT is suggestive of occult GI blood loss. Thus, a full evaluation should be performed to look for sources of GI bleeding, and reassurance is inappropriate. The next best step for this particular case would be a video capsule endoscopy, which may be able to identify small bowel

lesions that could account for her blood loss. CT arteriography is unlikely to be helpful in this case, as this imaging modality depends on a bleeding rate of roughly 0.5 mL/min or more to detect bleeding from the culprit vessel. Because this patient has had no overt evidence of bleeding, it is unlikely that she is losing blood from a GI source at a rate >0.5 mL/min. A tagged WBC scan is a modality used to detect inflammation and does not help localize occult GI bleeding. A tagged RBC scan (radionuclide imaging) is the most sensitive radiographic test for GI bleeding; however, it requires ongoing bleeding at a rate of 0.3-0.5 mL/min. This exam is rarely performed given its limited accuracy in locating the source of bleeding compared with CT arteriography.

11. **The correct answer is: C. Chronic malabsorptive diarrhea.** The first step in determining the cause of a patient's diarrhea is to characterize it. Diarrhea is considered acute if the patient has had <2 weeks of symptoms and is often secondary to infection. Diarrhea is considered chronic if symptoms have lasted >4 weeks. (Symptoms lasting 2-4 weeks may be either acute or chronic.) This patient's symptoms have lasted several months, and the presentation is most consistent with chronic diarrhea. A history of foul-smelling, floating stools with an elevated fecal fat would be most consistent with either a malabsorptive or maldigestive diarrhea. The patient's presentation is most consistent with (but not limited to) an etiology such as celiac disease or small intestinal bacterial overgrowth. Fecal fat would not be expected to be elevated in chronic secretory diarrhea, and typically this type of diarrhea does not improve with fasting.

12. **The correct answer is: C. CT of the abdomen and pelvis.** This patient has several risk factors for *C. difficile* infection, including age and recent antibiotic use. A history of recent antibiotic exposure may be lacking when *C. difficile* infection occurs in an immunocompromised or elderly patient but increases the pretest probability of the infection. Based on the patient's vital signs—tachycardia, hypotension, and fever—in conjunction with her leukocytosis, she has evidence of severe disease. Abdominal and pelvic CT should be performed given her diffusely tender abdomen and lack of bowel sounds to rule out life-threatening complications of the infection, including toxic megacolon, colonic perforation, and peritonitis. Pending the results of the CT, surgery may need to be consulted for consideration of colectomy. Bezlotoxumab, a monoclonal antibody that binds to the *C. difficile* toxin B, is used as an adjunctive therapy in patients with recurrent *C. difficile* infection. Fidaxomicin can be considered for the treatment of nonfulminant *C. difficile* infection if fulminant disease has been excluded.

13. **The correct answer is: A. Discontinue the MiraLAX.** The next most appropriate step is to decrease or discontinue MiraLAX and monitor the patient clinically. The stool testing results likely represent *C. difficile* colonization rather than *C. difficile*–associated diarrhea (CDAD). This conclusion is supported by the absence of fever, absence of leukocytosis, presence of an alternative explanation for loose stools, and a negative *C. difficile* toxin result. Up to 20% of hospitalized patients who receive antibiotics may have asymptomatic *C. difficile* colonization (as determined by positive *C. difficile* PCR testing) without clinical CDAD. Therefore, the likely culprit for her loose stools, laxative use, should be addressed first, and she should be monitored clinically. Treatment of *C. difficile* infection should not be implemented at this time. Glutamate dehydrogenase testing would not yield additional clarity to the question of colonization versus CDAD.

14. **The correct answer is: B. Immunocompromised patients.** In patients with a nontoxic examination and normal PO intake, conservative measures (adequate hydration, PRN antidiarrheal medications) can be employed for nontyphoidal *Salmonella* infection. Immunocompromised patients represent a group of patients that should be considered for antibiotic treatment (typically with a fluoroquinolone antibiotic). Young age and prior exposure to *Salmonella* do not impact treatment decisions for a subsequent episode.

15. **The correct answer is: A. Cessation of marijuana.** The patient's history of recurrent, stereotypic episodes of acute vomiting in the setting of heavy marijuana use raises concern for cannabinoid hyperemesis syndrome. Alleviation of symptoms with hot showers is a typical feature of this syndrome. IV fluids, antiemetics, and benzodiazepines may be used to control acute symptoms. However, agents such as ondansetron and lorazepam are not recommended for long-term use because of their risk and side-effect profiles. The mainstay of treatment of this disorder is cessation of marijuana use. For refractory symptoms, tricyclic antidepressants can be considered. Given the self-limited nature of the patient's episodes and history consistent with cannabinoid hyperemesis syndrome, an EGD is not needed at this time.

16. **The correct answer is: A. MiraLAX.** This patient is presenting 1 month after initial diagnosis of IBS-C. She has initiated conversative measures with exclusion of gas-producing foods, psyllium, and a high-fiber diet. Physical activity is also an important component of the management of IBS, with the current guidelines suggesting 30 minutes of exercise five times a week. In patients who fail to improve with psyllium alone, polyethylene glycol, or MiraLAX, is advised as add-on therapy. MiraLAX should be trialed for at least 6 to 8 weeks before other agents are considered. Adjunctive pharmacologic therapies are then added for patients with moderate-to-severe symptoms felt to impair their quality of life. Lubiprostone acts locally on the chloride channel activator and enhances chloride-rich intestinal fluid secretion, providing relief to patients with IBS-C despite polyethylene glycol. Linaclotide is another option in patients with moderate-to-severe disease refractory to initial laxative therapy. Linaclotide is a guanylate cyclase agonist that stimulates intestinal fluid secretion and transit. Both lubiprostone and linaclotide would be appropriate adjunctive therapies for patients with IBS-C; however, this patient has not yet had an adequate trial of conversative measures and has only mild symptoms. Alosetron is a pharmacologic option for patients with diarrhea-predominant IBS and would not be clinically appropriate in this case.

17. **The correct answer is: D. All of the above.** This critically ill patient has developed paralytic ileus of the colon, sometimes called colonic pseudo-obstruction or Ogilvie syndrome (although the latter designation was originally applied to paraneoplastic colonic pseudo-obstruction). Risk factors for colonic pseudo-obstruction in this patient include critical illness, pancreatitis, hospitalization, and opioid administration. Management of colonic pseudo-obstruction is centered around bowel rest, bowel decompression, and restoring normal intestinal peristalsis. Conservative measures such as making the patient NPO and discontinuing offending medications should be employed first. Bowel decompression can be attempted with either nasogastric tube or rectal tube placement (or both). For patients receiving narcotics, methylnaltrexone, a peripheral μ-opioid antagonist that acts locally in the gut without causing systemic withdrawal symptoms, can be attempted to reverse the bowel-slowing effects of opioids. Finally, treatment with neostigmine, a cholinesterase inhibitor that results in parasympathomimetic activity, can also be attempted.

18. **The correct answer is: A. Begin enteral nutrition.** At this point, more aggressive nutritional support should be attempted because the patient is not meeting her caloric needs on peripheral IV D5NS alone. Enteral nutrition is the preferred route of nutritional support in the absence of a contraindication. The colonic pseudo-obstruction has resolved, as evidenced by the spontaneous passage of stool and flatus and ability for the rectal tube to be discontinued. Therefore, enteral nutrition should be attempted first, and the patient should be monitored closely. Should she be unable to tolerate enteral nutrition because of nausea, vomiting, or recurrence of colonic pseudo-obstruction, alternative forms of nutritional support such as peripheral parenteral nutrition and total parenteral nutrition should then be considered.

19. **The correct answer is: C. Outpatient therapy with PO metronidazole and cip-rofloxacin.** The patient has risk factors for diverticulosis (age, obesity) and presents with symptoms of diverticulitis. Cross-sectional imaging confirms this diagnosis and demonstrates lack of complications (abscess, perforation, or fistula). The episode can be characterized as mild in severity, because he has few comorbidities, is able to tolerate PO intake, has pain that is well controlled with acetaminophen, and has uncomplicated disease on CT. Therefore, it is reasonable to pursue outpatient therapy with PO antibiotics for a 7- to 10-day course. Antibiotic regimens may include metronidazole with a fluoroquinolone or amoxicillin/clavulanic acid. Hospitalization should be considered for patients who appear toxic, cannot tolerate PO intake, require narcotics for pain, have significant medical co-morbidity, or have complicated disease. Surgery would not be indicated because this is the patient's first presentation of diverticulitis and his disease is uncomplicated. Surgical resection can be considered for multiple episodes of recurrent diverticulitis. Finally, interventional radiology consultation for drain placement is not needed at this time because he demonstrates no evidence of abscess formation.

20. **The correct answer is: D. The risk of recurrence within 10 years is approximately 20%.** After a first episode of diverticulitis, the 10-year risk of recurrent diverticulitis is approximately 20% (range, 10%-30%). Choice A is incorrect because the risk of complicated diverticulitis increases with a second episode. Choice C is incorrect because there is no evidence to support the use of amoxicillin/clavulanic acid in the prevention of recurrent disease; there is weak evidence for mesalamine and rifaximin (*Cochrane Database Syst Rev.* 2017;10:CD009839; *Am J Gastroenterol.* 2016;111:579; *Ann Gastroenterol.* 2016;29:24). Choice B is incorrect because there is no specific number of episodes above which surgical resection should be considered; surgical resection should be considered on a case-by-case basis.

21. **The correct answer is: C. Fecal DNA testing every 3 years.** Currently, colonoscopy is the gold standard for colon cancer screening. Based on both the American Gastroenterological Association and U.S. Preventive Services Task Force guidelines, the screening regimens listed further are considered acceptable in patients who decline colonoscopy. When discussing the risks and benefits of the different screening modalities, however, it is important to inform patients that if one of these noninvasive tests is positive, they will need to undergo colonoscopy for further workup.

- FOBT or fecal immunochemical test (FIT) yearly
- Flexible sigmoidoscopy every 5 years or flexible sigmoidoscopy every 10 years with a yearly FIT test
- Fecal DNA test (eg, Cologuard) every 3 years
- CT colonography every 5 years

22. **The correct answer is: B. Family history of colorectal cancer in her mother.** Her family history of colorectal cancer in a first-degree relative places her at increased risk of colon cancer. Guidelines recommend that persons with a family history of colorectal cancer in a first-degree relative begin colorectal cancer screening at 40 years of age, or 10 years before the earliest age of colorectal cancer diagnosis in the family member, whichever comes first. (This patient should have begun screening at 40 years of age.) There are no data to suggest that a personal history of hypertension or ulcerative colitis in a cousin increases a patient's risk of colorectal cancer. Finally, aspirin use is not associated with increased risk of colorectal cancer; in fact, some data suggest that aspirin use may be a protective factor against colorectal cancer.

23. **The correct answer is: C. Mucosal inflammation in the rectum and extending proximally.** In a patient with ulcerative colitis, colonoscopy would be expected to show continuous mucosal inflammation beginning in the rectum and extending proximally. Deep cobble-stoning ulceration with skip lesions is a feature seen in Crohn colitis. With this patient's degree of symptoms, including grossly bloody diarrhea, one would not generally expect a grossly normal-appearing colonoscopy if the diagnosis is ulcerative colitis. Finally, pseudomembranes are a feature typical of *C. difficile* infection.

24. **The correct answer is: B. He has an increased risk of colorectal cancer compared with the baseline population.** The patient should be informed that he is at increased risk of colorectal cancer with his diagnosis of left-sided ulcerative colitis, and he should undergo a more aggressive colorectal cancer screening strategy compared with persons at average risk of colorectal cancer. A typical screening strategy would be to perform a surveillance colonoscopy 8 to 10 years after the initial diagnosis of ulcerative colitis and then every 1 to 3 years thereafter. Active smoking is actually associated with a lower risk of ulcerative colitis (it is, however, associated with a higher risk of Crohn disease). Persons with ulcerative colitis have a normal life expectancy when compared with persons without ulcerative colitis. Patients with recurrent inflammation because of ulcerative colitis can develop strictures, typically in the rectosigmoid colon, although less frequently than those with Crohn disease.

25. **The correct answer is: D. All of the above.** This patient is at risk for all of the complications listed. Patients with extensive ileal disease or ileal resection experience both fat malabsorption and impaired bile acid reabsorption. Fat malabsorption leads to excess fat in the intestinal lumen, which binds calcium. Binding of calcium to fat leaves an excess of oxalate available for colonic absorption, which can then lead to urinary calcium oxalate stones. Intestinal fat malabsorption also leads to impaired reabsorption of fat-soluble vitamins, including vitamin D, which can lead to osteopenia and osteoporosis. Finally, an increased risk of gallstone formation in those with Crohn disease is not completely understood, although it is thought to be related to impaired bile reabsorption and circulation, leading to hypersaturation of bile with cholesterol; however, about half of the gallstones are bilirubin stones, so other mechanisms are involved.

26. **The correct answer is: B. Infliximab.** This patient has clinical, endoscopic, and histologic findings consistent with severely acute ulcerative colitis. She has responded to IV glucocorticoids, and once remission is achieved, she will need to be transitioned to an agent for long-term maintenance of remission. For severe disease, many clinicians will choose a biologic agent. This is in contrast to the "step-up" approach, which begins with the least toxic regimen (typically a nonbiologic agent). From the list provided, infliximab is the best treatment option for maintenance of remission in those presenting with severe acute ulcerative colitis (*Lancet.* 2017;389:1218; *NEJM* 2016;374:1754; *Ann Rheum Dis.* 2017;76:1723; *JAMA.* 2019;321:156). Oral prednisone is incorrect, as the goal should be to transition patients to a glucocorticoid-sparing agent for maintenance of remission, given the adverse effects of long-term glucocorticoid use. Methotrexate is incorrect, as this therapy is approved for Crohn disease and not for ulcerative colitis. Cyclosporine is an incorrect choice, as it is used for the management of acute severe ulcerative colitis and not as a long-term maintenance therapy.

27. **The correct answer is: A. CT angiography of the abdomen.** This elderly patient who is not anticoagulated for AF is at risk for arterial embolism. The "pain out of proportion to physical examination findings" is classic for acute mesenteric ischemia. The elevated lactate and WBC count are likely due to bowel infarction. Of the possibilities listed, CT angiography (arterial phase) is the noninvasive test of choice (the venous phase is used for

the diagnosis of mesenteric venous thrombosis). Invasive angiography is the gold standard, can be potentially therapeutic (eg, embolectomy), and would be the next step if CT angiography is suggestive of vascular occlusion.

28. **The correct answer is: A. Decreased blood flow to the gut because of mesenteric atherosclerosis.** The presentation is classic for "intestinal angina," which is characterized by postprandial abdominal pain, early satiety, and weight loss because of fear of eating. The pathophysiologic basis is decreased blood flow to the gut because of mesenteric atherosclerosis, and the syndrome of chronic mesenteric ischemia can often be seen in patients with vascular disease elsewhere (such as CAD, carotid artery disease, peripheral artery disease). The pain is intermittent (postprandial), but if the pain becomes constant, acute mesenteric thrombosis should be considered. The other choices are more often associated with constant pain, rectal bleeding, abdominal tenderness, and an elevated lactate level or WBC count depending on whether there is bowel infarction.

29. **The correct answer is: D. Ultrasonography with Doppler ultrasound of the mesenteric vessels.** Ultrasonography with Doppler ultrasound or CT angiography (with arterial, not venous, phase contrast) is a reasonable first step in the diagnosis of chronic mesenteric ischemia. Although invasive angiography is the gold standard, it is reasonable to obtain imaging with ultrasonography first, especially because the patient has a history of chronic kidney disease and should avoid a contrast agent. If ultrasonography is negative but clinical suspicion for mesenteric ischemia is high, CT angiography should be pursued. A possible role for tonometry, spectroscopic oximetry, and MR angiography in the diagnosis of chronic mesenteric ischemia has been suggested, but the clinical usefulness of these studies, which are still under investigation, has not been established.

30. **The correct answer is: A. IV lactated Ringer's solution and pain management.** The patient has alcohol-related acute pancreatitis. She has a history of multiple prior episodes of acute pancreatitis, which explains why the lipase level is normal (because of chronic loss of functioning pancreatic cells). Her story of epigastric acute pain radiating to the back associated with nausea and vomiting is classic. She has signs of volume depletion on examination. It is likely too early for alcohol withdrawal, given that she had multiple drinks on the day of presentation. The mainstay of treatment for pancreatitis is aggressive fluid resuscitation in the first 24 hours. A 10-20 mL/kg IV bolus should be followed by 1.5-3 mL/kg/h depending on the patient's volume status. Lactated Ringer's solution may be superior to normal saline.

31. **The correct answer is: A. Consult GI for endoscopic retrograde cholangiopancreatography (ERCP).** This patient presents with clinical evidence most suggestive of gallstone pancreatitis and choledocholithiasis. Treatment for choledocholithiasis is with ERCP and stone extraction followed by cholecystectomy once the pancreatitis has subsided. Intermittent postprandial abdominal pain leading up to this presentation is most consistent with biliary pain associated with gallstones. If pancreatitis is mild, cholecystectomy during the initial hospitalization for gallstone pancreatitis can reduce the risk of recurrence, but would not be the immediate next step in management. Although early enteral feeding is encouraged, this should not be trialed until the patient is clinically stable and the choledocholithiasis has been addressed. MRCP can be a useful imaging modality to exclude bile duct stones, but because a bile duct stone was seen on CT this test would not be necessary.

32. **The correct answer is: D. Percutaneous drainage.** The patient has infected pancreatic necrosis (5% of all cases, 30% of cases of severe acute pancreatitis), which is associated with high mortality. This should be treated with a carbapenem or metronidazole plus

a fluoroquinolone. She is clinically unstable and should undergo percutaneous drainage (often followed by minimally invasive surgical debridement) or endoscopic necrosectomy; these management options have been shown to be superior to open necrosectomy. IV fluids and antibiotics may temporize but are not definitive management strategies.

33. **The correct answer is: A. Antinuclear antibody and immunoglobulin (Ig)G subtypes.** This patient presents with steatorrhea and abdominal pain, which are likely a result of chronic pancreatitis and the inability of the pancreas to secrete normal digestive enzymes. Edema of the pancreas may cause compression of the bile duct, leading to cholestatic liver biochemical levels. The patient's HbA_{1c} is also elevated because the pancreas has lost the ability to secrete insulin as a result of chronic inflammation. The next best step in laboratory workup in this young, otherwise healthy patient would be antinuclear antibody and IgG subtypes to assess for autoimmune pancreatitis (IgG4-related autoimmune pancreatitis). There is no evidence of infection, so cultures are not warranted. HIV, *H. pylori* testing, and a serum alcohol level are unlikely to help elucidate the etiology of chronic pancreatitis in this case. Glucocorticoids would be first-line treatment for autoimmune pancreatitis, and immunomodulators (azathioprine, mycophenolate mofetil, cyclophosphamide, rituximab) may be used if the patient relapses.

34. **The correct answer is: B. Azithromycin.** Of the options given, azithromycin is the most likely drug to cause a pure cholestatic pattern of abnormal liver chemistries, as may other macrolide antibiotics, azathioprine, chlorpromazine, estrogens, and 6-mercaptopurine. Acetaminophen classically causes hepatocellular injury with "towering" aminotransferase elevation after an overdose. Hydralazine may also cause hepatocellular injury. Nitrofurantoin, amoxicillin-clavulanic acid, azathioprine, carbamazepine, mirtazapine, and penicillin may cause a "mixed" pattern with elevated AST, ALT, and alkaline phosphatase levels. The next best step would be to discontinue the culprit medication (azithromycin) and consider liver imaging if the abnormalities do not resolve.

35. **The correct answer is: C. Review prior lab results and ask about a current illness or stressor.** This patient likely has Gilbert syndrome, as demonstrated by an elevated unconjugated bilirubin with normal liver enzymes, normal liver synthetic function, and no symptoms, medications, or alcohol use. In this patient, review of prior lab work would reveal previous elevated indirect bilirubin levels, which improved after a period of illness or stress. Gilbert syndrome is the most common inherited disorder of bilirubin glucuronidation and is a benign condition (present in 4%-16% of the population). It is characterized by recurrent episodes of jaundice and may be triggered by, among other things, dehydration, fasting, intercurrent disease, menstruation, and overexertion. Other than jaundice, patients are typically asymptomatic. The diagnosis is made by excluding other causes of unconjugated hyperbilirubinemia, although genetic testing is available. A presumptive diagnosis can be made in patients with the following features:

- Unconjugated hyperbilirubinemia on repeated testing
- A normal CBC, blood smear, and reticulocyte count
- Normal serum aminotransferase and alkaline phosphatase levels

36. **The correct answer is: C. γ-Glutamyl transpeptidase.** This patient has an isolated elevated alkaline phosphatase, which may or may not relate to her itching. The first step in working up an isolated elevated alkaline phosphatase is to repeat the test fasting (a level 1.5-2 × upper limit of normal [ULN] can be seen postprandially). Pregnancy and medications are other common causes of an elevated alkaline phosphatase, but when these causes have been ruled out, the next best step is to establish whether the alkaline phosphatase is of bone or liver origin. Checking a γ-glutamyl transpeptidase would be the test of choice.

If the γ-glutamyl transpeptidase level is elevated, ultrasonography should be done to look for bile ductal dilatation, and testing for antinuclear and antimitochondrial antibodies should be done for primary biliary cholangitis. This patient is the right demographic for primary biliary cholangitis, but the first step is to establish whether this is a bone or liver source of alkaline phosphatase. Antioxidants are not indicated.

37. **The correct answer is: C. IgM anti–hepatitis A virus (HAV).** This patient has a story typical for an acute hepatitis as demonstrated by the extremely high aminotransferase levels (ALT > AST) and acute presentation with nausea, vomiting, jaundice, and RUQ pain. He had sick contacts who may have been in day care centers (over the incubation period of 2-6 weeks) and may have acquired hepatitis A via the fecal-oral route. HBV or HCV infection is less likely, given the lack of IV drug use or other bloodborne exposures. Alcohol-associated hepatitis is even less likely, especially given the pattern and degree of aminotransferase elevations (typically AST > ALT and AST <400 U/L in alcohol-associated hepatitis).

38. **The correct answer is: B. Ischemic hepatitis.** The differential diagnosis of acute severe elevations in ALT/AST levels includes ischemia, toxins, medications, acute viral infections (such as acute viral hepatitis or reactivation of Epstein-Barr virus or cytomegalovirus infection), acute biliary obstruction, and rhabdomyolysis. This patient's clinical history is significant for a ventricular fibrillation cardiac arrest because of acute myocardial ischemia from acute coronary thrombosis. Because he was found down by EMS providers, it is unclear how long he experienced poor perfusion, which resulted in hypotension and ischemic injury to the liver. An ALT:LDH ratio <1.5 is particularly sensitive for distinguishing ischemic from viral hepatitis given the elevation in LDH associated with ischemia. Alcohol intoxication typically does not cause AST/ALT elevations >400, and the patient has no clinical history to suggest acute viral hepatitis or acetaminophen toxicity, although routine serologic workup and an acetaminophen level on admission would be appropriate in this case.

39. **The correct answer is: B. Begin tenofovir.** This patient has HBeAg-positive chronic HBV (immunoreactive phase). This is demonstrated by the fact that he is HBeAg-positive (anti-HBe negative) and has an elevated ALT level. On a liver biopsy specimen, he would likely have moderate-to-severe inflammation. The HBV DNA level is over 20 000 IU/mL. Chronic HBV infection should be treated in the immunoreactive and immune reactivation phases and in patients with cirrhosis with an elevated HBV DNA level or decompensation. First-line treatment is with a nucleo(s/t)ide analog, entecavir or tenofovir, which are well-tolerated and, unlike lamivudine, are associated with a low rate of resistance at 5 years. HBeAg seroconversion occurs in 30% to 40% of treated patients, with loss of HBsAg in 5% to 10%. Tenofovir is also preferred if there is a history of lamivudine resistance.

40. **The correct answer is: A. IV ceftriaxone.** The patient has alcohol-associated hepatitis and a high Maddrey discriminant function (>32); therefore, his mortality rate is high (1-month mortality of 35%-45%). It is worth considering oral glucocorticoids, but he has ongoing SBP and an active infection is a contraindication to prednisolone (contraindications include active bacterial or fungal infection, chronic HCV infection, or HBV infection). Although pentoxifylline would be a therapeutic possibility in a patient with a contraindication to glucocorticoids, it would not be recommended in conjunction with glucocorticoids and is no longer considered effective in alcohol-associated hepatitis. He has had multiple admissions for alcohol-associated hepatitis and evidence of an active infection and would not be accepted for liver transplantation at this time. Instead, he should be managed by treating his SBP, optimizing hydration, nutrition, stress ulcer prophylaxis, and abstinence from alcohol.

41. **The correct answer is: D. Suggest treatment with glecaprevir-pibrentasvir (a direct-acting antiviral regimen).** Treatment with direct-acting antiviral therapy should be made available to all patients with chronic HCV infection, unless life expectancy is short, in order to prevent complications such as cirrhosis and HCC. The direct-acting antivirals can achieve sustained virologic responses, or cure, in a high (>95%) proportion of patients and have few adverse events. HCV treatment with direct-acting antivirals has been shown to improve mortality, even in the absence of cirrhosis (*Lancet.* 2019;393:1453), and the World Health Organization (WHO) has set an elimination target for HCV by 2030.

    In patients with an eGFR <30 mL/min or on dialysis, the most robust data are for the direct-acting antivirals glecaprevir-pibrentasvir (Mavyret) and elbasvir-grazoprevir (Zepatier). Recent data suggest that sofosbuvir/velpatasvir (Epclusa) can also be used in this population. Glecaprevir-pribrentasvir is a pangenotypic regimen that has been shown to have excellent sustained viral response rates with 8 weeks of treatment in patients with chronic kidney disease or end-stage renal disease (including those on dialysis).

    Treatment with pegylated interferon and ribavirin is rarely used, as it has a worse side-effect profile and lower sustained viral response rate than direct-acting antivirals. There is no need to perform a liver biopsy to confirm absence or presence of cirrhosis, given that there is no evidence of fibrosis or cirrhosis on imaging and vibration-controlled transient elastography. Moreover, compensated cirrhosis would not change treatment recommendation in this case.

42. **The correct answer is: A. 10% loss of the patient's total body weight through diet and exercise.** This patient presents with a new diagnosis of NAFLD. Her risk factors for this disease include obesity, diabetes mellitus, hypertension, obstructive sleep apnea, and hyperlipidemia. Based on her liver biopsy she does not have evidence of advanced fibrosis (stage F3-F4) at this time, and aggressive lifestyle intervention is important to prevent progression to cirrhosis. Currently, there are no Food and Drug Administration (FDA)-approved pharmacologic therapies for NAFLD. Lifestyle intervention with weight loss and physical activity is crucial to disease management. Several studies have demonstrated that a 5% total body weight loss can reduce a patient's degree of steatosis, and 7% to 10% total body weight loss can improve fibrosis. Based on the patient's morbid obesity, increased risk of fibrosis progression with diabetes mellitus, and liver biopsy finding of established fibrosis, a 7% to 10% total body weight loss would be an ideal, though difficult to achieve, goal. Vitamin E supplementation was found in the PIVENS trial to improve histologic outcomes in patients without diabetes mellitus; however, vitamin E is not currently recommended in patients with diabetes mellitus. Metformin is frequently used as an off-label therapy for weight loss and improvement in insulin resistance in patients with NAFLD. Both medical therapies and referral for bariatric surgery should not be considered until an initial trial of lifestyle therapy with weight loss and physical activity is initiated.

43. **The correct answer is: A. Screening EGD for esophageal varices, biannual RUQ ultrasound ± alpha fetoprotein (AFP) to screen for hepatocellular carcinoma (HCC), and hepatitis A and B vaccination.** Once a patient is determined to have a new diagnosis of cirrhosis based on liver histology, several screening tests should be performed. Based on the current American College of Gastroenterology (ACG) guidelines, all patients should undergo an EGD to screen for esophageal varices. Based on the findings on endoscopy, the frequency of screening and need for further intervention (such as a nonselective β-blocker or variceal band ligation) will be determined. Additionally, once a diagnosis of cirrhosis is made, patients should undergo biannual RUQ ultrasound to screen for HCC. The utility of combined ultrasound and AFP testing compared with ultrasound alone is controversial. Lastly, given the significant increase in severity of disease in patients

with cirrhosis who acquire viral hepatitis, all patients should receive vaccination against hepatitis A and B; there is no vaccine for hepatitis C virus.

44. **The correct answer is: B. N-acetylcysteine.** Adult patients who present soon (within 4 hours) after a potentially toxic ingestion of acetaminophen (single dose ≥7.5 g) are likely to benefit from GI decontamination with activated charcoal. Charcoal should be withheld in patients who are sedated and may not be able to protect their airway unless they undergo intubation. This patient's presentation is too delayed and she is too lethargic for administration of charcoal. Acetaminophen is not removed by hemodialysis, and pentoxifylline is not useful in the treatment of acute liver failure because of acetaminophen. N-acetylcysteine is the accepted antidote for acetaminophen poisoning and is given to all patients at significant risk for hepatotoxicity. Although the acetaminophen level is not yet back, she has evidence of liver damage and a history of acetaminophen ingestion.

   Indications for N-acetylcysteine therapy include:

   - Serum acetaminophen concentration drawn at 4 hours or more following acute ingestion of an immediate-release preparation is above the "treatment" line of the treatment nomogram for acetaminophen poisoning
   - A suspected single ingestion of >150 mg/kg (7.5 g total dose regardless of weight) in a patient for whom the serum acetaminophen concentration will not be available until >8 hours from the time of ingestion
   - An unknown time of ingestion and a serum acetaminophen concentration >10 µg/mL
   - A history of acetaminophen ingestion and any evidence of liver injury
   - A delayed presentation (>24 hours after ingestion) of laboratory evidence of liver injury (ranging from mildly elevated aminotransferase levels to acute liver failure) and a history of excessive acetaminophen ingestion

45. **The correct answer is: C. IV mannitol.** The patient has developed grade 3 encephalopathy (somnolence to stupor, confusion, gross disorientation) requiring intubation for airway protection. Acute hyperammonemia (as in acute liver failure) induces accumulation of glutamine inside astrocytes and causes cerebral edema, a common cause of death in this patient population. Although the evidence is mixed for routine intracranial pressure monitoring in acute liver failure, it should be considered in patients with grade 3 or 4 encephalopathy. If intracranial pressure is found to be elevated, mannitol, 0.5 to 1.0 mg/kg IV, should be given. In patients with grade 3 or 4 encephalopathy, acute kidney injury, or on a vasopressor, consider prophylactic 3% hypertonic saline with a goal of a serum sodium concentration of 145 to 155 mEq/L. In patients with refractory elevated intracranial pressure despite these measures, consider initiation of a barbiturate and therapeutic hypothermia. Lactulose should generally be avoided in patients with acute liver failure and an elevated ammonia level because of the risk of volume depletion from a high stool output.

46. **The correct answer is: C. Platelets.** Patients with acute liver failure are at risk for bleeding because of multiple hematologic abnormalities including thrombocytopenia, elevated prothrombin time [PT] and partial thromboplastin time, decreased fibrinogen, decreased synthesis of coagulation factors (although this is somewhat balanced by decreased protein C and S levels), and disseminated intravascular coagulation. The INR is not helpful for determining the bleeding risk because of the decrease in protein C and S production, which are not directly measured. Neither fresh frozen plasma nor cryoprecipitate is administered to "correct" the PT/INR prior to a procedure, because several large reviews of available evidence have shown no clinical benefit. In this patient, an INR of 1.5 would not be significantly changed by fresh frozen plasma administration (studies have shown that transfusions of fresh frozen plasma will not reliably decrease the INR below about 1.7).

Cryoprecipitate should be given to patients who are bleeding and who have a fibrinogen level of $\leq$100 to 120 mg/dL. Vitamin K can be given if there is concern for vitamin K deficiency to assess whether the INR corrects, but IV vitamin K takes 6 to 8 hours to be effective and would not be useful right before a procedure. It is reasonable to aim for a platelet count of 50 000/mm^3 in the setting of bleeding or prior to a procedure (as in this case), but in the absence of bleeding or an imminent procedure, platelet administration should be avoided unless the platelet count is <10 000 to 15 000.

47. **The correct answer is: A. IV ceftriaxone.** Empiric antibiotic therapy for SBP pending culture results include third-generation cephalosporin, such as ceftriaxone, or amoxicillin-clavulanic acid for 5 days. In cases that occur in areas with high fluoroquinolone resistance or when the patient is already taking a fluoroquinolone for SBP prophylaxis, it is better to avoid this class of antibiotic. There are increasing rates of extended-spectrum β-lactamase (ESBL) infections and infections caused by other resistant organisms. Therefore, if the patient has a history of infections caused by a resistant organism, has had multiple recent hospitalizations, or is systemically unwell, it is reasonable to consider broader empiric coverage such as a fourth-generation cephalosporin or a carbapenem.

48. **The correct answer is: B. Hold diuretics and give IV albumin 1 g/kg.** The patient may have hepatorenal syndrome. Common precipitants include GI bleeding, overdiuresis, infection, serial large-volume paracenteses, and drugs such as NSAIDs. In suspected hepatorenal syndrome, the first step is to rule out prerenal acute kidney injury with volume expansion by holding diuretics and giving IV albumin 1 g/kg/d for 2 days. In this case, it would also be appropriate to discontinue the β-blocker (rather than simply reduce the dose). If the renal function and MAP do not improve with an albumin challenge, a trial of midodrine and octreotide or a vasopressor to raise the patient's BPs and improve renal perfusion would be appropriate. There is no clear evidence of infection, so an empiric treatment for sepsis is not necessarily indicated.

49. **The correct answer is: A. Endoscopic variceal ligation and nonselective β-blocker.** Secondary prevention for all patients after a first variceal bleed includes β-blocker and endoscopic variceal ligation (rather than either alone) because of the ~50% risk of rebleeding and ~30% mortality rate. Primary prevention for medium-to-large esophageal varices that have not yet bled includes a β-blocker or endoscopic variceal ligation (usually not both). TIPS can also be considered in patients with Child class B or class C cirrhosis within 72 hours of admission for a variceal bleed (less rebleeding, more encephalopathy, no change in mortality) (*Hepatology.* 2016;63:581) or for refractory bleeding not controlled with endoscopic therapy. In this case, choice D is not the most appropriate next management step, because the patient is not currently bleeding, and therapy with endoscopic variceal ligation and nonselective β-blocker should first be attempted. A Sengstaken-Blakemore tube may be placed in a patient with uncontrollable bleeding, often followed by TIPS placement.

50. **The correct answer is: D. EGD screening for varices and initiation of anticoagulation.** Treatment of acute portal vein thrombus in a noncirrhotic patient includes low-molecular-weight heparin, followed by warfarin for 6 months, or indefinitely if the cause is irreversible. In a patient with cirrhosis, anticoagulation increases the rates of recanalization of the portal vein without increasing the risk of bleeding (*Gastroenterology.* 2017;153:480). The patient should be screened for high-risk varices prior to initiation of anticoagulation (*Nat Rev Gastroenterol Hepatol.* 2014;11:435) and, if identified, variceal bleeding prophylaxis is initiated. For chronic portal vein thromboses, anticoagulation should be initiated if the patient is noncirrhotic or has a hypercoagulable state. If the patient is cirrhotic, anticoagulation may be considered if the patient is symptomatic or is demonstrated to have progression of

the thrombus on follow-up imaging. Anticoagulation options for patients both with and without cirrhosis include direct-acting oral anticoagulants (DOACs), heparin, and warfarin. At this time, the data on whether DOACs are safe and efficacious for patients with cirrhosis remain unclear, although they are increasingly used in clinical practice given the unreliability of INR monitoring in patients with cirrhosis.

51. **The correct answer is: A. Abdominal ultrasonography with Doppler ultrasound.** The presenting features are suggestive of Budd-Chiari syndrome (BCS, a rare disorder, occurring in one per million people). BCS should be suspected in patients with a history of oral contraceptive pill (OCP) use, prior venous thrombosis, myeloproliferative disorder such as polycythemia rubra vera, or malignancy. In 25% of cases, BCS is idiopathic. The presentation often consists of RUQ abdominal pain, ascites, and hepatomegaly. Serum AST, ALT, and alkaline phosphatase levels are often elevated. Acute liver failure may be present. The diagnosis is generally made using abdominal ultrasonography with Doppler ultrasound, which shows an occlusion in the hepatic veins or inferior vena cava (IVC). Alternative approaches include MRI and MRV or CT of the abdomen and pelvis with IV contrast. In this patient's case, MRI with gadolinium should be avoided because of the risk of nephrogenic systemic fibrosis associated with end-stage renal disease.

52. **The correct answer is: D. Sinusoidal obstruction syndrome.** Sinusoidal obstruction syndrome (formerly known as hepatic veno-occlusive disease) results from the occlusion of hepatic venules and sinusoids because of a toxic insult to hepatic vein endothelium. The syndrome is associated with a 20% mortality rate. It is characterized by hepatomegaly, RUQ pain, jaundice, and ascites, most often occurring in patients undergoing HSCT and less commonly following the use of certain chemotherapeutic agents in nontransplant settings, ingestion of alkaloid toxins, high-dose radiation therapy, or liver transplantation. Treatment is supportive and consists largely of fluid management with diuretics.

53. **The correct answer is: C. Portal hypertension.** The serum-ascites albumin gradient equals the serum albumin concentration minus the ascites albumin concentration (in g/dL). A serum-ascites albumin gradient ≥1.1 signifies portal hypertension with ~97% accuracy. If portal hypertension plus another cause of ascites (seen in ~5% of cases) coexist, the serum-ascites albumin gradient is still ≥1.1. In this patient's case, the serum-ascites albumin gradient is 2.5, suggestive of portal hypertension (most likely because of cirrhosis). The other causes would typically present with a serum-ascites albumin gradient of <1.1.

54. **The correct answer is: A. CT of the abdomen and pelvis.** The patient has secondary bacterial peritonitis, which may be due to an intra-abdominal abscess or perforation and should be suspected in a patient who has recently undergone laparotomy. Runyon criteria include the following: ascitic fluid total protein >1 g/dL, glucose <50 mg/dL, and LDH >ULN for serum. Cultures may reveal polymicrobial growth. Treatment is with a third-generation cephalosporin and metronidazole. Urgent abdominal imaging with CT is most appropriate in this case, and the patient may require an exploratory laparotomy.

55. **The correct answer is: D. IV vancomycin and gentamicin.** Peritonitis in the setting of peritoneal dialysis is usually caused by intraluminal contamination (suboptimal sterile technique when handling the catheter, or "touch contamination"). Approximately 45% to 65% of cases are caused by gram-positive organisms and 15% to 35% by gram-negative organisms. In up to 40% of cases, a causative organism is never found, and empiric antibiotics should cover both gram-negative and gram-positive organisms. Coagulase-negative staphylococcus will cause the majority of infections, and some will be methicillin resistant. Of the antibiotic choices, vancomycin and gentamicin cover methicillin-resistant gram-positive organisms as well as gram-negative organisms effectively.

56. **The correct answer is: C. ERCP.** This patient has acute ("ascending") cholangitis, likely because of a bile duct stone (although this is not seen on the ultrasonography, the bile duct is dilated, which is suggestive of choledocholithiasis in the right clinical setting). She has "Reynolds pentad," which is a syndrome of RUQ pain, jaundice, and fever and chills (Charcot triad) plus shock and confusion (present in ~15% of patients). Antibiotics should be initiated as soon as possible and should be broad in spectrum to cover common bile pathogens (eg, ampicillin + gentamicin [or levofloxacin] with or without metronidazole [if severe]; carbapenems; piperacillin-tazobactam). If there is a history of resistant organisms, carbapenem can be used initially. Approximately 80% of patients respond to conservative treatment with antibiotics, in which case biliary drainage can be performed on an elective basis. Approximately 20% require urgent biliary decompression via ERCP (papillotomy, stone extraction, and/or stent insertion), as in this case.

57. **The correct answer is: D. Transabdominal ultrasonography.** This patient has many of the risk factors for cholelithiasis (female, obese, pregnant, age >40 years). She is presenting with symptoms typical of biliary pain ("colic"): episodic RUQ or epigastric abdominal pain that begins abruptly, is continuous, resolves slowly and lasts for 30 minutes to 3 hours, with or without radiation to scapula, and is associated with nausea and belching. Although it is possible that she has GERD, gastritis, and/or peptic ulcer disease, the symptoms are typical of biliary pain related to gallstones, which should be explored first with abdominal ultrasonography. Management of biliary pain is usually supportive in pregnant women, but if bouts of biliary pain are frequent, primary surgical management during pregnancy is reasonable because recurrence is common with conservative therapy and surgical therapy appears to be safe for mother and fetus. The preferred time for surgery is the second trimester.

58. **The correct answer is: A. Cholecystectomy.** Acalculous cholecystitis is caused by gallbladder stasis and ischemia (in the absence of cholelithiasis), resulting in a necroinflammatory response, and occurs mainly in critically ill or hospitalized patients. Acalculous cholecystitis often occurs after major surgery and may be associated with total parenteral nutrition, sepsis, trauma, burns, opiates, immunosuppression, and infections such as cytomegalovirus, candidiasis, cryptosporidiosis, campylobacteriosis, and typhoid fever. Although gallbladder abnormalities such as biliary sludge are present in many critically ill patients, gas in the gallbladder wall or lumen, lack of gallbladder wall enhancement, and edema around the gallbladder have the highest specificity for acalculous cholecystitis (99%, 95%, and 92%, respectively). In this patient with a persistent fever and shock, acalculous cholecystitis may be the source of sepsis. Indications for an emergency cholecystectomy include gallbladder necrosis, emphysematous cholecystitis (as in this case) because of a gas-forming organism, and gallbladder perforation. In acalculous cholecystitis without these features, a trial of a cholecystostomy tube would be the appropriate initial treatment.

4

NEPHROLOGY

QUESTIONS

1. A 25-year-old man with type 1 diabetes mellitus is admitted with lethargy and altered mental status. His roommate reports that the patient recently lost his job, started drinking again, and has been rationing his insulin. He takes topiramate for seizure disorder. On examination, the patient is barely arousable to stimuli. His blood pressure (BP) is 90/50 mmHg and his pulse is 120/min. Laboratory studies show: Na 128 mEq/L, K 5.3 mEq/L, Cl 94 mEq/L, HCO_3 14 mEq/L, glucose 560 mg/dL, serum osmolality 303 mmol/kg, and serum lactate 2.5 mmol/L. Arterial blood gas (ABG) shows a pH of 7.20, $PaCO_2$ of 23 mmHg, and PaO_2 of 88 mmHg. Urinalysis is positive for ketones and glucose, and a urine toxicology screen is positive for ethanol and cannabinoids.

   What is the cause of metabolic acidosis in this patient?

   A. Alcohol intoxication
   B. Diabetic ketoacidosis
   C. Lactic acidosis
   D. Renal tubular acidosis

2. A 35-year-old man with a history of alcohol use disorder complicated by seizures is brought into the emergency department (ED), as he was found stumbling in the park by pedestrians. He is afebrile, with heart rate (HR) in the 90s and BP 120/70s. His labs are notable for pH 7.20, PCO_2 32 mmHg (ABG) with Na 125 mEq/L, Cl 90 mEq/L, HCO_3 15 mEq/L, and albumin of 3.0 g/dL with a lactate elevated at 6 mmol/L and no serum ketones. The ED orders 2 L lactated Ringer's, and repeat labs show pH 7.18 with Cl 89 mEq/L, HCO_3 20 mEq/L, and repeat lactate 7 mmol/L.

   What is the most likely cause of this patient's acid-base disturbance?

   A. Alcoholic ketosis
   B. Hypovolemia
   C. Sepsis
   D. Thiamine deficiency
   E. Vomiting

3. A 38-year-old man with unknown past medical history is brought into the ED after he was found lying on the sidewalk. He is disoriented but reports intermittent blurry vision. He is afebrile with a pulse rate of 105/min, BP of 128/80 mmHg, and respiratory rate (RR) of 28 breaths/min. Examination is notable for pupillary dilation, poor dentition, and mild diffuse abdominal pain. Labs reveal Na 132 mEq/L, Cl 92 mEq/L, HCO_3 22 mEq/L, blood urea nitrogen (BUN) 30 mg/dL, Cr 1.2 mg/dL, Ca 7.4 mg/dL, glucose 160 mg/dL, and albumin 3 g/dL. Liver enzymes are normal. The measured serum osmolality is 350 mOsm/kg.

   What is the most likely ingestion that caused this patient's presentation?

   A. Aspirin toxicity
   B. Ethylene glycol
   C. Isopropyl alcohol
   D. Methanol
   E. Propylene glycol

4. A 38-year-old man comes to the hospital after a fall. He is found to have an ankle fracture, which is managed conservatively. He admits to extensive alcohol use and reports he would like to quit. He develops symptoms of alcohol withdrawal 48 hours into the hospitalization and is treated with intravenous (IV) diazepam per the Clinical Institute Withdrawal Assessment for Alcohol (CIWA) scale; 36 hours later, he develops worsening confusion and respiratory failure. Medications at this time include high-dose IV diazepam drip, IV thiamine, multivitamin, and acetaminophen. BP is 160/80 mmHg and his pulse is 108/min. On examination, he is somnolent and responds only to pain. Labs show an Na of 145 mEq/L, K of 3.8 mEq/L, Cl of 101 mEq/L, and HCO_3 of 20 mEq/L. Serum osmolality is 390 mOsm/kg, glucose 130 mg/dL, creatinine 1.6 mg/dL, and lactate 5 mmol/L. ABG shows a pH of 7.30, $PaCO_2$ of 42 mmHg, and PaO_2 of 88 mmHg. Urinalysis is mildly positive for ketones. Ethanol level is 2 mg/dL.

What is the most likely cause of this patient's metabolic abnormalities?

A. Alcoholic ketoacidosis
B. Diazepam
C. Ethylene glycol
D. Infection
E. Isopropyl alcohol

5. An 82-year-old female is evaluated in the ED for encephalopathy. One month prior to admission, she sustained a fall and had a vertebral fracture that was managed conservatively with pain control with an acetaminophen-oxycodone preparation as well as "around the clock" acetaminophen. Because of pain and decreased mobility, her functional status as well as her nutritional status had worsened progressively. Her laboratory results on presentation to the ED showed an arterial pH of 7.30, a PCO_2 of 21 mmHg, and a HCO_3 of 10 mEq/L. Serum chemistry revealed a creatinine of 1.7 mg/dL, sodium of 145 mEq/L, potassium of 3.4 mEq/L, and chloride of 110 mEq/L. Albumin was 3.5 g/dL and lactic acid 0.6 mmol/L. Serum osmolarity was measured at 298 mOsm/kg and calculated at 295 mOsm/kg, with a glucose of 110 mg/dL and no urinary ketones.

What test would most likely reveal the diagnosis of this patient's metabolic acidosis?

A. Measurement of EtOH levels in the blood
B. Urinary free cortisol to urinary free cortisone ratio
C. Serum salicylate levels
D. Serum β-hydroxybutyrate
E. Urine 5-oxoproline

6. A 55-year-old woman presents with weakness after 3 days of abdominal pain, diarrhea, and poor PO intake. She ate at a restaurant and 8 hours later developed crampy abdominal pain followed by multiple episodes of watery nonbloody diarrhea. She presents with weakness and inability to stand. In the ED, she is afebrile with HR 108/min, BP 100/60 mmHg, and RR 22 breaths/min. She has dry mucous membranes and no lower extremity edema. Labs are notable for pH of 7.18 with a PCO_2 of 28 mmHg on an ABG with Na 130 mEq/L, Cl 108 mEq/L, HCO_3 12 mEq/L, K 3.0 mEq/L, and albumin 4.0 g/dL.

What is the most likely cause of this patient's acid-base disorder?

A. Diarrhea
B. Hyperventilation
C. Lactic acidosis
D. Starvation ketosis
E. Vomiting

7. A 48-year-old woman with recently diagnosed rheumatoid arthritis is referred to a nephrologist for a low bicarbonate level. On evaluation, she has no complaints. Labs reveal Na 138 mEq/L, K 3.2 mEq/L, Cl 118 mEq/L, HCO_3 8 mEq/L, and albumin 4 g/dL with a serum pH of 7.28 and a PCO_2 of 24 mmHg. Urine studies are notable for Na 40 mEq/L, K 20 mEq/L, and Cl 30 mEq/L with urinalysis notable for trace blood, no protein, and a pH of 6.0. You suspect that she has type 1 renal tubular acidosis associated with rheumatoid arthritis.

   What is the most likely complication if this condition is left untreated?

   A. Hyperkalemia
   B. Kidney stones
   C. Osteomalacia
   D. Sepsis
   E. Venous thromboembolism

8. A 69-year-old man presents to the hospital with difficulty breathing. He reports that he has had trouble "catching his breath," especially when he walks up the stairs. He was previously very active and regularly played tennis with friends, which he is no longer able to do. He has a recent history of bladder cancer and underwent a cystoprostatectomy and ileal neobladder creation 2 months ago. He reports that, recently, he has had to change his urine bag less frequently but does not report any abdominal pain or blood in the urine. He takes calcium, vitamin D, and docusate. On examination, his BP is 110/75 mmHg, pulse rate is 110/min, and RR is 24 breaths/min. His lungs are clear to auscultation. Chest radiograph (CXR) and electrocardiogram (ECG) are normal. Laboratory studies show an Na of 135 mEq/L, K of 3.7 mEq/L, Cl of 110 mEq/L, and HCO_3 of 14 mEq/L. ABG shows a pH of 7.28, PCO_2 of 30 mmHg, and PO_2 of 78 mmHg. Urinalysis shows 20 to 50 red blood cells (RBCs) and 20 to 50 white blood cells (WBCs) per high-power field (hpf).

   What is the cause of this patient's acid-base abnormalities?

   A. Neobladder dysfunction
   B. Pulmonary embolism
   C. Renal tubular acidosis
   D. Type B lactic acidosis
   E. Urinary tract infection (UTI)

9. A 32-year-old man presents to the ED with nausea and vomiting after eating sushi the night prior. Vitals include a pulse rate of 108/min, BP of 110/74 mmHg, and RR of 20 breaths/min. Examination is notable for dry mucous membranes and epigastric tenderness. Labs reveal Na 126 mEq/L, K 3.2 mEq/L, Cl 87 mEq/L, and HCO_3 20 mEq/L with albumin 2 g/dL. An ABG shows a pH of 7.38 and a PCO_2 of 36 mmHg.

   What is the cause of the patient's acid-base disturbance?

   A. High anion gap metabolic acidosis
   B. High anion gap metabolic acidosis, metabolic alkalosis with compensatory respiratory alkalosis
   C. Metabolic alkalosis and non–gap metabolic acidosis with compensatory respiratory acidosis
   D. No acid-base abnormality
   E. Non–gap metabolic acidosis

10. A 28-year-old woman presents to the ED with 3 days of emesis with inability to tolerate PO intake. She ate at a seafood restaurant 8 hours prior to symptom onset. Vitals are notable for HR 115/min, BP 92/52 mmHg, and RR 12 breaths/min. She is found to have dry

mucous membranes with no lower extremity edema. Labs are notable for pH 7.50, $PaCO_2$ 48 mmHg with Na 130 mEq/L, Cl 88 mEq/L, HCO_3 30 mEq/L, and K 2.8 mEq/L.

What is the best treatment for this patient?

A. Acetazolamide
B. Hemodialysis
C. Intubation for mechanical ventilation
D. IV normal saline
E. Observation

11. An ABG shows pH 7.15, PCO_2 20 mmHg, PO_2 80 mmHg, and HCO_3 12 mEq/L and a chemistry panel shows an anion gap of 16 mEq/L (normal 10-12 mEq/L).

What is the acid-base disturbance here?

A. Anion gap metabolic acidosis
B. Anion gap metabolic acidosis + non–gap metabolic acidosis
C. Anion gap metabolic acidosis + non–gap metabolic acidosis + respiratory alkalosis
D. Anion gap metabolic acidosis + respiratory alkalosis
E. Respiratory acidosis + metabolic alkalosis

12. A 34-year-old man presents to the ED after he was found to be confused by his friend at home. He is alert but disoriented and unable to answer questions. His friend relays that he was recently fired from his job and has been at home for the last week drinking 3 to 4 six-packs of beer per day. Vitals: he is afebrile, pulse 68/min, and BP 140/86 mmHg. Examination is notable for moist mucous membranes with normal capillary refill and skin turgor. Serum sodium is found to be 126 mEq/L with a glucose level of 120 mg/dL. Urine studies are sent. Urine osmolality is 75 mOsm/kg.

What is the next best step in management?

A. Administer loop diuretic
B. Restrict fluids
C. IV normal saline
D. Tolvaptan

13. A 76-year-old woman with a history of lung cancer presents to the ED with weakness 2 days following outpatient chemotherapy treatment. Vitals are notable for pulse 80/min, BP 110/70 mmHg, and RR 20 breaths/min. Labs are notable for Na 120 mEq/L. She receives 2 L of normal saline over 1 hour. She suffers a tonic-clonic seizure 30 minutes later. Repeat labs show Na 116 mEq/L.

What is the most likely etiology of this patient's hyponatremia?

A. Acute kidney injury (AKI)
B. Chemotherapy
C. Hypovolemia
D. Inappropriate antidiuretic hormone (ADH) release
E. Vomiting

14. A 72-year-old woman with hypothyroidism presents to the ED after her family found her confused in her apartment. She weighs 65 kg, is afebrile, with a pulse rate of 108/min, BP 122/74 mmHg, and RR 18 breaths/min. She does not require supplementary oxygen. She is complaining of nausea and headache but is arousable. In the ED, she has an episode of vomiting. Examination is notable for moist mucous membranes. Labs are notable for Na 118 mEq/L, BUN 18 mg/dL, and glucose 87 mg/dL with a serum osmolality of 250 mOsm/kg. UNa is 35 mEq/L and urine osmolality 450 mOsm/kg.

What is the next best step in management?

A. Bolus 2 L normal saline
B. Check thyroid-stimulating hormone (TSH) and free thyroxine (T4) levels
C. Give 3% hypertonic saline as a 100 mL bolus in 10 minutes, then recheck labs
D. Restrict free water and check labs in 4 hours
E. Start IV normal saline at 250 mL/h and recheck labs in 4 hours

15. A 37-year-old man with a history of alcohol use disorder and alcoholic hepatitis presented to the ED after he was found somnolent in the street by a friend. Physical examination reveals a HR of 102/min, BP of 100/60 mmHg. He is unable to provide further history. Laboratory results show a serum sodium of 120 mEq/L, potassium of 5.3 mEq/L, and creatinine of 1.1 mg/dL. His measured serum osmolality is 272 mOsm/kg. Urine sodium is <20 mEq/L, urine osmolarity is 400 mOsm/kg, and urine creatinine is 100 mg/dL. You suspect that his neurologic symptoms are related to hyponatremia and decide to aim for an increase of 6 mEq of sodium in the first 24 hours with IV sodium replacement.

Which of the following is NOT a risk factor for the development of osmotic demyelination syndrome (ODS) in patients with chronic hyponatremia?

A. Alcohol use
B. Hyperkalemia
C. Malnutrition
D. Liver disease
E. Rapid correction of hyponatremia

16. A 76-year-old woman with a history of Alzheimer disease and amyloidosis presents to the ED accompanied by her family, who noticed that she has been more confused and lethargic in the last few weeks. She is incontinent at baseline and the family does not think she has had any change in her urine output. Vitals are notable for HR 98/min, BP 118/76 mmHg, and RR 18 breaths/min. On examination, she is somnolent but easily arousable, with dry mucous membranes. Serum sodium is 156 mEq/L with glucose 140 mg/dL. Urine osmolality is found to be 225 mOsm/kg with a serum osmolality of 335 mOsm/kg. A Foley catheter is placed, and an IV of normal saline is started. Over the next 12 hours, she voids 1.5 L and repeat serum Na is 154 mEq/L and urine osmolality is 255 mOsm/kg. Desmopressin (DDAVP) is administered, and urine osmolality increases from 285 to 310 mOsm/kg.

What is the most likely diagnosis?

A. Central diabetes insipidus
B. Gastrointestinal (GI) free water loss
C. Lack of access to free water
D. Nephrogenic diabetes insipidus
E. Osmotic diuresis

17. A 26-year-old pregnant woman is admitted at 32 weeks of gestation with suspected pre-eclampsia. She reports increased thirst and urinary frequency in the last few weeks. She has a history of bipolar disorder, which was managed with lithium in the past. Her BP is 155/80 mmHg, and her physical examination is unremarkable. Her blood counts and liver function tests are normal. She is treated with bed rest, IV magnesium, and labetalol. When her polyuria persists despite fluid restriction, a DDAVP challenge is administered.

	Baseline	6 hours of fluid restriction	2 hours after DDAVP challenge
Sodium	138 mEq/L	143 mEq/L	141 mEq/L
Serum osmolality	287 mOsm/kg	295 mOsm/kg	290 mOsm/kg
Urine osmolality	90 mOsm/kg	95 mOsm/kg	310 mOsm/kg
Urine volume	8 L/24 h	3 L/6 h	300 mL/2 h

What is the cause of her polyuria?

A. Central diabetes insipidus
B. Gestational diabetes insipidus
C. Nephrogenic diabetes insipidus
D. Preeclampsia
E. Primary polydipsia

18. A 38-year-old man presents to the ED with palpitations and diarrhea. The evening prior, he participated in an eating contest and ate a large quantity of black licorice, after which he has felt ill and has developed diarrhea. Vitals are notable for a pulse rate of 90 to 95/min (frequent premature ventricular contractions), BP 172/102 mmHg, and RR 22 breaths/min. Examination is notable for an anxious man without distress; mucous membranes are moist; and abdomen is mildly tender. Labs are notable for Na 142 mEq/L, Cl 102 mEq/L, HCO_3 18 mEq/L, K 2.8 mEq/L, WBC 9000/μL, urine Na 10 mg/dL, K 40 mg/dL, Cl 60 mg/dL, and Cr 2 mg/dL.

What is the most likely etiology for this patient's hypokalemia?

A. Diarrhea
B. Licorice ingestion
C. Renal tubular acidosis
D. Thiazide
E. Vomiting

19. A 70-year-old woman is admitted to the intensive care unit (ICU) after an out-of-hospital cardiac arrest. She undergoes coronary revascularization and is then started on a therapeutic hypothermia protocol. Her temperature is 32.5°C after 12 hours. She is intubated, sedated, and receiving vasopressin and norepinephrine infusions. The resident on call notices that the patient's potassium has fallen from 3.9 mEq/L at admission to 2.8 mEq/L. The urine output recorded over the last 24 hours is about 3.5 L and the serum creatinine is normal. Stool output is 200 mL.

What is the cause of this patient's hypokalemia?

A. Cardiac revascularization
B. Diarrhea
C. Hypoaldosteronism (type IV) renal tubular acidosis
D. Hypothermia
E. Mechanical ventilation

20. A 72-year-old man with a history of chronic lymphocytic leukemia presents to his oncologist for follow-up. He has been doing well and has no complaints. Labs show Na 132 mEq/L, K 8.2 mEq/L, HCO_3 26 mEq/L, BUN 28 mg/dL, Cr 1.2 mg/dL, glucose 220 mg/dL, and WBC 372/μL. ECG shows normal sinus rhythm and no peaked T waves. Ca gluconate, insulin, and dextrose are administered. Repeat potassium is 8.5 mEq/L and repeat ECG shows no changes.

What is the most likely etiology of this patient's hyperkalemia?

A. Hyperglycemia
B. Hyporeninemic hypoaldosteronism
C. Pseudohyperkalemia
D. Renal failure
E. Tumor lysis syndrome

21. A 52-year-old man with a history of diabetes, hypertension, chronic kidney disease (CKD; baseline Cr 1.5), and chronic obstructive pulmonary disease (COPD) is admitted to the hospital with a COPD exacerbation. He is on day 3 of his hospitalization and is being treated for COPD with short-acting bronchodilators and oral prednisone. Today, his labs are notable for pH 7.32 with Na 130 mEq/L, K 5.5 mEq/L, HCO_3 28 mEq/L, BUN 30 mg/dL, Cr 1.7 mg/dL, and glucose 450 mg/dL.

    What is the most likely cause of this patient's hyperkalemia?

    A. Acidemia
    B. AKI
    C. Excessive dietary intake
    D. Hyperglycemia
    E. Medications

22. A 68-year-old man with hypertension, diabetes, and end-stage renal disease (ESRD) on hemodialysis on the surgical service is post-op day 2 from a small bowel resection after presenting to the ED with a small bowel obstruction. The patient is anuric at baseline. Vitals are notable for a HR of 86/min and BP 150/80 mmHg. On examination, mucous membranes are moist, jugular venous pressure (JVP) is 8 cm, and abdomen is mildly tender with a well-healing vertical midline incision. He has a right brachiocephalic fistula with a palpable thrill. Labs are notable for Na 134 mEq/L, K 5.8 mEq/L, and BUN 50 mg/dL. ECG is reviewed, which shows a normal sinus rhythm with stable T-wave inversions in V_4 to V_6. The patient is scheduled to have dialysis in 2 days, so you decide to give 10 U regular insulin IV with two amps of D50W and would like to give sodium polystyrene sulfonate (SPS) (Kayexalate).

    What is a contraindication to SPS administration?

    A. COPD
    B. Hyperglycemia
    C. Hyponatremia
    D. Recent bowel surgery
    E. Sepsis

23. A 60-year-old man with a history of coronary artery disease (CAD) s/p coronary artery bypass grafting (CABG) is found down at home by his family members. Emergency Medical Services (EMS) is called; when they arrive, he is found pulseless and cardiopulmonary resuscitation (CPR) is initiated, achieving return of spontaneous circulation. He receives fluid resuscitation in the ED with 4 L of isotonic fluid and is admitted to the ICU. After 12 hours in the ICU, his hemodynamics have improved but he now has evidence of pulmonary edema in the CXR and progressive difficulty with the ventilator. He remains anuric despite a dose of furosemide 120 mg IV. Laboratory results are notable for a creatinine of 1.4 mg/dL, bicarbonate of 14 mEq/L, and potassium of 6.9 mEq/L with a widened QRS relative to his baseline.

30. A 55-year-old woman with a history of hypertension, diabetes mellitus, and CKD stage 4 is admitted with chest pain. Initial ECG was negative for ST abnormalities, but subsequent ECGs a few hours later showed ischemic ST segment changes. A myocardial infarction is suspected, and a cardiac catheterization is planned. Medications include lisinopril, torsemide, aspirin, carvedilol, and insulin. BP is 110/66 mmHg and pulse is 60/min. There is no peripheral edema, and the lungs are clear to auscultation.

What is the best intervention to reduce the risk of contrast-associated AKI in this patient?

A. Hemodialysis immediately after the procedure
B. IV N-acetylcysteine
C. IV normal saline
D. Oral fluids

31. A 63-year-old man with hypertension, diabetes mellitus, and end-stage kidney disease on hemodialysis three times a week is admitted from the dialysis unit with shortness of breath and chest discomfort. He presented to the dialysis unit with these symptoms and was immediately sent to the ED without the initiation of dialysis. He denies fever, chills, cough, or dizziness. BP is 160/70 mmHg, pulse is 110/min, and weight is 73 kg. He is 1 kg above his dry weight. Physical examination shows clear lungs and a normal JVP. On admission, his high-sensitivity troponin T level is 135 ng/L and his second troponin T level, a few hours later, was 405 ng/L (reference <9 ng/L). CXR shows clear lung fields. ECG shows signs of left ventricular hypertrophy (LVH) and new, nonspecific ST segment abnormalities.

What is the most appropriate next step in management?

A. Aspirin, nitrates, and cardiology consult for cardiac catheterization
B. CT pulmonary embolism study
C. Observation
D. Repeat troponin levels a few hours later
E. Urgent hemodialysis and ultrafiltration

32. A 68-year-old man with a history of heart failure with reduced EF (last known LV EF 40%) is admitted to the hospital for a weight gain of 15 kg despite increasing doses of home diuretics. He is warm and well perfused on examination with 2+ bilateral lower extremity pitting edema as well as bilateral crackles in the lung bases. A transthoracic echocardiogram shows similar findings to his prior study with an LV EF of 40% and biatrial dilation. Cr is only slightly above his baseline at 1.4 (baseline 1.1). He is started on a furosemide infusion at 10 mg/h. Urine output only increases a small amount and after 1 day on the infusion he has only lost 0.2 kg.

What is the best next step in management?

A. Switch to bumetanide
B. Start dobutamine
C. Start milrinone
D. Start metolazone
E. Start renal replacement therapy

33. A 65-year-old man is admitted with decompensated congestive heart failure after failing outpatient diuresis. He reports a gain of 25 lb over the last 3 to 4 weeks and dyspnea at rest. He has been on torsemide 60 mg twice a day during that period. A furosemide bolus of 100 mg IV is administered, and he is started on an infusion at 10 mg/h. He responds well and loses 10 lb in the first 5 days but continues to require supplemental oxygen (2 L/min nasal cannula), has dyspnea on walking, and has bilateral crackles. On day 6, his HCO_3 on the chemistry panel is noticed to be 45 mEq/L and an ABG drawn shows pH of 7.51 and $PaCO_2$ of 52 mmHg. In a team meeting, it is decided that IV diuresis needs to be continued.

What is the most appropriate treatment?

A. Add acetazolamide
B. Add amiloride
C. Add spironolactone
D. Infuse normal saline
E. Insist that the furosemide be stopped

34. A 60-year-old woman with hypertension presents to the clinic with persistently high home BP readings. She is currently on lisinopril 40 mg daily, amlodipine 10 mg daily, and chlorthalidone 12.5 mg daily. She follows a strict salt-restricted diet, exercises every day, and does not drink alcohol or smoke tobacco. Her home BP measurements are in the 150-165/85-95 mmHg range. Her comorbidities include CAD and well-controlled diabetes mellitus. Her lab work shows an estimated glomerular filtration rate (eGFR) of 40 mL/min/1.73 m^2 and a potassium of 4.9 mEq/L.

What is the next best step in management?

A. Add carvedilol
B. Add spironolactone
C. Change chlorthalidone to furosemide 40 mg daily
D. Increase chlorthalidone to 25 mg daily
E. Increase lisinopril to 60 mg daily

35. A 33-year-old gravida 2 para 1 with a history of preeclampsia in her previous pregnancy and is currently 33 weeks pregnant is admitted with a BP of 170/95 mmHg. She has no symptoms.

Which of the following medications should be avoided in this patient?

A. Hydralazine
B. Labetalol
C. Lisinopril
D. Methyldopa
E. Nifedipine

36. A 60-year-old woman is just admitted to the medical ICU with septic shock secondary to a foot infection that was left untreated. She is on 6 µg/kg/min norepinephrine and 0.04 U/min vasopressin, and her lactate is 3 mmol/L. She is intubated and initiated on mechanical ventilation. An ABG reveals a pH of 7.29 and a PO_2 of 104 mmHg on 30% FiO_2 and a positive end-expiratory pressure (PEEP) of 5 mmHg. A CXR reveals mild pulmonary edema. Her BUN and Cr are 63 mg/dL and 4.2 mg/dL, respectively. Her urine output is 25 mL/h.

What is the next best step in management?

A. Give IV sodium bicarbonate
B. Monitor closely with IV furosemide as needed
C. Start continuous renal replacement therapy
D. Start intermittent hemodialysis

37. A 59-year-old woman with type 2 diabetes mellitus comes to the hospital with complaints of cough, congestion, and fever for the last 2 weeks. Her BP is 85/50 mmHg and a CXR showed right lower lobe pneumonia. Her admission creatinine was 11 mg/dL (baseline

2.6 mg/dL), and her potassium was 6.5 mEq/L. Nonspecific ST segment abnormalities are seen on her ECG. A Foley catheter is inserted with no return of urine. She is started on IV antibiotics and IV fluids. One hour later, she continues to have no urine output and her potassium rises to 7 mEq/L. She is started on emergent hemodialysis. Over the next week, she received three dialysis sessions and her infection has resolved. Her urine output has progressively increased, and she now makes around 2.1 L of urine a day. Her BUN is 65 mg/dL, creatinine is 4.1 mg/dL, and potassium is 4.3 mEq/L. Her last dialysis session was 48 hours ago. Her postdialysis BUN was 55 mg/dL and her creatinine was 3.3 mg/dL.

What is the next best step in management?

A.   Dialysis today
B.   Dialysis until serum creatinine is <2 mg/dL
C.   IV furosemide to augment urine output
D.   Observation only

38. A 32-year-old woman is admitted to the ICU for distributive shock and hypoxemic respiratory failure. She is intubated and her BP requires the support of three vasopressors to maintain mean arterial pressure (MAP) >65. She is also being treated with vancomycin, cefepime, and metronidazole for sepsis of unknown origin. Her obligate intake from infusions, tube feeds, and antibiotics totals about 3.5 L/day. On hospital day 2 her creatinine begins to rise, and her urine output abruptly decreases to 25 cc/h despite maximum dose of loop diuretics and augmentation with a thiazide diuretic. Other labs are currently unremarkable including a K of 4.1 mEq/L, BUN of 35 mg/dL, phosphate of 3.5 mEq/L, and Na of 136 mEq/L. On hospital day 3, her oxygen requirement and PEEP increase to 90% and 15 cm H_2O, respectively.

What is the next best step in management?

A.   Continue current management
B.   Add spironolactone
C.   Start intermittent hemodialysis
D.   Start continuous renal replacement such as continuous veno-venous hemofiltration (CVVH)
E.   Stop tube feeds

39. A 45-year-old woman with ESRD on three times weekly hemodialysis is admitted to the hospital with cellulitis. While she is admitted, the team notices that she has a left brachiocephalic fistula with a good thrill and bruit but has been receiving dialysis through a central venous catheter. The patient reports that the fistula was placed 3 months ago. The fistula is examined, is deemed to have matured well, and is used for hemodialysis that day with full blood flow rates (400 mL/min). Immediately on return to the inpatient unit, the patient complains of numbness and severe pain in her left hand. The radial pulse is nonpalpable and the fingers are cold to the touch. Her vital signs are stable.

What is the next best step in management?

A.   Elevate the arm
B.   Observe
C.   Perform surgical evaluation
D.   Prescribe high-dose gabapentin
E.   Reduce blood flow rates during next dialysis session

40. A 73-year-old woman with ESRD complicated by severe calciphylaxis, type 2 diabetes mellitus, and prior stroke is brought to the ED for worsening pain of her wounds. In the ED

she is incidentally found to be in atrial fibrillation. Vitals are HR 89/min, BP 125/79 mmHg, RR 18 breaths/min, and O_2 sat 96% on room air. She is admitted for IV pain medication and for management of atrial fibrillation.

What mediation should be AVOIDED in this patient?

A. Metoprolol
B. Apixaban
C. Amiodarone
D. Heparin
E. Warfarin

41. A 62-year-old man with CKD stage 5 is admitted to the surgical unit of the hospital with severe acute-on-chronic leg ischemia. He has been feeling more fatigued and has had poor appetite for the past 6 months because of nausea. A leg angiogram revealed severe calcification bilaterally of the iliac arteries. Laboratory results showed a sodium of 131 mEq/L, potassium of 5.7 mEq/L, creatinine of 4 mg/dL, calcium of 9.1 mg/dL (corrected for albumin), phosphorus of 9 mg/dL, and parathyroid hormone (PTH) 400 pg/mL.

Which of the following would be recommended first to address this patient's mineral bone disease (MBD)?

A. Noncalcium phosphate binders
B. Calcitriol
C. Cinacalcet
D. Low-calcium diet

42. A 72-year-old Hispanic man who recently immigrated to the United States from Colombia is seen at the outpatient primary care clinic 4 weeks after a recent hospital admission for pneumonia. At admission, his creatinine was found to be elevated (6 mg/dL). With fluids and supportive care, his creatinine trended down quickly to 3.1 mEq/L within 48 hours of admission and stayed at that level at hospital discharge. A repeat renal panel shows a creatinine of 3.2 mEq/L, which equates to an eGFR of 18 mL/min/1.73 m². His blood group type is A, and his body mass index (BMI) is 31 kg/m². He reveals that he has had difficulty controlling his diabetes for 35 years and is on insulin. He was told he had diabetic kidney disease years ago and reports hypertension, for which he is on amlodipine. He then shows you a stack of papers from his home country, which indicate that he had surgery for a <1 cm basal cell carcinoma of the skin (forearm) 2 years ago. He has a supportive family and plays golf on the weekends. He wants to avoid dialysis as much as possible and asks you about the possibility of being listed for a deceased donor kidney transplant.

What should you tell him?

A. He does not qualify for a kidney transplant because of his age
B. He does not qualify for a kidney transplant because of his history of cancer
C. He should explore the option of a living donor because the wait time will be shorter
D. He should be evaluated and listed for a kidney transplant now
E. He will qualify for a kidney transplant once he is on dialysis

43. A 50-year-old woman with alcoholic cirrhosis is admitted with worsening abdominal pain because of progressive ascites and altered mental status. She just achieved 6-month sobriety and was listed for a liver transplant 12 days ago. Examination shows a tense and distended abdomen, and her BP is 95/56 mmHg. Her mental status improves with lactulose. Her serum creatinine on admission is 4.2 mg/dL from a baseline of 1.5 mg/dL

and her serum albumin is 2.6 m/dL. Her MELD (Model for End-Stage Liver Disease) score is 28. Her urine sediment is bland, and her fractional excretion of sodium is <1%. Despite resuscitation with IV fluids and albumin and treatment with midodrine and octreotide, her creatinine worsens over the next 72 hours to 6.2 mg/dL and her mental status worsens again. A discussion regarding the initiation of dialysis is held with her and her family.

What is her most favorable prognostic factor if she were to be initiated on dialysis?

A. Age
B. Etiology of AKI
C. Listed for liver transplant
D. MELD score

44. A 65-year-old man with stage 5 CKD (eGFR of 12 mL/min) presents at clinic for his usual monthly appointment. In your last appointment, you discussed with him the possibility of home renal replacement modalities including home hemodialysis and peritoneal dialysis. He was listed for transplant about 6 months ago, but he is becoming more edematous despite increased doses of loop diuretics. He has good health literacy and good support at home and is considering peritoneal dialysis but is worried about the sustainability of peritoneal dialysis as he gets older. His primary goal is to live as long as possible, so he is willing to go to in-center dialysis if there is a chance that it would improve his survival.

Which of the following statements is true?

A. Home hemodialysis is associated with similar survival compared with conventional in-center hemodialysis
B. Peritoneal dialysis is associated with poorer cognitive functions compared with hemodialysis
C. Quality of life in transplant recipients is similar in patients on dialysis
D. Survival on peritoneal dialysis and survival on home hemodialysis are comparable

45. A 35-year-old African American woman diagnosed with systemic lupus erythematosus at age 30 is seen by her primary care physician (PCP) during a routine visit. She has no complaints, except for a malar rash. She has no other signs of systemic lupus, and her BP is 145/92 mmHg. She is on oral contraceptive pills. A spot urine sample from a week ago showed 800 mg/g of proteinuria, which is increased from the last check 1 year ago. There is no hematuria on the urinalysis and her renal panel is normal with a creatinine of 0.7 mg/dL. Her complement levels are mildly low.

What is the next best step in management?

A. Initiate immunosuppression with steroids and mycophenolate mofetil
B. Obtain a 24-hour protein/creatinine ratio
C. Refer her for kidney biopsy
D. Repeat urine/protein creatinine ratio in a month
E. Start her on lisinopril

46. A 27-year-old Asian man presents to the outpatient clinic after experiencing recurrent episodes of gross hematuria. He reports one such recent episode this past winter after he had "flu-like" symptoms. He is not on any medications. His BP is 135/90 mmHg. A urinalysis shows hematuria, and he is found to have a urine microalbumin/creatinine ratio of 0.6 g/g. His serum creatinine is 0.9 mg/dL. Renal ultrasound is normal. A renal biopsy reveals findings consistent with immunoglobulin A (IgA) nephropathy.

With which of the following should he be treated?

A. Cyclophosphamide
B. Fish oil
C. Lisinopril
D. Prednisone

47. A 44-year-old Caucasian male with relapsed chronic myeloid leukemia is in clinical remission after an allogenic hematopoietic stem cell transplantation 15 months ago. His cyclosporine was tapered and discontinued 3 months before admission. He now presents with a rash on his face and forearms for 2 weeks along with lower extremity swelling. He is found to have nephrotic syndrome with 7.2 g of proteinuria and a serum albumin of 2.3 mg/dL. His creatinine was elevated at 1.4 mg/dL from 0.9 mg/dL a month ago. Hepatitis and human immunodeficiency virus (HIV) serologies were negative. Serum and urine electrophoresis, C3, C4, antinuclear antibody (ANA), and ANCA levels were normal. His hemoglobin is 13 g/dL, WBC count is 8000/μL, and platelet count is 176 500/μL.

What is the most likely diagnosis?

A. ANCA vasculitis
B. Focal segmental glomerulosclerosis
C. Membranous nephropathy
D. Minimal change disease
E. Thrombotic microangiopathy

48. A 65-year-old male with a history of hypertension is evaluated in the clinic for proteinuria. Five years before presentation, he was diagnosed with stage 3 CKD with moderately increased urine albumin (200 mg/g). He was managed with an angiotensin-converting enzyme (ACE) inhibitor and BP control. Two months before evaluation he developed new-onset bilateral leg edema and was noted to have a subacute worsening of renal function with increase in creatinine from 1.2 to 1.5 mg/dL (eGFR of 43 mL/min/1.73 m²) and worsening proteinuria to 700 mg/day. A renal biopsy revealed IgA nephropathy with secondary focal segmental glomerulosclerosis and about 70% interstitial fibrosis.

What is the next best step in management?

A. Corticosteroids
B. Mycophenolate
C. Sodium-glucose cotransporter 2 (SGLT-2) inhibitors
D. Angiotensin receptor blocker (ARB)

49. A 53-year-old woman presented with hematuria, nephrotic-range proteinuria (3.7 g/d), and elevated creatinine (1.9 g/dL). A kidney biopsy revealed monoclonal deposition disease with proliferative glomerulonephritis.

What is (are) the best test(s) to detect the monoclonal protein in the circulation?

A. Serum protein electrophoresis (SPEP) and urine protein electrophoresis
B. SPEP, serum immunofixation, and serum free light chain assay
C. Urine protein electrophoresis, urine immunofixation, and urine free light chain assay
D. Urine free light chain assay

50. A 38-year-old woman is admitted with abdominal pain and fevers for the past week. Her chemistry panel shows a serum creatinine of 4.1 mg/dL (1.0 mg/dL 1 month ago), and her urine sediment shows dysmorphic red cells. Serologies are sent and are pending. A kidney biopsy is done, and crescentic glomerulonephritis is seen on light microscopy.

What is the LEAST likely diagnosis in this patient?

A. ANCA vasculitis
B. Anti–glomerular basement membrane disease
C. Hemolytic uremic syndrome
D. IgA nephropathy
E. Lupus nephritis

51. A 45-year-old woman with hepatitis C presents to the ED with malaise, joint pain, and change in the color of her urine. She has been lost to GI follow-up and has not been treated for hepatitis C. Over the past week, she has developed worsening joint pain and swelling around her ankles. Vitals are notable for a BP of 164/98 mmHg. Examination is notable for moist mucous membranes, bibasilar crackles, no ascites, 1+ ankle edema, and purpura along her extremities. Labs are notable for a Cr of 2.4 mg/dL (baseline 1.2 mg/dL), decreased C3 and C4. A Foley catheter is placed, yielding 300 mL of tea-colored urine. A urinalysis shows 2+ blood and 1+ protein. A representative image from her urine sediment is displayed.

What is the most likely diagnosis?

A. Cryoglobulinemic glomerulonephritis
B. Henoch-Schönlein purpura
C. Hepatorenal syndrome
D. Postrenal AKI
E. Prerenal AKI

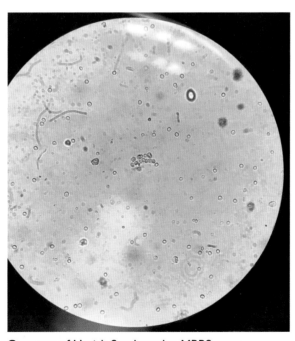

Courtesy of Harish Seethapathy, MBBS.

52. A 57-year-old man presents to an urgent care clinic because of a change in the color of his urine for a week. He describes his urine as looking "tea colored." He denies any recent trauma, kidney stones, or Foley catheter insertion. The patient has a history of diabetes and chronic back pain using ibuprofen as needed. Vitals are normal and physical examination is unremarkable. A serum chemistry panel shows normal creatinine.

What is the most appropriate next step in management?

A. CT urography
B. Observation
C. Renal ultrasound
D. Urinalysis + sediment
E. Urology referral

53. A 63-year-old man with a history of rheumatoid arthritis for 20 years, hypertension, heart failure with preserved EF, atrial fibrillation, alcohol use disorder, and benign prostatic hyperplasia is seen in nephrology clinic after being referred by his PCP for 3+ protein on routine urinalysis last month. He denies any worsening shortness of breath and endorses lower extremity edema, for which he takes furosemide daily. Other than 3+ proteinuria on his urinalysis, he had no other lab abnormalities. His serum creatinine is at his baseline of 1.2 mg/dL, and his BP taken in nephrology clinic was 145/85 mmHg.

What is the most likely diagnosis?

A. AA amyloidosis
B. Cardiorenal syndrome
C. Multiple myeloma cast nephropathy
D. Thrombotic microangiopathy
E. Urinary tract obstruction

54. A 58-year-old man with known IgG κ light chain multiple myeloma is sent to the ED from clinic after he is found to have a newly elevated Cr of 3.5 mg/dL from his baseline of 1.3 mg/dL. Urinalysis is bland, but a urine protein/creatinine is elevated at 5.6 g/g, and a urine albumin/creatinine is 0.8 g/g. He is started on IV fluids to maintain an hourly urine output of >100 cc/h.

What is the most likely etiology of his proteinuria?

A. Glomerular proteinuria
B. Tubulointerstitial proteinuria
C. Overflow proteinuria
D. Isolated proteinuria

55. A 45-year-old man is seen in nephrology clinic for recurrent kidney stones. His first kidney stone occurred in his 20s and he passed it without requiring further intervention. Since then, he has had two other kidney stones, both of which resolved and passed with conservative measures only. He has never had stone analysis done and has never had a 24-hour urine collection analysis.

Which of the following is appropriate information to share with this patient?

A. Knowing the composition of the stone or having urine chemistry analysis is not important in the management of nephrolithiasis
B. Dietary modification is unlikely to prevent another kidney stone
C. Most kidney stones <0.5 cm in diameter will pass spontaneously
D. Most patients who pass a kidney stone will never experience another one in their lifetime
E. Potassium citrate will prevent new uric acid and calcium phosphate stone formation

56. A 47-year-old man with Crohn disease is admitted to the hospital with severe diarrhea for the last 3 days. He reports that he has a history of chronic diarrhea and has intermittent bouts of severe diarrhea. He also has a history of diet-controlled diabetes mellitus, with his

last hemoglobin A_{1c} (HbA_{1c}) being 6.6%, and a history of hypertension, for which he takes 5 mg of amlodipine. He reports passing a kidney stone 3 years ago. His creatinine on admission was 4.5 mg/dL, which decreased to 3.8 mg/dL after fluid resuscitation. You notice that his creatinine was 0.5 mg/dL 5 years ago and 1.3 mg/dL 8 months ago when he was seen by his PCP. His urine protein:creatinine ratio is 0.2 g/dL. His renal ultrasound is normal.

What is the most likely etiology of his CKD?

A. Diabetic nephropathy
B. Hypertensive nephropathy
C. Oxalate nephropathy
D. Recurrent AKI

57. A 68-year-old man with a history of hypertension and end-stage liver disease is evaluated in the clinic for nephrolithiasis. He received a successful liver transplant 8 months prior to evaluation. Current medications include low-dose aspirin, labetalol, and cyclosporine. A noncontrast CT scan shows bilateral renal stones. Laboratory results are notable for a creatinine of 1.9 mg/dL. A 24-hour urine collection shows 1700 mg of urine creatinine (normal for weight), a urine volume of 1 L, calcium/creatinine excretion of 35 (normal range 34-196), and urine pH of 5.4. Urine sediment reveals rhomboid crystals with polychromatic birefringence under polarized light.

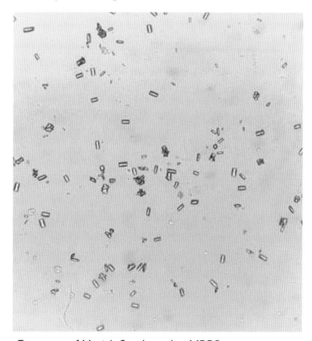

Courtesy of Harish Seethapathy, MBBS.

Which of the following would NOT be a recommendation to prevent further renal stones in this patient?

A. Increase fluid intake
B. Decrease calcium intake
C. Alkalinize urine
D. Consider switching his immunosuppressive medication

58. A 45-year-old woman is admitted with flank pain and hematuria. On imaging, she was found to have three kidney stones, one of which was obstructing the ureter. One day after admission, she passed the stone and her pain and hematuria resolved. Her serum creatinine has been between 1.3 and 1.6 mg/dL over the last few months. Her serum calcium is 9 mg/dL (normal 8.5-10 mg/dL), and her vitamin D level is 53 ng/mL (normal 30-60 ng/mL). She reports childhood asthma but no other medical conditions. She works a desk job and keeps herself well hydrated. She extensively researches health issues online and takes medications that she feels improve her health, including cholecalciferol 500 units daily; multivitamins, including vitamin B complex and vitamin C (2 g daily); aspirin 81 mg daily; and fish oil 1000 mg daily.

Which of the following is most likely contributing to kidney disease and formation of kidney stones in this patient?

A. Fish oil
B. Vitamin B
C. Vitamin C
D. Vitamin D

ANSWERS

1. **The correct answer is: B. Diabetic ketoacidosis.** This patient most likely has diabetic ketoacidosis with an anion gap metabolic acidosis, along with hyperglycemia, glucosuria, and ketonuria. Initially in the acute phase of diabetic ketoacidosis, while ketoacids build up, an anion gap metabolic acidosis becomes apparent; however, in patients with normal renal function, diabetic ketoacidosis can also cause normal gap metabolic acidosis later on when the ketoacids (which can potentially be converted to bicarbonate in the liver) are excreted in the urine, thereby causing loss of bicarbonate. Renal tubular acidosis because of topiramate usually causes a mild proximal renal tubular acidosis along with hypokalemia. Ethanol intoxication can lead to ketoacidosis because of starvation but hypoglycemia is usually present along with it. Mild lactate elevation, as seen in this patient, does not cause this degree of acidosis. Moreover, the overall picture fits diabetic ketoacidosis much better.

2. **The correct answer is: D. Thiamine deficiency.** This patient presents with a pH of 7.20 with a high anion gap metabolic acidosis, most likely because of type B lactic acidosis in the setting of thiamine deficiency. This patient has a metabolic acidosis given a pH <7.40 with an anion gap of 22 (125 − 90 − 15 + 2) with albumin of 3 g/dL. The change in anion gap over change in bicarbonate (ie, delta/delta) is 1:1, so there is no metabolic alkalosis (vomiting unlikely etiology). As this patient's lactic acidosis did not improve with 2 L of hypotonic IV fluid resuscitation and he is afebrile with a normal BP, type A lactic acidosis because of ischemia is unlikely (eg, hypovolemia, septic shock, hypoxemia). As such, type B (nonhypoxic) lactic acidosis is more likely. Etiologies of type B lactic acidosis include thiamine deficiency, seizures, metformin, propofol, niacin, and glycol intoxications. Thiamine is an essential cofactor for pyruvate dehydrogenase, which converts pyruvate to acetyl-CoA, which enters the Krebs cycle (aerobic metabolism). In thiamine deficiency, pyruvate is instead converted to lactate. Patients with alcohol use disorder are at risk for thiamine deficiency, which can be treated with IV thiamine.

3. **The correct answer is: D. Methanol.** This patient presents with altered mental status and blurry vision with an elevated anion and osmolar gap, which is most likely because of methanol (also known as wood alcohol) ingestion. He has vision changes with an anion gap of 20.5 (18 uncorrected for albumin) and an osmolar gap of 23. An elevated anion gap and osmolar gap is seen with methanol, ethylene glycol, propylene glycol, and diethylene glycol ingestion; however, blurry vision, pupillary dilation, and papilledema are seen specifically with methanol ingestion at doses as low as 10 mL. In terms of the other choices, isopropyl alcohol usually presents with normal anion gap and increased osmolar gap and typically causes pancreatitis. Aspirin toxicity is associated with fever, tinnitus, respiratory alkalosis (early), and metabolic acidosis (late) and does not increase the osmolar gap. Ethylene glycol causes heart failure with hypocalcemia, AKI, and calcium oxalate crystal formation. This patient had a normal BP, normal calcium (8.2 g/dL when corrected for albumin), and normal Cr. Propylene glycol can cause AKI and lactic acidosis, which are not noted here.

4. **The correct answer is: B. Diazepam.** This patient most likely has propylene glycol toxicity because of high doses of diazepam administration. He has an increased anion gap metabolic acidosis and an increased osmolar gap. Propylene glycol is the solvent used to administer IV diazepam, lorazepam, as well as phenobarbital. It can be toxic in high doses, leading to increased lactate levels and AKI. Treatment involves discontinuing the offending agent and dialysis in severe cases. Ethylene glycol can cause a similar picture with anion gap

acidosis and an increased osmolar gap. It is usually found in antifreeze solutions and causes profound acidosis and acute tubular necrosis (ATN) with calcium oxalate crystal formation in the urine. These manifestations are usually found at admission and not during hospitalization. Isopropyl alcohol can lead to an increased osmolar gap but not an anion gap acidosis.

5. **The correct answer is: E. Urine 5-oxoproline.** The etiology of anion gap metabolic acidosis can usually be found by using the mnemonic GOLD MARK. This acronym represents Glycols (ethylene and propylene), Oxoproline, L-lactate, D-lactate, Methanol, Aspirin, Renal failure, and Ketoacidosis. This patient had no osmolar gap, which argues against alcohol ingestion, and no lactic acidosis or ketones. Her history is notable for chronic use of acetaminophen and decreased food intake. Metabolic acidosis that is caused by 5-oxoproline results from disruption of the γ-glutamyl cycle. Hepatic glutathione stores are depleted in patients with acetaminophen toxicity, especially in malnourished and often female patients. Reduced glutathione levels increase the γ-glutamylcysteine synthetase activity, and γ-glutamylcysteine can be partially converted to 5-oxoproline. Medications that have been associated with increased 5-oxoproline generation (and hence higher levels detected in the urine) include acetaminophen, vigabatrin, and the antibiotics flucloxacillin and netilmicin.

6. **The correct answer is: A. Diarrhea.** This patient presents with a pH of 7.18 with a normal anion gap of 10, consistent with a non–gap metabolic acidosis in the setting of severe diarrhea. GI fluid above the ligament of Treitz (eg, stomach) is rich in acid, whereas GI fluid below the ligament of Treitz (small and large bowel) is rich in bicarbonate. As such, large-volume emesis causes a chloride depletion alkalosis because of loss of volume, chloride, and potassium, whereas diarrhea often causes a nongap acidosis because of loss of bicarbonate-rich fluid. Although severe hypovolemia can cause lactic acidosis and severe anorexia can cause starvation ketosis, this patient has a normal anion gap, so these choices are incorrect.

7. **The correct answer is: B. Kidney stones.** This patient's labs are suggestive of a distal (type I) renal tubular acidosis, which is likely acquired from her rheumatoid arthritis. She has a non–gap metabolic acidosis with appropriate respiratory compensation. The positive urine anion gap ($Na + K - Cl$) suggests ineffective secretion of NH_4^+ cations because one would expect a negative urine anion gap as NH_4^+ is secreted with Cl in a state of acidosis. Distal renal tubular acidosis is due to ineffective secretion of NH_4^+, resulting in an inappropriately higher urine pH >5.3 that distinguishes it from proximal renal tubular acidosis. Distal renal tubular acidosis is more prone to kidney stones because high urine pH favors precipitation of Ca phosphate and proximal reabsorption of citrate, which typically prevents Ca stone formation. In terms of the other options, osteomalacia is more commonly seen in proximal renal tubular acidosis because of concurrent proximal phosphate wasting. Venous thromboembolism is not associated with any renal tubular acidosis. Hyperkalemia is associated with type IV renal tubular acidosis in the setting of hypoaldosteronism. Proximal and distal renal tubular acidosis are both prone to hypokalemia because of distal K^+ secretion in lieu of NH_4^+. Patients with renal tubular acidosis are not at increased risk for infection.

8. **The correct answer is: A. Neobladder dysfunction.** This patient has a normal anion gap metabolic acidosis with appropriate respiratory compensation. He most likely has a neobladder dysfunction. An ileal conduit has an abundance of Na^+-H^+ exchangers. Urea traveling through the neobladder is metabolized to NH_4^+ and HCO_3^-. The NH_4^+ competes with Na^+ at the Na^+-H^+ exchanger and is reabsorbed in exchange for H^+. Cl^- in the urine

is also absorbed in exchange for HCO_3^- at the Cl^-/HCO_3^- exchanger. The absorbed NH_4^+ is metabolized in the liver to urea and H^+, resulting in the gain of a proton. Under well-functioning conditions, this is not an issue; however, if the transit time increases, as in the case of a neobladder dysfunction, the urine stays in contact with the intestinal luminal wall for a longer period and a normal anion gap acidosis develops. These patients require chronic bicarbonate replacement and sometimes revision of the conduit. Other causes, such as sepsis secondary to a UTI or type B lactic acidosis that occurs in short gut syndrome, produce an anion gap acidosis. This patient does not have any major reasons to suspect renal tubular acidosis. Most cases of renal tubular acidosis are mild and do not produce sudden severe acidosis.

9. **The correct answer is: B. High anion gap metabolic acidosis, metabolic alkalosis with compensatory respiratory alkalosis.** This patient presents with a normal pH but with multiple acid-base disturbances. The patient's can be calculated as $Na - Cl - HCO_3$, which is $126 - 87 - 20 = 19$; however, one needs to correct for albumin, by adding 2.5 to the anion gap for each 1 g/dL decrease in albumin below 4 g/dL. Hence, the corrected anion gap is $19 + 2.5 \times 2 = 24$. He has a 4 mEq/L decrease in HCO_3 whereas one would expect a decrease in HCO_3 of 12 mEq/L; hence, he has an additional metabolic alkalosis (delta-delta 3). His PCO_2 is slightly low, suggestive of a respiratory alkalosis. Using Winter's formula ($1.5 \times HCO_3^- + 8 \pm 2$), the expected PCO_2 is 36 to 40 mmHg, so his low PCO_2 is the expected respiratory compensation for his metabolic acidosis. He likely has an elevated anion gap from lactic acidosis and/or ketosis in the setting of poor oral intake and metabolic alkalosis from vomiting. Treatment should involve resuscitation with isotonic fluid and aggressive potassium repletion, as the alkalemia will persist in a state of hypochloremia and hypokalemia. In terms of the other choices, while the pH is normal, there is an abnormality, as this is a triple acid-base disturbance that is masked by concurrent metabolic acidosis and alkalosis. The patient has high anion gap metabolic acidosis, but one would expect a pH ~7.25 with HCO_3 12 mEq/L and PCO_2 28 mmHg if he has a pure high anion gap metabolic acidosis. This patient has an anion gap of 24 when corrected for albumin, so a non–gap metabolic acidosis is incorrect.

10. **The correct answer is: D. IV normal saline.** This patient presents with emesis, resulting in loss of Cl-rich fluids and therefore a hyperchloremic, hypokalemic metabolic alkalosis. The treatment of choice for saline-responsive metabolic alkalosis is IV saline. Normally, the kidneys can easily handle bicarbonate excess; however, after loss of HCl, volume, and K (the generation phase of the metabolic alkalosis), the kidney will preferentially prioritize volume retention at the expense of persistent alkalemia (the maintenance phase). The macula densa senses low Cl and stimulates renin-angiotensin-aldosterone system and aldosterone secretion, which leads to not only Na retention but also H^+ and K secretion in principal cells. In addition, low potassium stimulates H^+ secretion in α-intercalated cells. As such, correction of metabolic alkalosis requires volume resuscitation with chloride-rich isotonic fluid (eg, normal saline) with aggressive potassium repletion (K > 4.0 mEq/L). As the alkalemia is corrected, potassium will shift extracellularly as well.

11. **The correct answer is: C. Anion gap metabolic acidosis + non–gap metabolic acidosis + respiratory alkalosis.**

Step 1: Evaluate the pH: This patient has an acidosis with a pH of 7.15.

Step 2: Identify whether it is respiratory or metabolic: PCO_2 here is 40 mmHg and the HCO_3 is 12 mmol/L; hence, it is metabolic.

Step 3: Look at the anion gap: The anion gap is elevated in this case; hence, the patient has an anion gap metabolic acidosis.

Step 4:   Check whether the respiratory response is adequate: The expected PCO_2 by Winter's formula should be (1.5 × [serum HCO_3] + 8 ± 2); the expected PCO_2 is 26 ± 2 mmHg. However, the patient's PCO_2 is 20 mmHg; hence, there is a coexistent respiratory alkalosis.

Step 5:   Calculate Δanion gap/ΔHCO₃ (delta/delta): Does the rise in anion gap match the fall in HCO_3? In this case the delta/delta is 4/12, which is <1; hence, there is a concomitant non–gap metabolic acidosis.

12. **The correct answer is: C. IV normal saline.** This patient presents with euvolemic hyponatremia with a history concerning for low-solute diet (alcohol intake without food) because of beer potomania. Administration of IV saline would provide solute, enabling free water excretion. Free water clearance (CH_2O) = solute excretion/UOsm. A normal US dietary solute load is 750 mOsm/day and the kidney's maximum diluting capacity is 50 mOsm/L, so under normal circumstances, we can drink about 15 L of free water prior to holding on to free water and developing hyponatremia. In beer potomania, daily solute intake ranges from 200 to 300 mOsm, so patients are only able to drink 4 to 6 L of free water (or beer) prior to developing hyponatremia. A six-pack is 72 ounces or ~2100 mL, so drinking 2 six-packs would overwhelm this patient's diluting capacity, after which he would hold on to free water. As he is maximally diluting his urine, his urine osmolality is <100 mOsm/kg. Administration of solute should increase this patient's serum sodium, so C is the correct answer. It is very important to note that these patients are at high risk of rapid correction because they will excrete free water once they are provided back with solute, and so frequent sodium monitors are critical here. In terms of other options, answer choices A and B do not increase solute intake, and thus are not good choices for this patient. ADH activity would be low as serum Osm <300 mOsm/kg. Tolvaptan is a vasopressin receptor (and therefore ADH) antagonist used as second line in syndrome of inappropriate antidiuretic hormone secretion (SIADH) and hypervolemic hyponatremia.

13. **The correct answer is: D. Inappropriate antidiuretic hormone (ADH) release.** This patient's hyponatremia worsened from 120 to 116 mEq/L, resulting in a seizure after normal saline resuscitation suggestive of SIADH. Inappropriate ADH release is seen in many disorders, including stroke, malignancy, carbamazepine, selective serotonin reuptake inhibitors (SSRIs), and pneumonia. This patient has a history of lung cancer, which is associated with inappropriate ADH release. Typically, urine Na is >20 mEq/L, suggestive of euvolemia, and urine osmolality is >100 mOsm/kg, suggestive of ADH activity and free water reabsorption. With normal saline administration, sodium levels can decrease if the urine osmolarity is higher than serum osmolarity. In this patient, aggressive IV normal saline administration decreased her Na to a dangerously low level, resulting in seizure. At this point, hypertonic saline should be administered in consultation with nephrology.

14. **The correct answer is: C. Give 3% hypertonic saline as a 100 mL bolus in 10 minutes, then recheck labs.** This patient presents with severe hyponatremia (defined as serum Na <120 mEq/L) of unknown chronicity and is at risk of life-threatening symptoms (seizures, respiratory failure, coma) because of cerebral edema. Both European and American expert panel guidelines recommend aggressive therapy with 3% saline in the setting of severe symptoms, defined as vomiting, deep somnolence, seizures, or coma. Hypertonic saline should be administered in consultation with nephrology but is typically given as a 150 mL bolus over 20 minutes (EU guidelines) or 100 mL over 10 minutes (US guidelines). An increase of serum Na by ~3 mEq/L is sufficient to reverse severe symptoms. In terms of other options, although this patient's hyponatremia may be due to underlying

hypothyroidism, the risk of life-threatening symptoms warrants initial rapid correction. Isotonic saline is the treatment of choice for hypovolemic hyponatremia; however, the severity of symptoms warrants hypertonic saline. In addition, this patient appears euvolemic with UNa >20 mEq/L, so SIADH is the more likely diagnosis; 2 L of isotonic saline without rechecking serum Na could further worsen serum Na. Free water restriction would be warranted in SIADH and is the next step, but this patient warrants more rapid correction given the severity of symptoms.

15. **The correct answer is: B. Hyperkalemia.** Most patients evaluated for hyponatremia have chronic hyponatremia. This is defined as hyponatremia present for more than 48 hours. The cutoff 48 hours is used as this is approximately the time that it takes for the cells in the brain to adapt to the decreased tonicity encountered in hyponatremia. During hyponatremia, cells excrete osmolytes, which effectively lowers their osmolarity and prevents further cell swelling. Rapid increases in serum sodium lead to shrinking of the cells that had adapted and can result in the severe neurologic clinical syndrome of ODS. In addition to the rate of sodium correction, underlying conditions such as alcoholism, malnutrition, or liver disease increase the risk of developing ODS if the serum sodium is rapidly corrected. In fact, hypokalemia (not hyperkalemia) is a risk factor for ODS. Repletion of K to treat hypokalemia will promote aldosterone activity, allowing more Na absorption (in exchange for K excretion), hence increasing the rate of Na correction and potentially increasing the risk of ODS. It is important to note that correction of hypokalemia increases serum sodium in a similar mEq per mEq basis as hyponatremia correction with sodium, and thus this has to be considered when predicting the expected increase in sodium by IV fluids.

16. **The correct answer is: D. Nephrogenic diabetes insipidus.** This patient presents with hypernatremia of unknown chronicity and is found to have symptomatic hypernatremia. The patient's serum osmolality is very high (335 mOsm/kg) and her urine osmolality is <300 mOsm/kg, suggesting insufficient ADH. After resuscitation with normal saline, she remains polyuric with ~675 mOsm/day, suggesting water diuresis as opposed to osmotic diuresis, so diabetes insipidus is most likely. Administration of DDAVP will differentiate central from nephrogenic diabetes insipidus. As she has less than a 50% increase in urine osmolality with DDAVP, she likely has nephrogenic diabetes insipidus. Answer A is incorrect, as DDAVP administration increased urine osmolality by <50%, so production of DDAVP is not the main etiology behind her diabetes insipidus. Answer B is incorrect as GI free water loss would be expected from significant watery diarrhea.

    Answer C is incorrect because although lack of free water would cause hypernatremia, this patient has adequate access to free water and remains polyuric because of inability to concentrate her urine. Answer E is incorrect, as this patient is below the threshold for glycosuria and polyuria with ~675 mOsm/day consistent with a water diuresis, whereas one would expect a urine osmolality >1000 mOsm/day with very high serum glucose levels in osmotic diuresis.

17. **The correct answer is: B. Gestational diabetes insipidus.** This patient most likely has gestational diabetes insipidus caused by the production of placental vasopressinase, which degrades normally produced vasopressin. It usually presents in the third trimester and resolves over weeks in the postpartum period. Diagnosis and treatment are with DDAVP, which is resistant to endogenous vasopressinase and is effective in raising the urine osmolality. Central diabetes insipidus is another possibility in this patient, who responds to DDAVP; however, the more obvious cause in this patient is gestational diabetes insipidus. Lithium can cause nephrogenic diabetes insipidus, sometimes after treatment

cessation, but nephrogenic diabetes insipidus is unlikely since the polyuria responded to DDAVP. Primary polydipsia resolves with fluid restriction, which was not the case here. Preeclampsia is a risk factor for gestational diabetes insipidus since the liver, which is the site of vasopressinase degradation, may be affected, but preeclampsia by itself does not lead to diabetes insipidus.

18. **The correct answer is: B. Licorice ingestion.** This patient presents with hypokalemia with urine K/Cr ratio >13 and high BP in the setting of large ingestion of black licorice. Glycyrrhizic acid, an ingredient in licorice, inhibits 11-β-hydroxysteroid dehydrogenase, the enzyme responsible for inactivating cortisol in the adrenal glands. Black licorice, ingested in large quantities, can result in hypercortisolism. In states of cortisol excess, cortisol activates mineralocorticoid receptors in the principal cell, causing sodium retention and potassium excretion and resulting in severe hypokalemia. Both salt retention and hypercortisolism contribute to elevated BP. In terms of other options, although this patient has diarrhea, which can cause extrarenal losses of potassium, the $U_{K/Cr}$ is >13. If this patient's hypokalemia were because of diarrhea, the $U_{K/Cr}$ would be <13. Thiazides cause renal losses of potassium; however, this patient does not take a thiazide and his BP is high. Hypokalemia is frequently associated with proximal (type II) and distal (type I) renal tubular acidosis; however, this patient's urine anion gap is −10. This patient does not have a history of vomiting and one would expect metabolic alkalosis with hypochloremia and elevated bicarbonate, whereas this patient has normal chloride and low bicarbonate.

19. **The correct answer is: D. Hypothermia.** Therapeutic hypothermia can cause intracellular shift of potassium by increased activity of the Na^+-K^+-ATPase and can also cause some urinary loss of potassium because of cold-induced diuresis; hence, this patient's hypokalemia is consistent with the initiation of therapeutic hypothermia. Serum electrolytes should be closely monitored during rewarming since rebound hyperkalemia can occur. The other causes are not consistent with this presentation. Mechanical ventilation and cardiac revascularization do not cause hypokalemia. The patient's stool output is not high enough for diarrhea to be a cause of hypokalemia, and hyperaldosteronism would have been apparent on presentation and is unlikely to present acutely.

20. **The correct answer is: C. Pseudohyperkalemia.** This patient, who presents with persistent severe hyperkalemia on a serum chemistry panel without ECG changes, most likely has pseudohyperkalemia in the setting of leukocytosis. A clue to pseudohyperkalemia is the unchanged serum potassium despite hyperkalemia treatment and a normal ECG. Various leukemias (eg, acute myeloid leukemia and chronic lymphocytic leukemia) have been associated with pseudohyperkalemia. In leukemias, fragile cell membranes are prone to cell lysis during transportation and processing, resulting in falsely high potassium levels. Chronic lymphocytic leukemia with WBCs in the 400s has been shown to falsely increase the measured serum potassium by approximately 4 mEq/L. A strategy to determine the true plasma potassium is to check the potassium level on a venous blood gas where handling and processing are minimized and cells are less prone to lysis. In terms of other options, although this patient is hyperglycemic, it is mild and unlikely to cause significant hyperkalemia. Tumor lysis syndrome is most common with solid tumors during induction chemotherapy. In addition, true serum potassium levels in the range of 8.2 to 8.5 mEq/L should cause ECG changes. Hyporeninemic hypoaldosteronism can cause hyperkalemia and can be caused by diabetes mellitus, NSAID use, HIV, and multiple myeloma. His lack of response to hyperkalemia treatment and ECG changes make this unlikely, and this patient has an elevated bicarbonate and so is unlikely to have hypoaldosteronism. This patient has a normal creatinine and is unlikely to have hyperkalemia because of renal failure.

21. **The correct answer is: D. Hyperglycemia.** This patient has developed mild hyperkalemia from transcellular shifts in the setting of hyperglycemia. With his underlying diabetes, he likely has type IV renal tubular acidosis, in which he is prone to hyperkalemia with an inability to secrete K^+ because of aldosterone resistance. With treatment for his COPD exacerbation, he has become significantly hyperglycemic. Hyperglycemia is associated with extracellular increased osmolality, which promotes passive movement of potassium from the intracellular to the extracellular fluid. As such, his glucose of 450 mg/dL and high serum osmolality have resulted in mild hyperkalemia. Correction of his hyperglycemia with insulin should correct his hyperkalemia.

22. **The correct answer is: D. Recent bowel surgery.** SPS is a GI cation exchanger that is used to remove potassium in hyperkalemia. In a retrospective study involving 501 patients who received SPS for hyperkalemia, serum potassium decreased by a mean of 0.93 mEq/L within 24 hours (*Clin Nephrol.* 2016;85:38); however, there were two cases (0.04%) of bowel necrosis related to administration. As such, experts recommend avoiding SPS in postoperative patients who have undergone bowel surgery.

23. **The correct answer is: A. Consult nephrology for renal replacement therapy.** This patient is anuric despite IV diuresis, so the next best step is to initiate renal replacement therapy for hyperkalemia with ECG changes and hypoxemic respiratory failure because of pulmonary edema. He most likely is anuric from ATN, as he suffered a cardiac arrest with prolonged renal ischemia. Normal saline would not be beneficial in a patient who is hypoxemic from pulmonary edema and unlikely to have prerenal AKI. Repeating a basic metabolic panel or giving a different loop diuretic is not adequate for this patient with progressive difficulty on the ventilator from pulmonary edema. Potassium binding resins would help with GI removal of potassium but are not likely to be fast-acting enough or sufficient in an anuric patient with multiple indications for renal replacement therapy.

24. **The correct answer is: C. Heart failure.** This patient presents with a congestive heart failure exacerbation with AKI, most likely because of hypervolemia causing a cardiorenal syndrome. Cardiorenal syndrome is a type of prerenal AKI that results from venous congestion and decreased renal perfusion. As there is no intrinsic injury, a urinalysis should have no blood or protein present, as would be seen with contrast or vasculitis. Treatment includes decongestion with IV diuretics.

25. **The correct answer is: D. Continue supportive measures.** Proteinuria is usually a sign of renal injury (either tubular or glomerular injury), whereas albuminuria reflects glomerular dysfunction. Use of spot urine checks to calculate the protein:creatinine ratio as a surrogate marker of 24 hours urine protein excretion has become well accepted and is widely used to monitor patients with CKD. The assumption is that a given patient excretes about 1000 mg of creatinine in the urine in a day, and thus using a urine sample with measured protein and creatinine can serve to estimate daily urine protein excretion. However, this assumption is inaccurate in AKI. During AKI, the urinary creatinine excretion is decreased until a new steady state is achieved. If the urine creatinine is very low, then the protein/creatinine ratio will overestimate 24-hour protein excretion. This may result in misclassification of patients with AKI as having nephrotic-range proteinuria, confounding the diagnostic process. In this patient with otherwise classic features of AKI in the form of ATN, the best course is to continue guideline-directed management of septic shock and severe AKI. If an exact measurement of urine protein was desirable, a 24-hour urine collection for measurement of urine protein could be considered.

26. **The correct answer is: C. Place a Foley catheter.** The patient most likely has postobstructive AKI given his diagnosis of benign prostatic hyperplasia as inferred from his prescription for tamsulosin, his physical examination, as well as his proportionally higher potassium than one would predict from his AKI. Although renal ultrasound or other imaging and IV fluids would also be reasonable, the first step is to place a Foley catheter that would be both diagnostic and therapeutic. Furosemide would also be reasonable after the obstruction has been relieved if the patient had signs of volume overload, but would not be part of the initial management.

27. **The correct answer is: C. Kidney biopsy.** This patient most likely has AKI with symptoms (diarrhea, poor oral intake) and examination (hypotension) suggestive of prerenal kidney injury. His kidneys were normal at baseline; however, his creatinine has not significantly improved with IV hydration. This is highly suggestive of acute interstitial nephritis as a cause of his AKI. Checkpoint inhibitors (pembrolizumab, nivolumab, ipilimumab) are a class of drugs that ramp up the native immune response against tumor antigens. This can have adverse consequences on normal tissue such as the kidneys, thyroid, adrenals, and intestines. Checkpoint nephritis can present variably, and WBCs/WBC casts in the urine may or may not be present. A kidney biopsy should be considered in patients at low risk for bleeding and in whom the diagnosis is not obvious. Empiric prednisone can be considered in patients at high risk of bleeding from a kidney biopsy, but steroids have adverse effects, and a false diagnosis of acute interstitial nephritis can have important implications for therapy going forward. A Foley catheter is not indicated in patients with no signs of obstruction and reasonable urine output. In addition, medications, such as proton pump inhibitors, have been associated with checkpoint nephritis and should be stopped or switched to H_2 blockers.

28. **The correct answer is: D. IV crystalloid at 200 mL/h.** Individuals with rhabdomyolysis are volume depleted because of sequestration of fluid within the muscles. Aggressive fluid resuscitation with crystalloid is key in helping prevent the occurrence or worsening of AKI; hence, isotonic crystalloid administration is recommended in severe cases of rhabdomyolysis. There is no evidence for colloid use in rhabdomyolysis. In patients with AKI who become volume overloaded, furosemide may be used to augment urine flow and decrease overload, but it should not be used in isolation as initial therapy. Isotonic IV sodium bicarbonate may be used in severe rhabdomyolysis after volume repletion with isotonic saline, but there is scant evidence that alkaline diuresis improves renal outcomes, and it may be harmful in patients with hypocalcemia, such as in this patient. Frequent monitoring of arterial pH and ionized calcium is recommended. Dialysis may be necessary if patients do not respond to initial fluid resuscitation and develop severe AKI but should not be instituted as initial therapy.

29. **The correct answer is: A. Increased risk of CKD, ESRD, and mortality.** A meta-analysis comprising 2 million patients found individuals with AKI at an increased risk of new or progressive CKD (hazard ratio 2.67, 95% confidence interval [CI] 1.99-3.58), ESRD (hazard ratio 4.81, 95% CI 3.04-7.62), and death (hazard ratio 1.80, 95% CI 1.61-2.02) *(Kidney Int. 2019;95:160)*. The risk of CKD, ESRD, and death increased with the severity of AKI, with patients sustaining AKI stage 3 having the highest risk for all outcomes. The risk of death in patients who developed AKI compared with those who did not was notably higher for patients undergoing limb or coronary angiography or transcatheter aortic valve replacement (hazard ratio 3.07, 95% CI 2.12-4.46) than in patients undergoing cardiovascular surgery (hazard ratio 1.75, 95% CI 1.55-1.98), who were in intensive care (hazard ratio 1.47, 95% CI 1.32-1.65), or who were in a general hospital setting (hazard ratio 1.41, 95% CI 1.26-1.56).

30. **The correct answer is: C. IV normal saline.** Contrast-associated AKI is typically mild and occurs 48 to 72 hours after the procedure. In most patients, the kidney function recovers to baseline and dialysis is almost never required. Although there is some controversy regarding the cause-and-effect relationship between contrast agents and AKI, there are sufficient data to suggest that severe kidney injury leading to serious adverse events, such as requiring dialysis, is extremely rare. Preexisting kidney disease is the strongest risk factor for the development of AKI. Isotonic saline has been shown in multiple studies to reduce the incidence of AKI, whereas N-acetylcysteine has not been shown to be beneficial. Hemodialysis does not help prevent contrast-associated AKI. In low-risk patients who are not expected to have adverse effects from minimal volume expansion, IV saline, or IV isotonic bicarbonate, is recommended to reduce the risk of contrast-associated AKI.

31. **The correct answer is: A. Aspirin, nitrates, and cardiology consult for cardiac catheterization.** Symptoms of acute coronary syndrome in patients with ESRD are frequently misjudged to be secondary to inadequate dialysis or volume removal. The presentation is often atypical in these patients, and a high degree of suspicion is required. Typical ST changes on ECG are often absent. The pathophysiology behind increased troponin levels in ESRD is not well understood. It may be secondary to chronic structural heart disease with troponin release rather than reduced renal clearance. This patient has gained just 1 kg after his last dialysis session and does not have major signs of volume overload. His troponin levels have tripled since admission; hence, dialysis should be deferred until an evaluation for acute coronary syndrome has been performed. Acute coronary syndrome is more likely than a pulmonary embolism in this setting and a CT scan is not necessary at this stage.

32. **The correct answer is: D. Start metolazone.** This patient is chronically on loop diuretics and has gained weight despite increasing doses, including IV furosemide. Since his Cr is near to his baseline, the most likely cause of his resistance to diuretics is hypertrophy of the distal convoluted tubule and collecting duct that has developed in the setting of long-term diuretic use. Thus, the best approach is to block the Na^+-Cl^- cotransporter with a thiazide diuretic to augment the effect of a loop diuretic. Inotropes are sometimes useful to support diuresis in patients in cardiogenic shock, but this patient is normotensive and warm on examination, making shock an unlikely cause of his resistance to diuretics. There is no evidence that one loop diuretic is better than another one, so switching to bumetanide would not be the best next step. Hemodialysis is not indicated yet since he has not failed aggressive augmentation of diuresis until after a thiazide is given.

33. **The correct answer is: A. Add acetazolamide.** This patient has diuretic-induced sodium and chloride loss. The increased sodium delivery to the distal tubule leads to increased absorption of the sodium through the ENaC channel and increased H^+ secretion into the urine from the intercalated cells in compensation. Chloride depletion also leads to bicarbonate retention in the distal tubule, thereby causing metabolic alkalosis. Acetazolamide inhibits carbonic anhydrase in the proximal tubule and leads to loss of bicarbonate; it also promotes further diuresis, although it is a weak diuretic by itself. This leads to lowering of the serum bicarbonate concentration and betterment of the diuretic-induced metabolic alkalosis. Typical doses include 250 to 500 mg twice or thrice a day until the pH improves to normal levels. Infusion of normal saline may help replete the sodium and chloride and reverse the alkalosis but would be counterproductive in this patient with significant volume overload. Stopping the loop diuretic would do the same. Spironolactone and amiloride are not used for this purpose.

34. **The correct answer is: D. Increase chlorthalidone to 25 mg daily.** Resistant hypertension indicates uncontrolled hypertension on optimal doses of three drugs, one of which should be a diuretic. This patient has uncontrolled hypertension, but the dose of one of the drugs is not optimized, so the best option would be to increase chlorthalidone to 25 mg daily. Adding a fourth drug, such as carvedilol (a good choice with her history of CAD) or spironolactone, may be considered if her BP remains uncontrolled after uptitration of the chlorthalidone dose. Lisinopril is already at the maximum dose and an increase may lead to adverse effects, such as hyperkalemia. Changing to a loop diuretic may be required when her eGFR drops below 20 to 25 mL/min/1.73 m^2, but it is not necessary at this time.

35. **The correct answer is: C. Lisinopril.** Methyldopa, labetalol, nifedipine, and hydralazine are the most studied antiteratogenic drugs that can be safely used during pregnancy. Labetalol and hydralazine are commonly used in hypertensive crises. These drugs are also compatible with lactation. ACE inhibitors and ARBs are teratogenic, especially during the second and third trimester of pregnancy, and can lead to fetal pulmonary hypoplasia, malformations, fetal renal failure, growth retardation, and miscarriages; hence, these drugs should be switched during pregnancy planning or at conception.

36. **The correct answer is: B. Monitor closely with IV furosemide as needed.** The IDEAL-ICU study showed no mortality benefit for early (within 12 hours of AKI) versus late (after 48 hours of AKI) renal replacement therapy in patients with septic shock. This is consistent with the published results of the AKIKI trial. Notably, 38% of the patients in the delayed group did not receive renal replacement therapy, and only 17% of the patients in the delayed group required emergency renal replacement therapy. Although there was prevailing thought that early dialysis initiation may improve acid-base, electrolyte, and fluid balance and potentially avoid adverse outcomes, that has been proven not to be the case. Initiating renal replacement therapy early may unnecessarily expose patients to the risks associated with dialysis, such as access complications and prolonged ICU stay; hence, close monitoring and use of IV diuretics to maintain fluid balance is recommended in the early period of AKI, unless there is an emergent indication for renal replacement therapy, such as severe volume overload, metabolic acidosis (pH < 7.15), and hyperkalemia (>6 mEq/L) refractory to medical therapy. If dialysis were to be initiated in this patient, continuous renal replacement therapy would be the preferred choice because of hemodynamic instability. Although indications for bicarbonate therapy are controversial, it is not recommended for patients with an arterial pH >7.2. There are some data that suggest it may prevent the need for renal replacement therapy and potentially improve survival in patients with severe AKI.

37. **The correct answer is: D. Observation only.** It can be particularly challenging to decide when to stop or interrupt dialysis in patients with an underlying CKD and an acute insult. Studies have shown that having a robust urine output is a strong predictor of dialysis discontinuation. There is no specific laboratory threshold where dialysis is not indicated. Patients with AKI should be evaluated daily for renal replacement therapy needs, including metabolic derangements and volume overload. IV furosemide is not required unless volume removal takes precedence. In patients outside the critical care setting, volume removal is not an overwhelming issue; hence, furosemide can be avoided with a urine output >2 L. In this patient, therefore, it is prudent to wait and watch to see if she recovers enough kidney function to stay off dialysis. The increase in BUN and creatinine from postdialysis levels is expected with equilibration postdialysis since these concentrations are lowered rapidly by dialysis and then slowly increase during equilibration when dialysis is discontinued.

38. **The correct answer is: D. Start continuous renal replacement such as continuous veno-venous hemofiltration (CVVH).** This patient has severe oliguric AKI, likely from ischemic ATN, and worsening gas exchange as evidenced by her increased need for PEEP and FiO_2. She has high obligate intake from infusions and tube feeds, and has failed attempts to use diuretics to augment urine output, thus she has an indication to start renal replacement therapy for volume management. Although there is no evidence that intermittent hemodialysis is better than continuous renal replacement therapy such as CVVH, or vice versa, slow continuous fluid removal is often better tolerated in patients in severe shock with the need for several liters/day of volume removal. Further augmentation of diuresis with an aldosterone inhibitor is unlikely to improve urine output enough to keep up with her daily intake. Patients who are critically ill should receive adequate nutrition so stopping tube feeds is never indicated. However, one should always ensure patients with high obligate intake are on the most concentrated formula of tube feeds available to minimize further fluid overload.

39. **The correct answer is: C. Perform surgical evaluation.** This patient has steal syndrome, which diverts blood away from the arteries of the hand and can lead to ischemia. It requires immediate surgical evaluation and, potentially, ligation of the fistula if severe. Mild steal syndrome can be managed with lowering dialysis blood flow rates if the symptoms are manageable; however, in this patient with severe pain and a nonpalpable pulse, a surgical evaluation is paramount. Some patients experience mild numbness for months to years before steal syndrome becomes apparent, whereas in others it becomes apparent with the first use of a fistula. Risk factors for steal syndrome in dialysis patients include smoking, diabetes, hypertension, and peripheral vascular disease.

40. **The correct answer is: E. Warfarin.** Calciphylaxis results from ischemia in the small blood arterioles secondary to calcification of the tunica media and subsequent thrombosis, leading to painful skin lesions. Warfarin use is a risk factor for calciphylaxis and should be avoided in patients who are at risk for and/or already have calciphylaxis. All the other medications listed are not contraindicated in calciphylaxis and could be used to manage this patient's atrial fibrillation. She should also be treated with sodium thiosulfate and ensure that her PTH, phosphorous, and calcium are at the appropriate levels. Pain control is usually achieved with opioids.

41. **The correct answer is: A. Noncalcium phosphate binders.** The patient presents with advanced CKD with clinical and laboratory findings attributable to the MBD present in patients with CKD, also called CKD-MBD. Vascular calcification is common in patients with CKD and is associated with significant morbidity and mortality. A key element in the pathogenesis of vascular calcification is hyperphosphatemia. Hyperphosphatemia can contribute to uncontrolled secondary hyperparathyroidism, and phosphorus may also directly contribute to injure vascular smooth muscle cells, which leads to a pro-osteogenic phenotype in the arteries with subsequent deposition of calcium phosphate crystals. Hyperphosphatemia control includes diet counseling, use of phosphate binders (preferably noncalcium binders), and consideration of renal replacement therapies in patients with advanced CKD with other indications for dialysis such as uremia, uncontrolled hyperkalemia, or uncontrolled metabolic acidosis. Cinacalcet is an allosteric activator of the calcium-sensing receptor in the parathyroid cells, which reduces PTH secretion and thus is frequently used in secondary hyperparathyroidism, especially after other measures, such as phosphorus control, have been taken. Cinacalcet use might be limited by GI side effects and hypocalcemia. Although vitamin D analogs such as calcitriol can also decrease PTH secretion, such analogs

should not be used in the presence of uncontrolled hyperphosphatemia, especially with clinical evidence of vascular calcification, because vitamin D analogs can further increase the absorption of calcium and phosphorus. Low-phosphorus diet counseling is advised, rather than low-calcium diet, in cases of CKD-MBD.

42. **The correct answer is: D. He should be evaluated and listed for a kidney transplant now.** As of the end of 2021, there were close to 93 000 patients on the kidney transplant waiting list, with 20% being Hispanics. There is no age limit for a candidate to be listed. For most malignancies, a period of 2 to 5 years before transplantation is recommended. No waiting period is required for cancers such as nonmelanomatous skin cancers, in situ bladder and cervical cancers, or small (<7 cm) and incidentally discovered renal cancers that are removed. A wait time of more than 2 years is required for melanomas and breast, colorectal, and uterine cancers to account for recurrence risk. The median wait times according to blood group type are as follows: 2 years for AB, 3 years for A, and 5 years for B and O. This patient is 72 years old but leads an active life and seems to have adequate family support. With a blood group type that has a lower-than-average wait time, he should undergo a recipient evaluation and get listed for a transplant. Although he is undergoing workup, he should attempt to lose weight and lower his BMI, as obesity is associated with delayed graft function. The current eGFR cutoff to be listed is ≤20 mL/min/1.73 m^2, and he does not have to wait until he is on dialysis. In fact, listing him as soon as possible is paramount given he can accrue time on the transplant list now and, potentially, get a transplant before he is on dialysis. He should be encouraged to look at potential living donors since they are associated with better patient and graft survival; however, that should not delay him being listed on the deceased donor transplant list.

43. **The correct answer is: C. Listed for liver transplant.** A study showed that cirrhotic patients requiring renal replacement therapy had an extremely poor prognosis with a median survival of around 2 to 3 weeks in the absence of liver transplant (*Clin J Am Soc Nephrol.* 2018;13:16). There was no difference in mortality if the AKI was secondary to ATN or because of hepatorenal syndrome. Patients of older age with higher MELD scores and indicators of critical illness, such as vasopressor initiation, mechanical ventilation, or continuous renal replacement therapy, had a worse outcome. Being listed for a liver transplant was associated with mortality at 6 months. Almost half the subjects (48%) listed for a liver transplant obtained a transplant, and mortality was also much lower in the group listed for transplant (45%) compared with those who were not (84%). Our patient is not young and has a high MELD score. Although her overall prognosis is poor, her transplant listing status is associated with a more favorable prognosis compared with not being listed.

44. **The correct answer is: D. Survival on peritoneal dialysis and survival on home hemodialysis are comparable.** Transplant recipients report a superior quality of life compared with patients on any modality of dialysis. Overall, peritoneal dialysis has not shown to have a mortality benefit over hemodialysis, although it has been shown to be associated with better cognitive function. Although there are no randomized trials, observational data suggest a survival benefit with home hemodialysis compared with in-center hemodialysis.

45. **The correct answer is: C. Refer her for kidney biopsy.** A kidney biopsy should be considered for all patients with suspected lupus nephritis. This includes patients with the following:

1. urine protein creatinine excretion of >0.5 g/day
2. abnormal kidney function
3. findings on urine sediment indicating active kidney involvement, such as persistent hematuria or RBC casts

Patients with no signs of systemic lupus disease and normal creatinine may have active renal involvement. Immune complex–mediated glomerulonephritis is the most common cause of lupus nephritis, and most forms of immune complex–mediated disease respond to mycophenolate and steroids; however, it is important to define the extent and chronicity of injury, both of which may modify the intensity and duration of treatment. This patient with 800 mg/g of proteinuria, active complements, and hypertension could have mesangioproliferative (class II), focal proliferative (class III), or diffuse proliferative (class IV) lupus nephritis. In addition to immunosuppression, intensive BP control is important. Since she is of childbearing age, she should also undergo contraceptive and preconception counseling. Although spot urine testing is not as reliable as using a 24-hour urine collection for testing proteinuria, obtaining the results should not delay the referral for a kidney biopsy. Patients in whom diagnosis and treatment of active renal lupus are delayed are at a much higher risk of progressing to ESRD.

46. **The correct answer is: C. Lisinopril.** IgA nephropathy, the most common glomerular disease in the developed world, most often presents with gross or microscopic hematuria. Gradual progression to ESRD over 15 to 20 years occurs in 50% of patients. Elevated creatinine, persistent urine protein creatinine ratio >1 g/day, and high BP (>140/90 mmHg) are markers of progressive loss of kidney function. The mainstays of IgA nephropathy treatment are BP control (<130/80 mmHg) and proteinuria reduction (<500 mg/g) with ACE inhibitors or ARBs. Fish oil may be used as an add-on therapy in patients with persistent proteinuria despite ACE inhibitors or ARBs. Immunosuppression, with either prednisone or cyclophosphamide, is suggested for patients with one or more of the following:

    1. persistent and progressive proteinuria >1 g/day after maximal medical therapy
    2. necrotizing glomerulonephritis on kidney biopsy
    3. acutely rising serum creatinine

    Immunosuppression is not recommended for patients without active inflammatory changes on a kidney biopsy or those with a stable CKD. Recurrent hematuria, by itself, is a nonspecific marker and is not an indication to treat unless there is a concurrent significant rise in creatinine and/or proteinuria.

47. **The correct answer is: C. Membranous nephropathy.** This patient, with recent discontinuation of immunosuppression and skin findings, most likely has chronic graft-versus-host disease. Chronic graft-versus-host disease can affect multiple organs, with skin, liver, and mucosal surfaces most often involved. Since 2000, there has been increasing recognition that nephrotic syndrome could be the renal manifestation of chronic graft-versus-host disease. Although this has not been proven conclusively, the temporal relationship between discontinuation of immunosuppression and presentation of nephrotic syndrome, as well as the coexistence of graft-versus-host disease involving other organs, suggest that is the case. The loss of immune tolerance as a result of decreased immunosuppression may result in reactivity of donor lymphocytes to the native kidney. Membranous glomerulonephritis is the most common lesion seen (~60%), whereas minimal change disease (20%-25%) and focal segmental glomerulosclerosis (<10%) are less common. Immunosuppression with a combination of steroids, cyclophosphamide, and rituximab is most commonly used in managing these patients. Thrombotic microangiopathy is unlikely in this patient with no anemia or thrombocytopenia. Although posttransplant ANCA vasculitis has been reported in the literature as a manifestation of chronic graft-versus-host disease, it usually presents with a nephritogenic pattern and, added to that, our patient's ANCA levels are normal.

48. The correct answer is: C. Sodium-glucose cotransporter 2 (SGLT-2) inhibitors. IgA nephropathy is a common type of glomerulonephritis. The spectrum of clinical presentation varies from asymptomatic microscopic hematuria to rapid progressive glomerulonephritis (RPGN). For most patients with IgA nephropathy without RPGN, BP control with ACE or ARB medications has been the mainstay of treatment to delay progression of disease. Recently, the DAPA-CKD trial, which included patients who had IgA nephropathy without diabetes, demonstrated a benefit of SGLT-2 inhibitors in delaying the progression of renal disease. Answer choices A and B are incorrect because immunosuppression is not advised in patients with IgA nephropathy with extensive fibrosis, such as in this patient. Given that the patient is already on an ACE inhibitor, the addition of an ARB is not recommended.

49. The correct answer is: B. SPEP, serum immunofixation, and serum free light chain assay. Monoclonal gammopathy of renal significance is the name assigned to a group of disorders in which patients have renal manifestations because of immunoglobulins produced by a B-cell or plasma cell clone but do not have sufficient circulating immunoglobulins to meet the criteria for MGUS (monoclonal gammopathy of unclear significance). Monoclonal gammopathy of renal significance comprises a spectrum of diseases, including monoclonal Ig deposition disease, proliferative glomerulonephritis with monoclonal Ig deposits, C3 glomerulonephritis (C3 with masked Ig deposits), amyloidosis, fibrillary glomerulonephritis, cryoglobulinemia, and immunotactoid glomerulopathy. These diseases have various rates of detection of monoclonal protein in the peripheral blood or urine, with light chain deposit disease having detection rates of 65% to 100%, whereas proliferative glomerulonephritis with monoclonal Ig deposit has the lowest detection rates (20%-30%). Evaluation of patients with monoclonal gammopathy of renal significance involves various tests to detect the monoclonal protein, including SPEP, urine protein electrophoresis, serum immunofixation, and serum free light chain assay. Among these tests, the combination of SPEP (monoclonal spike), serum immunofixation (to confirm monoclonality and type of protein), and serum free light chain assay (abnormal κ/λ ratio inferring monoclonality) has the highest sensitivity to detect a monoclonal protein. The addition of urine tests fails to improve diagnostic sensitivity. A bone marrow biopsy should be considered in those in whom a monoclonal protein is not detected using the aforementioned methods.

50. The correct answer is: C. Hemolytic uremic syndrome. This patient has a rapidly progressive glomerulonephritis, with crescent formation seen on a kidney biopsy. Anti–glomerular basement membrane disease and ANCA-associated glomerulonephritis are the most common causes of crescentic glomerulonephritis, with 85% of anti–glomerular basement membrane disease and 50% of ANCA disease presenting in this manner (>50% crescents on a kidney biopsy). Lupus nephritis and IgA nephropathy can also rarely present with crescentic glomerulonephritis. Kidney biopsy in hemolytic uremic syndrome typically demonstrates endothelial injury and thrombi/fibrin deposition in the glomerular capillaries and arterioles.

51. The correct answer is: A. Cryoglobulinemic glomerulonephritis. This patient, who presented with gross hematuria, hypertension, and AKI, was found to have protein and blood on urinalysis, with RBC casts most concerning for acute glomerulonephritis. Cryoglobulinemia results from deposition of cold-sensitive antibodies and complement proteins within blood vessels, causing decreased perfusion and ischemia. Cryoglobulinemia is associated with untreated hepatitis C and can cause membranoproliferative glomerulonephritis with a reduction in C3 and C4. Her urinalysis is active with protein and blood with an RBC cast shown on her urine sediment. Treatment involves treating hepatitis C with direct-acting antiviral therapy, avoidance of cold temperatures, and consideration of plasmapheresis and immunosuppression (eg, steroids) for rapidly progressive glomerulo-nephritis. Although Henoch-Schönlein purpura presents with palpable purpura and can cause glomerulonephritis, one would expect a normal C3. This patient does not have a history of cirrhosis, and hepatorenal syndrome is a diagnosis of exclusion with no signs of intrinsic kidney injury. This patient does not have significant urinary retention, and one would expect a bland urinalysis and sediment with postrenal AKI. This patient has moist mucous membranes and an active sediment. One would expect bland urinalysis and sediment with prerenal AKI.

52. **The correct answer is: D. Urinalysis + sediment.** This patient presents with gross hematuria without a recent history of trauma or suspected kidney stone. The next best step in management to differentiate intrarenal from extrarenal etiologies is a urinalysis with sediment. If glomerular in etiology, one may expect dysmorphic RBCs or RBC casts. As there is no history of flank pain, recent kidney stone, or trauma, CT urography would not be indicated. Gross hematuria should be initially worked up with CT urography in case of suspected stone or history of trauma; otherwise, urinalysis is appropriate. Renal ultrasound is indicated in the evaluation of AKI/CKD but would not help significantly in workup for gross hematuria. Urology referral at this time is not appropriate as the etiology should first be evaluated by urinalysis.

53. **The correct answer is: A. AA Amyloidosis.** Many conditions can produce a urinalysis that appears relatively normal with little or no cells, casts, or protein. Vascular injuries, such as thrombotic microangiopathies and malignant hypertension, can rarely produce red cells in the urine, but the urine is most often clear. Patients with conditions that obstruct the tubules (like cast nephropathy), externally obstruct the flow of urine (such as benign prostatic hypertrophy), or compress the vasculature (such as abdominal compartment syndrome) have a normal urinalysis. A decrease in effective circulating volume, such as in hepatorenal syndrome or cardiorenal syndrome, also produces benign-appearing urine. Other conditions that produce AKI and a normal urinalysis include hypercalcemic ne-phropathy, phosphate nephropathy, and tumor lysis syndrome. Amyloidosis, a primarily glomerular process, usually presents with glomerular proteinuria (albuminuria), which would be present on urinalysis. AA amyloidosis is a subtype of amyloidosis seen in patients with chronic inflammatory conditions, such as autoimmune diseases.

54. **The correct answer is: C. Overflow proteinuria.** Proteinuria in light chain nephropa-thy is due to light chains that are filtered by the glomerulus and then usually reabsorbed in the proximal convoluted tubule. However, in light chain disease, high levels of light chains exceed the transport maximum capacity of the proximal tubule cells and excess light chain is excreted in the urine. Glomerular proteinuria results from damage to the glomerular basement membrane and podocytes that enables proteins like albumin, which are normally excluded from diffusion out of the capillary, to enter the urinary space of Bowman's cap-sule. Light chains are normally filtered even with intact glomerular basement membranes, so this is not an example of glomerular proteinuria. Tubulointerstitial proteinuria is usually mild ($<$2 g/day), and results from damage to the tubular cells that normally reabsorb the small amount of protein that is filtered in the glomerulus, such that none of it is excreted in the urine. Isolated proteinuria is also mild ($<$1 g/day), and usually is in response to a functional change in systemic physiology such as exercise or standing.

55. **The correct answer is: C. Most kidney stones <0.5 cm in diameter will pass spontaneously.** Most stones ($>$80%) $<$0.5 cm in size pass spontaneously. The chances of spontaneously passing a stone decrease with increase in size after that, with only 25% of stones $\geq$9 mm passing without intervention. Stone passage is also affected by location,

with proximal stones having lower chances of spontaneously passing compared with distal stones at the ureterovesical junction. One-third of patients experience a recurrence of a kidney stone in 5 years, and the rate of recurrence increases to almost 50% in 10 years. It is important to perform a stone compositional analysis or a 24-hour urine metabolic profile to evaluate the type of stone a patient is at risk for and instill management appropriately. With regard to the type of stones, calcium stones account for almost 80%, with calcium oxalate being the most common. Uric acid, cystine, struvite, and mixed-composition stones are less common. In a patient with calcium oxalate stones and low fluid intake, increasing the fluid intake in addition to dietary modification (low sodium, high potassium, low oxalate, low nondairy animal protein, increased fruit and vegetables, supplemental vitamin C) decreases the chances of new calcium stone formation by half. A low-calcium diet is not recommended. Alkalinizing the urine (pH > 6) with citrate helps prevent new uric acid stone formation but can conversely increase the risk of calcium phosphate stones.

56. **The correct answer is: C. Oxalate nephropathy.** Enteric hyperoxaluria is the most common cause of secondary hyperoxaluria and occurs in malabsorptive states, such as inflammatory bowel disease, pancreatic insufficiency, and bowel resections, or after bariatric surgery, such as Roux-en-Y gastric bypass. Chronic malabsorption leads to increased fatty acids in the intestinal lumen, which then binds the calcium that would otherwise bind with dietary oxalate. The high quantities of soluble oxalate then get absorbed and can lead to nephrolithiasis and oxalate nephropathy. Renal biopsy shows extensive tubular and interstitial damage, reflecting the direct toxicity of oxalate to the tubular epithelial cells, while the glomerulus is not typically affected. A 24-hour urine collection reveals high urinary oxalate levels, whereas urine calcium and citrate are low. Management includes dietary modification to include a diet low in fat and oxalate and relatively high in calcium. Liberal fluid intake is also recommended.

57. **The correct answer is: B. Decrease calcium intake.** The clinical vignette describes a patient with renal stones, which by urine sediment are consistent with uric acid crystals. Patients that receive a transplant and are treated with calcineurin inhibitors, particularly cyclosporine, are at higher risk for developing hyperuricemia and gout. In addition, in the presence of risk factors such as low urine volume and an acidic pH, hyperuricemia can favor the formation of uric acid crystals in the urine. The most important treatment in patients with uric acid stones is urine alkalinization, for example, with potassium citrate and increasing fluid intake. In this patient, the urine creatinine excretion is close to what is expected, meaning that he had an adequate 24-hour urine collection, and despite this his urine volume is low. Decreasing calcium intake should not influence the risk of uric acid stones.

58. **The correct answer is: C. Vitamin C.** This patient most likely has calcium oxalate nephrolithiasis and oxalate nephropathy. Oxalate nephropathy can be an inborn error of metabolism that manifests at birth or can be secondary to excessive oxalate consumption or absorption. Ingestion of high-dose vitamin C (1-2 g/day), an oxalate precursor, is associated with formation of calcium oxalate stones and oxalate deposition in the kidney. A large study showed that individuals taking vitamin C had twice the risk of kidney stones as individuals not taking vitamin C. Vitamin D intake with normal calcium levels does not lead to a higher stone risk. B6 supplementation lowers urinary oxalate and may reduce the risk of kidney stones.

HEMATOLOGY-ONCOLOGY

QUESTIONS

1. A 92-year-old woman with depression presents with fatigue and dyspnea. She lives alone, and her diet consists primarily of tea and toast. Examination is notable for body mass index (BMI) of 17, normal deep tendon reflexes, and a steady gait. Labs reveal hemoglobin (Hb) 9 g/dL, mean corpuscular volume (MCV) 108 fL/red cell, indirect bilirubin 1.5 mg/dL (normal <1 mg/dL), lactate dehydrogenase (LDH) 315 U/L (normal 140-280 U/L), homocysteine 75 µmol/L (normal <13 µmol/L), and methylmalonic acid 0.3 µmol/L (normal <0.4 µmol/L). Peripheral smear shows neutrophil hypersegmentation and macro-ovalocytes.

   What is the most likely etiology of her anemia?
   A. Anemia of chronic disease
   B. Folate deficiency
   C. Iron deficiency
   D. Vitamin B12 deficiency

2. A 39-year-old man presents with new bilateral hand and foot numbness. He is a vegan who regularly practices yoga but has noticed worsening imbalance during yoga recently. Examination reveals absent deep tendon reflexes in the upper and lower extremities. Labs are notable for Hb 10 g/dL, MCV 111 fL/red cell, indirect bilirubin 1.8 mg/dL (normal <1 mg/dL), LDH 332 U/L (normal 140-280 U/L), homocysteine 101 µmol/L (normal <13 µmol/L), and methylmalonic acid 75 µmol/L (normal <0.4 µmol/L). Peripheral smear shows neutrophil hypersegmentation and macro-ovalocytes.

   After confirmatory diagnostic tests, what is the most appropriate treatment?
   A. Folate 5 mg oral daily for 3 months
   B. Levothyroxine 50 µg daily
   C. Oral ferrous gluconate three times daily
   D. Vitamin B12 1 mg intramuscular (IM) weekly and then monthly

3. A 66-year-old man presents with fatigue and dyspnea. He does not like to see doctors and does not have a primary care physician (PCP). His wife notes that, over the past few weeks, he has started eating ice frequently. Examination is notable for angular cheilitis, atrophic glossitis, and guaiac positive stool. Labs reveal Hb 9.2 g/dL and MCV 75 fL/red cell.

   What will his iron studies likely show (normal iron 60-170 µg/dL, normal total iron binding capacity [TIBC] 240-450 µg/dL, normal ferritin 12-250 ng/mL)?
   A. Iron 132 µg/dL, TIBC 299 µg/dL, ferritin 204 ng/mL
   B. Iron 210 µg/dL, TIBC 350 µg/dL, ferritin 375 ng/mL
   C. Iron/TIBC <18%, ferritin 5 ng/mL
   D. Iron/TIBC >18%, ferritin 314 ng/mL

4. A 21-year-old man presents with fatigue and gum bleeding. He has no past medical history (PMH), and he is not taking any medications, including supplements and over-the-counter (OTC) medications. Labs are notable for white blood cell (WBC)

1100/µL, Hb 7.3 g/dL, platelets 15 000/µL, and reticulocytes 1%. Viral studies, including human immunodeficiency virus (HIV), Epstein-Barr virus, parvovirus B19, and human herpesvirus 6 (HHV-6), are negative. A bone marrow biopsy shows hypocellularity.

What is the most appropriate management?

A. Allogeneic stem cell transplant
B. Immunosuppression
C. Supportive care
D. Thrombopoietin mimetics

5. A 46-year-old woman with lupus on hydroxychloroquine presents with increasing fatigue, painful arthralgias, and oral ulcers. She takes no other medications, denies alcohol use, and lives in a home constructed in the last 5 years. Labs show Hb 8.9 g/dL from 12.2 mg/dL last year, transferrin saturation 16%, ferritin 350 ng/mL (normal 12-250 ng/mL), MCV 82 fL/red cell, and normal creatinine.

What is the most likely diagnosis?

A. Anemia of chronic inflammation
B. Anemia of chronic kidney disease
C. Iron deficiency anemia
D. Sideroblastic anemia

6. A 74-year-old woman recently diagnosed with pneumonia treated with levofloxacin presents with dyspnea and jaundice. Examination shows tachycardia to 110s, splenomegaly, and cervical lymphadenopathy. Labs are notable for WBC 15 800/µL, absolute lymphocyte count 7500/µL (normal <5000/µL), Hb 6.9 g/dL, platelets 160 000/µL, direct bilirubin 0.2 mg/dL, indirect bilirubin 2.6 mg/dL (normal <1 mg/dL), reticulocytes 11% (normal 0.5%-2.5%), LDH 511 U/L (normal 140-280 U/L), haptoglobin undetectable (normal 30-200 mg/dL), and a positive Coombs test. Peripheral smear shows spherocytic red blood cells (RBCs) and no schistocytes.

What is the most likely diagnosis?

A. Autoimmune hemolytic anemia
B. Drug-induced hemolytic anemia
C. Hereditary spherocytosis
D. Microangiopathic hemolytic anemia (MAHA)

7. A 35-year-old woman presents for evaluation of acute fatigue over the past week. She states that 2 weeks ago, her two children, ages 7 and 9, developed a febrile illness associated with prominent redness of the cheeks. They recovered well and have returned to school. A few days later, the patient developed a low-grade fever, which resolved spontaneously, and she is not sure whether she also had the redness of the cheeks. Her laboratory workup is shown below:

Laboratory studies	
WBC count	8500/µL
Hb	8.4 g/dL (previously 12.1 g/dL)
MCV	89 fL/red cell
Platelets	255 000/µL
Total bilirubin	0.8 mg/dL

Which of the following is the most likely diagnosis?

A. Anemia of chronic disease
B. Aplastic anemia
C. Folate deficiency
D. α-Thalassemia
E. Pure red cell aplasia

8. A 55-year-old woman presents for a routine annual physical and to establish care with her new provider. Her PCP sends basic laboratory studies, which reveal evidence of anemia with Hb 10.1 g/dL, MCV 70 fL/red cell, and transferrin saturation 35%. At the next follow-up visit, the patient brings her medical records from the time of her first pregnancy at age 29, which are shown below:

Laboratory studies	
WBC count	7200/µL
Hb	9.8 g/dL
MCV	69 fL/red cell
Platelets	255 000/µL
Total bilirubin	0.8 mg/dL
Transferrin saturation	29% (normal >18%)
Hb electrophoresis	
HbA2	<2.0% (normal 2%-3%)
HbA	95% (normal 95%-98%)
HbF	<1.0% (normal 0.8%-2%)
HbH	2.5% (normal 0%)

Which of the following is the correct diagnosis?

A. Iron deficiency anemia
B. α-Thalassemia major
C. α-Thalassemia minor
D. β-Thalassemia major
E. β-Thalassemia minor

9. A 42-year-old woman with sickle cell disease presents with a vaso-occlusive pain episode requiring admission for intravenous (IV) pain medications. Social history is notable for current smoking. On hospital day 2, she develops cough, dyspnea, fever, and a new 4 L nasal cannula oxygen requirement. Physical examination reveals tachypnea, intercostal retractions, diffuse wheezing, and bibasilar rales. Chest x-ray (CXR) shows new bilateral lower lobe opacities.

Labs show hematocrit 22%, WBC 12 000/µL with 80% neutrophils, and reticulocytes 8%. Blood and sputum cultures are sent. Electrocardiogram (ECG) shows sinus tachycardia with heart rate (HR) 110 beats/min and no ST or T-wave changes. She is started on broad-spectrum antibiotics for pneumonia. However, her oxygen saturation drops to 85% on 4 L nasal cannula, and she transiently requires a 100% nonrebreather before stabilization at oxygen saturations of 90% on 6 L nasal cannula. She is transferred to the intensive care unit (ICU) for closer monitoring of her tenuous respiratory status.

What is the most important next treatment step for this patient?

A. Albuterol nebulizer
B. Dexamethasone
C. Exchange transfusion
D. RBC transfusion

10. A 25-year-old man presents with fatigue, fevers, dyspnea on exertion, and a rash on his lower extremities for the past 4 days. Aside from a fever, his vital signs are normal. Initial examination reveals a normal neurologic examination and mental status. Labs show hematocrit 18%, platelets 13 000/μL, and creatinine 1.1 mg/dL (baseline 0.7 mg/dL), LDH 1122 U/L, total bilirubin 1.4 mg/dL, and direct bilirubin 0.2 mg/dL. Initial peripheral smear shows rare schistocytes.

    A few hours later, he develops altered mental status consisting of word salad speech and an inability to follow commands. Peripheral smear shows increased schistocytes.

    How should this be managed?

    A. Fresh frozen plasma followed by observation
    B. Plasma exchange
    C. Platelet transfusion
    D. RBC transfusion

11. A 32-year-old African American woman presents with fatigue and dyspnea on exertion. She was given trimethoprim-sulfamethoxazole (TMP-SMX) for a urinary tract infection (UTI) 5 days ago. She looks pale and has a HR of 105 beats/min. Complete blood count (CBC) reveals Hb 6.0 g/dL and hematocrit 19%.

    What diagnostic test should be performed next?

    A. Flow cytometry
    B. Glucose-6-phosphate dehydrogenase (G6PD) testing
    C. Hb electrophoresis
    D. Osmotic fragility

12. An 88-year-old woman with a history of coronary artery disease (CAD) for which she had undergone coronary artery bypass graft surgery 10 years ago, atrial fibrillation on chronic warfarin therapy, hypertension, heart failure with preserved ejection fraction, and chronic kidney disease is brought to the emergency room (ER) by her family after a mechanical fall at home with a complaint of altered mental status.

    On examination, she is somnolent, but arousable to voice. A noncontrast head computed tomography (CT) is performed and demonstrates a 2-cm subdural hematoma with associated midline shift.

Laboratory studies	
Creatinine	1.9 mg/dL
Hb	12.5 g/dL
Platelets	205 000/μL
PT-INR	3.9
PTT	30 sec

    In addition to discontinuing warfarin and any antiplatelet therapy that the patient is receiving, which of the following is the most appropriate next step in treatment?

    A. Administer 4-factor prothrombin complex concentrate (4F-PCC)
    B. Administer 10 mg oral vitamin K
    C. Administer fresh frozen plasma
    D. Administer platelet transfusion
    E. Transfuse 1 unit packed RBCs

13. A 65-year-old man with hypertension, type 2 diabetes mellitus (T2DM) on insulin, CAD, and chronic kidney disease on dialysis presents to his hemodialysis clinic for his

scheduled dialysis treatment after missing his preceding two dialysis runs. On sitting down in the dialysis chair, he develops spontaneous epistaxis. The bleeding continues even after 40 minutes despite holding pressure.

On examination, the patient is twitching intermittently and is slow to respond but is oriented to person, place, and time.

Laboratory studies	
BUN	85 mg/dL
Creatinine	6 mg/dL
Hb	12.5 g/dL
Platelets	205 000/μL
PT-INR	1.0
PTT	30 sec

Which of the following best describes the etiology of the patient's abnormal hemostasis and the appropriate intervention?

A. Acquired platelet disorder; DDAVP (desmopressin acetate)
B. Acquired platelet disorder; discontinue insulin
C. Acquired platelet disorder; transfuse platelets
D. Inherited platelet disorder; DDAVP
E. Inherited platelet disorder; transfuse platelets

14. A 27-year-old man presents to the emergency department (ED) with a complaint of abdominal pain and lower extremity rash for 2 to 3 days. Although he has been drinking adequate fluids, he has been urinating less frequently.

On examination, there is a raised, purpuric rash over the bilateral lower extremities. Temperature is 37°C (98.6°F), blood pressure (BP) is 122/84 mmHg, pulse rate is 90/min and regular, and respiration rate is 18/min. Pulmonary examination reveals decreased breath sounds at the bases, and abdominal examination shows diffuse tenderness without rebound or guarding.

Laboratory studies	
BUN	45 mg/dL
Creatinine	2.6 mg/dL
AST	22 U/L
ALT	23 U/L
Total bilirubin	0.3 mg/dL
Alkaline phosphatase	102 U/L
Hb	10.5 g/dL
WBC count	9200/μL
Platelets	200 000/μL

Which of the following is the most appropriate diagnostic test to perform next?

A. Antineutrophil cytoplasmic antibody (ANCA) titer
B. Peripheral blood smear to evaluate for schistocytes
C. Renal biopsy with direct immunofluorescence microscopy and serum anti–glomerular basement membrane antibody
D. Renal ultrasound with Doppler
E. Skin biopsy with direct immunofluorescence microscopy

15. A 38-year-old African American woman with no significant PMH other than hypothyroidism presents to urgent care after a 10-day trip to England with a complaint of several days of weakness, abdominal pain, nausea, and low-grade fever.

On physical examination, the patient appears fatigued and has scattered petechiae over her bilateral shins. Her cardiac and pulmonary examinations are normal.

Laboratory studies	
BUN	18 mg/dL
Creatinine	0.95 mg/dL
AST	22 U/L
ALT	23 U/L
Total bilirubin	1.8 mg/dL
Direct bilirubin	0.4 mg/dL
LDH	807 U/L
Hb	9.2 g/dL
Direct antiglobulin (Coombs) test (DAT)	Negative
WBC count	7200/μL
Platelets	12 000/μL
Peripheral smear	Few platelets, three schistocytes per high power field (hpf)
ADAMTS13 assay	Pending

Which of the following is the most likely diagnosis?

A. Drug-induced thrombocytopenia
B. Evan syndrome
C. Hemolytic uremic syndrome (HUS)
D. Primary immune thrombocytopenia
E. Thrombotic thrombocytopenic purpura

16. A 55-year-old woman with a recent admission 4 weeks ago for appendectomy, during which she received prophylactic subcutaneous (SC) heparin, was admitted 2 days ago with shortness of breath on exertion and chest tightness. She was found on workup to have newly elevated troponin and ECG changes, consistent with non–ST elevation myocardial infarction. She was started on a heparin drip and has been awaiting coronary angiogram.

This morning, she complained of new right lower extremity pain and swelling and was found to have a deep vein thrombosis (DVT). On examination, she has bruising over the bilateral arms, swelling of the right lower extremity, and pain with dorsiflexion of the right foot.

Laboratory studies	
BUN	18 mg/dL
Creatinine	0.95 mg/dL
Hb	12.8 g/dL (13.2 g/dL on admission)
WBC count	7200/μL
Platelets	65 000/μL (155 000/μL on admission)

Which of the following is the most appropriate next step?

A. Continue heparin, send platelet factor 4 (PF4)-heparin enzyme-linked immunosorbent assay (ELISA)
B. Continue heparin, send serotonin release assay
C. Stop heparin, send PF4-heparin ELISA, start bivalirudin
D. Stop heparin, send PF4-heparin ELISA, start warfarin
E. Stop heparin, send serotonin release assay, await results before resuming anticoagulation

17. A 24-year-old man presents to his PCP's office with 1 week of spontaneous nose and gum bleeding. He otherwise feels well and recalls having an upper respiratory tract infection 3 weeks prior for which he took OTC nonsteroidal anti-inflammatory drugs (NSAIDs) for 1 to 2 days. He has never had similar symptoms in the past, and there is no family history of any bleeding diathesis. On examination, he has petechiae in his oral mucosa. Two 0.5-cm blood blisters are noted on his buccal mucosa.

CBC reveals WBC 7000/μL, normal differential, Hb 14 g/dL, platelets 4000/μL. Remaining blood work including renal and liver function tests (LFT) were within normal limits. Peripheral blood smear shows normal RBCs, WBCs, and decreased albeit large platelets.

What is the diagnosis in this case?

A. Acute lymphoid leukemia
B. Acute myelogenous leukemia (AML)
C. Ehrlichiosis
D. Immune thrombocytopenic purpura
E. NSAID-induced thrombocytopenia

18. How would you treat the patient in Question 17 in the acute setting?

A. Emergent splenectomy
B. Intravenous immunoglobulin (IVIG) + steroids
C. Platelet transfusion
D. Thrombopoietin agonist therapy (eg, romiplostim)
E. Watchful waiting for platelet recovery

19. A 54-year-old woman with hepatitis C and compensated cirrhosis is involved in a motor vehicle accident (MVA) and suffers a left femoral fracture needing urgent surgical exploration and fixation. Her labs show WBC 7000/μL (normal differential), Hb 11 g/dL, and platelets 40 000/μL. International normalized ratio (INR) is 1.3. Both Hb and platelets have been stable on a few lab checks ranging back to the last 6 months.

What blood products does this patient need prior to proceeding with surgery?

A. 2 U fresh frozen plasma and 10 mg IV vitamin K
B. 2 U fresh frozen plasma and platelet transfusion with a platelet goal >50 000/μL
C. No blood products necessary. Proceed with surgery
D. Platelet transfusion with a platelet goal >50 000/μL
E. Thrombopoietin agonist: Romiplostim 10 mg/kg SC × 1

20. In which of the following situations will DDAVP (intranasal or IV) NOT be an appropriate therapy for controlling bleeding?

A. End-stage renal disease
B. Mild hemophilia A
C. Mild type I von Willebrand disease (vWD)
D. Type 3 vWD

21. A previously healthy 45-year-old man with no PMH and taking no medications presented to the ED with severe substernal chest pain and was diagnosed with an anterior ST elevation myocardial infarction for which he underwent immediate percutaneous intervention with a drug-eluting stent to the proximal left anterior descending coronary artery. His course was complicated by cardiogenic shock requiring inotropes and an intra-aortic balloon pump placement. He was started on dual antiplatelet therapy with aspirin and ticagrelor and an IV unfractionated heparin drip at the time of the percutaneous coronary intervention. On day 2 of his admission, his platelet count was noted to be 70 000/μL, down from 180 000/μL on admission. Other blood counts were normal.

What is NOT a possible etiology of his thrombocytopenia?

A. Disseminated intravascular coagulation (DIC)
B. Intra-aortic balloon pump
C. Type 1 heparin-induced thrombocytopenia (HIT)
D. Type 2 HIT

22. A 62-year-old woman presents with weakness, fatigue, recurrent epistaxis, and a recent UTI currently being treated with ciprofloxacin. Physical examination shows dried blood in bilateral nares and scattered ecchymoses on her trunk, arms, and legs. Labs are notable for WBC 1200/μL, Hb 8 g/dL, platelets 31 000/μL, prothrombin time (PT) 20 seconds (normal 16 sec), INR 1.7 (normal 1.1), partial thromboplastin time (PTT) 41 seconds (normal 25-35 sec), D-dimer >3.0 μg/mL (normal <0.5 μg/mL), and fibrinogen 2.2 g/L (normal >2 g/L). Peripheral smear shows very rare large myeloid precursors with a high nucleus to cytoplasmic ratio, fine chromatin, bilobed nuclei, prominent nucleoli, and cytoplasmic granules.

Which of the following agents is most appropriate to administer?

A. Cryoprecipitate
B. IV vitamin K
C. PCC
D. Platelet transfusion

23. A 77-year-old man with atrial fibrillation on dabigatran presents with new right-sided weakness. Labs are notable for normal creatinine and an elevated INR. A head CT shows an intracerebral hemorrhage in the left frontal lobe. He last took dabigatran 3 hours before presentation.

Which of the following agents is most appropriate to administer?

A. Andexanet-alfa
B. Factor VIII inhibitor bypassing activity (FEIBA)
C. Fresh frozen plasma
D. Idarucizumab

24. A 17-year-old boy with severe hemophilia A has been on prophylactic factor VIII infusions over the last decade to reduce bleeding complications. However, over the past year he had five episodes of spontaneous hemarthrosis and was diagnosed with a high titer of factor VIII inhibitor.

What is the best prophylactic therapy to reduce his risk of bleeding?

A. Aminocaproic acid
B. Emicizumab
C. High-dose recombinant factor VIII
D. Recombinant factor IX
E. Recombinant factor VIIa

25. A 38-year-old man presents with 2 days of intermittent periumbilical to right upper quadrant pain with associated nausea and vomiting. He also reports a few weeks of fatigue, a faint yellowing of his skin, and episodes of dark urine at night. Physical examination reveals abdominal tenderness and distention.

Labs show WBC 2000/μL, hematocrit 24%, platelets 80 000/μL, reticulocytes 8%, LDH 960 U/L, total bilirubin 4 mg/dL, direct bilirubin 0.3 mg/dL, and a negative Coombs test. Abdominal CT with contrast shows a filling defect in the superior mesenteric vein with mesenteric stranding and bowel wall enhancement with no evidence of collateralization.

What diagnostic test will reveal the most likely underlying disorder?

A. Activated protein C resistance assay
B. Antithrombin III levels
C. Flow cytometry for CD55 and CD59
D. Protein C and S levels

26. A 25-year-old woman with hypothyroidism presents with new persistent weakness of her right hand. She notes transient episodes of right hand weakness over the past few weeks as well as a new rash on her lower extremities. Her current episode of right hand weakness is similar to her prior episodes except that it has now lasted a few hours longer than the other episodes, which lasted only minutes. Physical examination reveals 0/5 strength of her right hand and reticular erythema on her bilateral lower extremities.

Labs are notable for WBC 8000/μL, 75% neutrophils, hematocrit 36%, and platelets 110 000/μL. A head CT shows no acute intracranial hemorrhage, and a brain magnetic resonance imaging (MRI) shows a small ischemic infarction in the left precentral gyrus and multifocal white matter lesions. She is initially treated with recombinant tissue plasminogen activator with improvement in her right hand strength. She is subsequently started on a heparin drip and aspirin. Further testing reveals significantly elevated anticardiolipin and β-2-glycoprotein antibodies that remain elevated on repeat testing 3 months later.

Which long-term anticoagulation option is most appropriate for this patient?

A. Apixaban
B. Dabigatran
C. Enoxaparin
D. Warfarin

27. A 36-year-old man presents to a hematologist after discovering he has factor V Leiden, which was diagnosed on a commercial genetic test. He asks about starting anticoagulation to minimize his risk of developing a blood clot. He has no history of blood clots.

Which anticoagulation plan is indicated for this patient?

A. 6 months' anticoagulation
B. 12 months' anticoagulation
C. Lifelong anticoagulation
D. No anticoagulation

28. A 73-year-old man is referred to hematology for a persistently elevated WBC count of 20 000/μL for the past year with an absolute lymphocyte count of 9000/μL. He takes aspirin and atorvastatin and is otherwise healthy. He has had no recent illnesses. His liver and kidney function are normal on recent blood work. Lymph node examination is normal. Flow cytometry and molecular diagnostics result in a diagnosis of chronic lymphocytic leukemia.

What treatment is indicated at this time?

A. Ibrutinib
B. No treatment
C. Steroids
D. Venetoclax

29. A 69-year-old man presents to the hospital for acute myocardial infarction, for which he undergoes emergent balloon angioplasty and subsequent stent placement. His presenting WBC count was 13 000/µL with no eosinophils, but the day after his arrival, he is noted to have eosinophils to 500/µL and a rise in his creatinine to 2.0 mg/dL from a baseline of 1.0 mg/dL. LFTs remain normal.

What is the most likely cause of this eosinophilia?

A. Drug rash with eosinophilia and systemic symptoms (DRESS)
B. Infection
C. Microscopic cholesterol emboli
D. Myeloproliferative neoplasm

30. A 36-year-old woman with a history of seizure disorder on phenytoin presents to the clinic with dysuria and urinary frequency. She is diagnosed with UTI and is started on a course of TMP-SMX. Five days later, she comes back to the clinic for ongoing urinary symptoms. You check a CBC with differential which shows: WBC count of 3400/µL, Hb 12.1 g/dL, platelets 324 000/µL, and absolute neutrophil count (ANC) 620/µL. Two months ago, her CBC was normal.

What is the most likely explanation for this patient's neutropenia?

A. Cytomegalovirus (CMV) infection
B. Myelodysplastic syndrome
C. Drug reaction
D. Cyclic neutropenia

31. A 19-year-old man with no PMH sustains severe burns over 40% of his body in a house fire. He is admitted to the burn unit for supportive care with fluids and debridement. On hospital day 3, you note that his WBC count is elevated at 14 500/µL with an ANC of 11 000/µL. The rest of his CBC is normal. He has been tachycardic since admission and his BP has consistently been around 90/60 mmHg. His lactate level is 2.7. You send a broad infectious disease workup including blood cultures, CXR, and urinalysis, which are unrevealing.

What is the most likely explanation for this patient's neutrophilia?

A. Tissue necrosis
B. Bacterial infection
C. Congenital
D. Fungal infection

32. A 52-year-old woman is sent to the ER after routine outpatient blood testing identified a WBC count of 100 000/µL. Her kidney function, liver function, and electrolytes are all normal. She is mentating well and breathing room air. Uric acid and coagulation tests are normal. Examination of her blood under the microscope identifies basophilia and numerous left-shifted neutrophils.

What is the most likely diagnosis?

A. AML
B. Chronic myelogenous leukemia
C. *Strongyloides* infection
D. Systemic mastocytosis

33. A 36-year-old man with chronic lower gastrointestinal (GI) bleeds because of internal hemorrhoids despite multiple banding attempts by gastroenterology presents to the ED with significant fatigue. He is found to have an Hb of 6.8 and receives a transfusion of 1 unit of packed RBCs that is run over 1 hour. At the end of the transfusion he develops hives. He has no shortness of breath, wheezing, lip swelling, or voice hoarseness. The patient receives IV diphenhydramine and the hives resolve. The patient asks whether this will happen again if he needs another blood transfusion.

What is the most appropriate modification to make to the patient's future blood transfusions?

A. Premedicate with IV diphenhydramine
B. Run the blood transfusion more slowly
C. Order irradiated blood products only
D. Order washed blood products only

34. A 57-year-old man with polycystic kidney disease requiring a renal transplant last year on tacrolimus, azathioprine, and prednisone presents with a diverticular bleed. Labs are notable for Hb 6.2 g/dL.

Which of the following types of RBCs is the most appropriate to administer?

A. CMV-negative
B. Irradiated
C. Irradiated, CMV-negative, and leukoreduced
D. Leukoreduced

35. A 32-year-old man with sickle cell disease presents with faint jaundice, dark urine, and a low-grade fever. A week earlier, he had been admitted for a vaso-occlusive pain crisis and treated with pain medications, as well as a unit of packed RBCs for symptomatic anemia below his usual baseline. Labs are notable for Hb 6.1 g/dL (baseline 7-8 g/dL), direct bilirubin 0.3 mg/dL, indirect bilirubin 2.5 mg/dL (normal <1 mg/dL), LDH 400 U/L (normal 140-280 U/L), haptoglobin 20 mg/dL (normal 30-200 mg/dL), a positive Coombs test, and urinalysis trace positive for RBCs. He is started on IV fluids.

What is the most appropriate next step?

A. Consult the blood bank
B. Discharge home
C. Obtain blood cultures
D. Transfuse 1 unit packed RBCs

36. An 86-year-old woman with chronic obstructive pulmonary disease (COPD) on 2 L home O_2 and heart failure with preserved ejection fraction presents with coffee ground emesis. Initial physical examination is notable for a weight of 89 lb and a height of 5 feet. Baseline Hb was 9.7 g/dL from recent clinic visit. At presentation, Hb was 7.8 g/dL with drop to 5.8 g/dL, so she was transfused 3 units packed RBCs with appropriate Hb response to 8.8 g/dL. Around 6 hours later, she developed respiratory distress with desaturations to the 70s and hypertension with systolic BPs in the 180s. CXR showed new perihilar

fullness, indistinct pulmonary vasculature, and bibasilar patchy opacities. She was treated with Nitropaste, IV Lasix, and bilevel positive airway pressure (BiPAP) but continued to desaturate and so was transferred to the ICU.

What is the most likely etiology of her respiratory distress?

A. Acute hemolytic reaction
B. Anaphylactic transfusion reaction
C. Transfusion-associated circulatory overload
D. Transfusion-related acute lung injury

37. A 66-year-old woman with hypertension presents with fatigue and a wound on her left arm. She reports tripping over furniture in her house and falling onto her left arm with a resulting wound a few days ago. Physical examination reveals a laceration with a 2-cm area of surrounding erythema and warmth though without purulence.

Labs are notable for hematocrit 24%, reticulocytes 2%, WBC 3500/μL, ANC 600/μL, and platelets 120 000/μL. Folate, vitamin B12, and copper levels are normal, and an HIV test is negative. Peripheral smear reveals macro-ovalocytes, myelocytes, promyelocytes, and rare myeloblasts, as well as neutrophils with bilobed nuclei. Bone marrow biopsy demonstrates hypercellularity, mild fibrosis, increased abnormal megakaryocytes, and 2% myeloblasts. Cytogenetics shows deletion 11q with no other abnormalities.

Which of the following is NOT an appropriate treatment for this patient?

A. Allogeneic stem cell transplant
B. Azacitidine
C. Epoetin alfa
D. Cephalexin

38. For the patient in Question 37, which of the following is indicated for infection prophylaxis?

A. Live attenuated zoster vaccine
B. Pegfilgrastim
C. Pneumococcal vaccine every 5 years
D. Prophylactic cephalexin

39. A 61-year-old man who runs marathons presents with new dyspnea after running 3 to 5 miles for the past few weeks. He also reports more bruises on his legs and more frequent episodes of epistaxis. Physical examination reveals clear lungs and scattered ecchymoses on his lower extremities.

Labs are notable for hematocrit 22%, reticulocytes 1%, WBC 2900/μL, ANC 400/μL, and platelets 25 000/μL. Peripheral smear reveals macro-ovalocytes, myeloblasts, and neutrophils with bilobed nuclei. Bone marrow biopsy demonstrates hypercellularity, moderate fibrosis, dysplastic erythrocytes, and 5% myeloblasts. Cytogenetics shows deletions 3q and 7q with no other abnormalities.

Which of the following is an appropriate treatment for this patient?

A. Allogeneic stem cell transplant
B. Hypomethylating agents
C. Intensive chemotherapy
D. Targeted therapy with ivosidenib

40. A 45-year-old man presents to the hematology clinic after being diagnosed with an unprovoked DVT, for which he is now on therapeutic low-molecular-weight heparin. Initial testing was notable for low protein C and protein S levels. In clinic, he describes a chronic headache and tinnitus. He also has a constant burning sensation in his palms and soles.

Physical examination is remarkable for a red tint to his neck and face, a systolic flow murmur, and a BP of 170/90 mmHg. Labs are notable for WBC 12 000 /μL, Hb 17.5 g/dL, and hematocrit 50%. Erythropoietin levels are sent and return low. Meanwhile, testing for JAK2 mutations has been sent, and results are pending.

Which of the following will NOT be indicated in the patient's subsequent therapy?

A. Aspirin
B. Clopidogrel
C. Hydroxyurea
D. Phlebotomy

41. A 70-year-old woman with PMH significant for lupus presents to her PCP with fatigue and abdominal pain.

On examination, she is diaphoretic and tender to right upper quadrant palpation. Her labs are significant for Hb 6 g/dL, platelets 450 000/μL, and WBC 10 000/μL. A bone marrow biopsy identifies extensive fibrosis. No BCL-ABL translocation is identified.

What is the next indicated course of treatment?

A. Allogeneic stem cell transplant
B. Hydroxyurea
C. Observation
D. RBC transfusion

42. A 43-year-old man is undergoing a preoperative evaluation for knee surgery, during which he has a CBC sent and is found to have a platelet count of 500 000/μL. Further workup rules out secondary causes of thrombocytosis, and he is diagnosed with essential thrombocytosis with a calreticulin mutation. He lives at home with his husband and continues to work as an accountant. He plays golf every Sunday and sleeps comfortably during the night.

What is the most appropriate treatment for the patient's essential thrombocytosis?

A. Allogeneic stem cell transplant
B. Hydroxyurea
C. Low-dose aspirin
D. Observation

43. A 66-year-old man with hyperlipidemia and hypertension was diagnosed with essential thrombocythemia (ET) 3 years ago. Testing for *JAK2* mutations was negative, and he has been managed with observation only. Today, he presents to the ED with left-sided facial droop and is found to have had a stroke. Examination is otherwise notable for splenomegaly. Labs show a platelet count of 850 000/μL, Hb 11.2 g/dL, and WBC 15 100/μL. Examination of the peripheral blood smear reveals large hypogranular platelets and no blasts. He is admitted for further management of stroke. You are consulted for management of ET.

What do you recommend?

A. Start aspirin 81 mg daily
B. Start hydroxyurea
C. Start aspirin 81 mg daily and anticoagulation with a factor X inhibitor
D. Start anticoagulation with a factor X inhibitor
E. Start hydroxyurea and aspirin 81 mg daily
F. Continue to observe

44. A 28-year-old woman presents to her PCP with 4 weeks of progressive fatigue, recurrent upper respiratory infections, and frequent bruising. A CBC is performed and demonstrates the following:

Hb	8.2 g/dL
WBC count	2000/μL
ANC	320/μL
Platelets	38 000/μL

She is sent to the ED, where a peripheral smear is reviewed and demonstrates circulating blasts, scarce platelets, and decreased RBC count. A bone marrow biopsy is performed and demonstrates 38% blasts. Blasts were positive for CD13, CD33, and myeloperoxidase on flow cytometry, and a diagnosis of AML was made.

Which of the following sets of laboratory results from the patient's bone marrow would be consistent with a favorable prognosis in this patient?

   A. Cytogenetics: deletion 5, FLT3 internal tandem duplication (FLT3-ITD)
   B. Cytogenetics: Monosomy 5, 7
   C. Cytogenetics: t(9;22)
   D. Cytogenetics: t(8;21), NPM1+

45. A 58-year-old woman with a history of breast cancer at age 49, treated with radiation and chemotherapy, presents to the ED with fatigue, recurrent fevers, and bruising following minimal injury over the past several weeks. On examination, she appears fatigued and has ecchymoses over her bilateral lower extremities. Her lungs are clear and cardiac examination is normal. A CXR shows clear bilateral lung fields without infiltrate or mediastinal adenopathy.

Her laboratory workup is notable for CBC with ANC 550/μL, platelets 45 000/μL, and Hb 9.8 g/dL. The differential shows 10% circulating blasts. A bone marrow biopsy confirms the diagnosis of AML. Cytogenetics and karyotype demonstrate intermediate prognosis.

Which of the following is the most appropriate choice for induction chemotherapy?

   A. Liposomal cytarabine and daunorubicin on days 1, 3, and 5
   B. Reduced intensity therapy with decitabine and 5-azacytidine
   C. Standard induction therapy, "7 + 3" with cytarabine for 7 days and idarubicin or daunorubicin for 3 days
   D. Standard induction therapy, "7 + 3" with cytarabine for 7 days and idarubicin or daunorubicin for 3 days, plus gemtuzumab ozogamicin on days 1, 4, and 7
   E. Standard induction therapy, "7 + 3" with cytarabine for 7 days and idarubicin or daunorubicin for 3 days, plus oral midostaurin on days 8 through 21

46. A 65-year-old man is noted on preoperative workup for hip replacement to have neutropenia, anemia, and thrombocytopenia, with atypical promyelocytes on his peripheral smear. A bone marrow biopsy is performed and demonstrates atypical promyelocytes with Auer rods. Cytogenetic studies on the bone marrow are sent for rush diagnostics and demonstrate translocation of the retinoic acid receptor, t(15;17), consistent with a diagnosis of acute promyelocytic leukemia (PML).

The patient is admitted to the hospital and treatment with all-*trans*-retinoic acid (ATRA) and arsenic trioxide (ATO) is initiated within 24 hours. He is monitored closely for DIC over the next week and remains hemodynamically stable. On the eighth day of treatment, he complains of increased shortness of breath, and his examination is notable for fever to 38.5°C and hypotension with BP 85/45 mmHg. CXR is performed and demonstrates bilateral pulmonary infiltrates.

What is the most likely diagnosis and most appropriate next step in management?

A. Acute respiratory distress syndrome; treat with antibiotics and diuresis

B. Acute respiratory distress syndrome; treat with intubation and low tidal-volume ventilation

C. Differentiation syndrome; treat with daunorubicin plus ATRA consolidation therapy and supportive care

D. Differentiation syndrome; treat with dexamethasone 10 mg twice daily and supportive care

E. Differentiation syndrome; treat with supportive care alone

47. A 28-year-old woman with a 7-year history of chronic phase chronic myelogenous leukemia is treated with imatinib at 400 mg/day. She feels fine, and you note that her quantitative polymerase chain reaction (QT-PCR) has been undetectable for more than 3 years. She recently got married and now wants to try and conceive and asks you about discontinuing the imatinib.

How would you advise her at this point?

A. If she discontinues the imatinib, she will have a 20% chance of recurrence in 24 months

B. If she discontinues the imatinib, she will have a 60% chance of recurrence in 24 months

C. If she discontinues the imatinib, she will have an 80% chance of recurrence in 24 months

D. She can never safely discontinue the imatinib and must continue indefinitely because she will surely relapse

E. She can safely stop the imatinib without worry of recurrence because she is cured

48. A 43-year-old woman was diagnosed with Ph-negative pre-B-cell acute lymphoblastic leukemia (ALL) in 2014. The presenting WBC was 45 000/μL; and the cytogenetics were normal (fluorescence in situ hybridization [FISH] and PCR for BCR-ABL negative). Cerebrospinal fluid (CSF) studies were negative. She was treated with hyper-CVAD (cyclophosphamide, vincristine, adriamycin, dexamethasone). She has two sibling donors. She unfortunately relapses following completion of maintenance therapy.

A repeat bone marrow biopsy shows 75% lymphoblasts; cytogenetics remain normal. Immunophenotype is CD45(dim), CD34, HLA-DR, TdT, CD123(dim; subset), B lymphoid markers CD19 (100%), CD20(dim), CD10, CD22 (15%), aberrant expression of CD33(dim), but negative for surface immunoglobulin light chain and other myeloid markers, including myeloperoxidase.

How would you treat this patient with relapsed disease?

A. Blinatumomab

B. High-dose cytarabine (HiDAC)-containing regimen (eg, FLAG-Ida [fludarabine, cytarabine, granulocyte-colony stimulating factor (G-CSF), idarubicin], HAM [high-dose cytosine arabinoside and mitoxantrone])

C. Inotuzumab ozogamicin

D. Liposomal vincristine plus corticosteroids

49. A 32-year-old man presents to the local ED with 2 weeks of increasing fatigue, anorexia, and fevers to 100.6°F. This morning, he noted bleeding from his gums and developed dyspnea on walking. His symptoms progressed rapidly during the day, with worsening dyspnea and new dizziness. His labs in the ED showed: WBC 210 000/μL, Hb 7 g/dL, platelets 11 000/μL; electrolytes showed a K of 5.9 mEq/L; blood urea nitrogen (BUN) 60 mg/dL and creatinine 2.0 mg/dL; LDH 1600 U/L; uric acid 18 mg/dL. Review of peripheral blood smear shows abnormal cells with large nuclei, multiple nucleoli with fine chromatin consistent with blasts without any granules. Peripheral blood flow cytometry is 50% blasts positive for CD13, CD117 and negative for CD3, CD4, CD19, CD20, and TdT.

What is the diagnosis?

A. AML
B. B-cell ALL
C. Chronic myelogenous leukemia
D. T-cell ALL

50. What complications of acute leukemia could the patient in Question 49 likely have?

A. Leukostasis
B. Sepsis
C. Spontaneous tumor lysis syndrome
D. All of the above

51. A 34-year-old man with HIV is brought to the ED after having a new seizure. He has been undomiciled for the past several years, and he has not had a recent CD4 check. CT of his head identifies a mass, and further diagnostic tests confirm a central nervous system (CNS) lymphoma.

What is the patient's CD4 count (cells/mm³) most likely to be?

A. <50
B. <100
C. <200
D. <400

52. A 73-year-old woman presents to her PCP for routine evaluation, during which she is found to have a white count of 23 000/μL with a lymphocyte count of 6000/μL. Peripheral smear shows smudge cells, and further workup confirms a diagnosis of chronic lymphocytic leukemia. Physical examination is unremarkable, and labs are otherwise normal.

What is the most appropriate therapy for this patient's chronic lymphocytic leukemia?

A. Chemotherapy
B. Ibrutinib
C. Observation
D. Splenectomy

53. A 73-year-old woman presents to the ED with fever, new weight loss, and dramatic lymphadenopathy, most prominent in her right groin. She has known chronic lymphocytic leukemia, for which she has been taking ibrutinib daily.

Labs show a WBC count of 50 000/μL, LDH 500 U/L, uric acid 9 mg/dL, potassium 6 mEq/L, phosphate 6 mg/dL, calcium 6 mg/dL, and creatinine 3 mg/dL.

What is the most likely diagnosis?

A. Acute CMV
B. AML
C. Diffuse large B-cell lymphoma (DLBCL)
D. Stage 4 chronic lymphocytic leukemia

54. A 29-year-old woman with a history of papillary thyroid carcinoma, for which she underwent total thyroidectomy 1 year earlier, presents to her PCP with a new right supraclavicular mass. A CT of the chest with contrast demonstrates a 1.5 × 3.2-cm enlarged right supraclavicular lymph node and multiple enlarged mediastinal lymph nodes, each measuring <2 cm without mass effect on the surrounding structures.

In addition to excisional lymph node biopsy, which of the following are required to complete staging?

A. CT abdomen/pelvis with contrast; bone marrow biopsy
B. CT abdomen/pelvis with contrast; bone marrow biopsy; head CT or MRI
C. Positron emission tomography (PET)-CT scan; bone marrow biopsy
D. PET-CT scan; bone marrow biopsy; head CT or MRI

55. The 29-year-old woman in Question 54 is found to have nodular sclerosis–type Hodgkin lymphoma on her excisional right supraclavicular lymph node biopsy. PET-CT demonstrates mediastinal involvement, with low-volume lymphadenopathy encasing several vascular structures, including the right pulmonary artery, without evidence of disease below the diaphragm. Bone marrow biopsy is negative for involvement with lymphoma. She has confirmed stage 2 disease.

Which of the following would be the most appropriate initial step in management?

A. ABVD (doxorubicin, bleomycin, vinblastine, dacarbazine) and repeat PET-CT after 2 cycles
B. Brentuximab-vedotin (antibody-drug conjugate against CD30) × 6 cycles
C. Escalated BEACOPP (bleomycin, etoposide, doxorubicin, cyclophosphamide, vincristine, procarbazine, and prednisone) for 6 cycles
D. Involved field radiation to neck
E. Pembrolizumab (anti–programmed cell death protein 1 [PD-1] monoclonal antibody [mAb]) × 6 cycles

56. A 55-year-old woman with a history of stage 4 Hodgkin lymphoma treated with 6 cycles of ABVD (doxorubicin, bleomycin, vinblastine, dacarbazine) at age 25 presents to establish care. She feels overall well, but complains of fatigue, slight dyspnea on exertion walking uphill, and weight gain of 15 lb over the past 6 weeks.

In addition to CBC with differential, which of the following would be the most appropriate initial workup specific to this patient's risk factors?

A. CXR, echocardiogram, pulmonary function tests
B. CXR, echocardiogram, pulmonary function tests, 8 AM cortisol
C. CXR, echocardiogram, thyroid-stimulating hormone (TSH), and free thyroxine (T4)
D. Mammography, CXR, pulmonary function tests
E. Mammography, echocardiogram, pulmonary function tests, TSH and free T4, 8 AM cortisol

57. A 47-year-old man with newly diagnosed diffuse large B-cell lymphoma presents to the oncology clinic for consideration of initial therapy options. He previously underwent an excisional lymph node biopsy of an enlarged axillary lymph node, prompted by cytopenias in routine blood work. Molecular studies show no rearrangements of MYC, BCL2, and BCL6. He underwent a staging PET-CT scan, which showed fluorodeoxyglucose (FDG)-avid disease only within lymph nodes in his right axillary and hilar mediastinal lymph nodes. His Eastern Cooperative Oncology Group (ECOG) performance status is 0. His LDH is 150 U/L.

Which of the following treatment regimens is the most appropriate initial therapy?

A. R-CHOP (rituximab, cyclophosphamide, doxorubicin, vincristine, prednisone)

B. DA-R-EPOCH (dose-adjusted rituximab, etoposide, prednisone, vincristine, cyclophosphamide, doxorubicin)

C. Chimeric antigen receptor T-cell (CAR-T) therapy (lisocabtagene, axicabtagene, or tisagenlecleucel)

D. ABVD (doxorubicin, bleomycin, vinblastine, dacarbazine)

58. A 76-year-old man presents to his PCP with fatigue, 20-lb unintentional weight loss, and several weeks of dark stool. He is found to have anemia with Hb of 8.8 g/dL. He is referred for endoscopy, which reveals a nonbleeding mass in the stomach. Biopsy reveals a clonal B-cell population with immunophenotype consistent with extranodal marginal zone lymphoma. *Helicobacter pylori* testing on the sample is positive.

Which of the following is the most appropriate next step in management?

A. Quadruple therapy for treatment of the *H. pylori* (bismuth, metronidazole, tetracycline, omeprazole)

B. Quadruple therapy for treatment of the *H. pylori* (bismuth, metronidazole, tetracycline, omeprazole) with concurrent involved-site radiation

C. Quadruple therapy for treatment of the *H. pylori* (bismuth, metronidazole, tetracycline, omeprazole) with concurrent rituximab plus bendamustine

D. Rituximab plus bendamustine followed by quadruple therapy for treatment of the *H. pylori* (bismuth, metronidazole, tetracycline, omeprazole)

E. Rituximab plus quadruple therapy for treatment of the *H. pylori* (bismuth, metronidazole, tetracycline, omeprazole)

59. A 78-year-old man presents to the ED with a complaint of severe left hip pain over the past 2 weeks. His family also reports that he has had decreased urine output, fatigue, and several episodes of confusion. On examination, the patient appears his stated age and is lying in bed, leaning to his right side because of pain in the left hip.

Laboratory studies	
BUN	45 mg/dL
Creatinine	3.5 mg/dL
Calcium	13.5 mg/dL
Hb	8.2 g/dL
WBC count	7200/μL
Platelets	185 000/μL
Serum free light chains	
κ	1500 mg/dL
λ	19.4 mg/dL
SPEP M-protein component	8 g/dL
Immunofixation	Monoclonal IgG-κ chain component of M spike

Which of the following are the next steps in diagnosis?

A. PET/CT chest/abdomen/pelvis

B. Bone marrow biopsy with cytogenetics and gene mutation analysis; skeletal survey

C. Peripheral blood cytogenetics; skeletal survey; PET/CT chest/abdomen/pelvis

D. Repeat serum protein electrophoresis (SPEP), serum free light chain assay, and immunofixation in 6 months

E. Repeat SPEP, serum free light chain assay, and immunofixation in 6 weeks

60. A 75-year-old man with a history of hypertension, T2DM, and hyperlipidemia undergoes preoperative laboratory workup prior to hernia repair. The complete metabolic panel demonstrates an elevated globulin gap, so his PCP sends serum free light chains, SPEP, and urine protein electrophoresis (UPEP) with immunofixation. On the SPEP, the M-protein spike is 0.8 g/dL; the serum free light chains show a $\kappa:\lambda$ ratio of 5, with elevated free κ light chain level. UPEP shows total protein <167 mg/24 hours and urine albumin <5 mg/dL. The creatinine is 0.8 mg/dL.

Which of the following most accurately represents this patient's risk of progression to multiple myeloma, Waldenström macroglobulinemia, or a malignant lymphoproliferative disease?

A. 0.5% per year; 10% lifetime risk
B. 1% per year; 25% lifetime risk
C. 4% per year; 50% lifetime risk
D. 10% per year; 80% lifetime risk
E. The patient already has multiple myeloma

61. A 68-year-old woman with no significant PMH is brought in by her husband to the ED for fatigue, mucosal bleeding, decreased appetite, new lower extremity rash, and decreased perfusion to her distal fingers and toes over the preceding 2 weeks. In addition, over the 2 days preceding admission, she developed headache, dizziness, blurry vision, decreased alertness, and shortness of breath. On physical examination, she is noted to have hepatomegaly extending 3 cm below the right costal margin. She is fatigued with decreased alertness and arousable only to loud sound or sternal rub. She is evaluated by dermatology for the lower extremity rash because of concern for vasculitis and is diagnosed with type I cryoglobulinemia.

Laboratory studies	
SPEP with immunofixation	IgM monoclonal spike 7 g/dL
UPEP	Negative
Creatinine	1.0 mg/dL
Hb	9 g/dL
Platelets	52 000/μL

Bone marrow biopsy shows increased plasmacytoid lymphocytes.

Which of the following is the most likely explanation for the patient's symptoms of confusion, headache, dizziness, blurred vision, and shortness of breath?

A. Amyloidosis secondary to immunoglobulin M (IgM) deposition
B. Anemia and hypercalcemia
C. Autoantibody activity of IgM
D. Hyperviscosity syndrome
E. Local tumor infiltration

62. A 75-year-old man with a history of CAD presents for follow-up after a recent diagnosis of anemia. In addition to fatigue related to his anemia, he complains of a tingling sensation and burning pain in the feet, extending up to the mid-calf. This discomfort limits his mobility, and he has difficulty sleeping because of the pain. Laboratory workup for his anemia is shown below:

Laboratory studies	
SPEP with immunofixation	IgM monoclonal spike 7 g/dL
UPEP	Negative
IgM	4895 mg/dL (normal 40-230 mg/dL)
Creatinine	0.8 mg/dL
Hb	10.2 g/dL
Platelets	105 000/µL
Viscosity	1.7 cP (normal 1.4-1.8 cP)

A bone marrow biopsy is performed and demonstrates 65% bone marrow involvement with monoclonal plasmacytoid lymphocytes. He is told that his overall presentation is consistent with a diagnosis of Waldenström macroglobulinemia.

Which of the following is the next best step in management?

A. Observation with repeat labs and clinical examination every 3 months

B. Start bendamustine + rituximab

C. Start bortezomib + dexamethasone + rituximab

D. Stem cell collection in preparation for autologous stem cell transplant

E. Urgent plasmapheresis

63. A 72-year-old woman presents for preoperative evaluation prior to left total hip arthroplasty. She has a long-standing history of osteoarthritis of the left hip after a skiing accident many years ago, and her most recent left hip x-ray demonstrates severe degenerative changes with joint space narrowing, without evidence of fracture. She has not seen a PCP in 4 years, so a comprehensive metabolic panel and CBC are performed. Pertinent results are shown below:

Laboratory studies	
Creatinine	0.8 mg/dL
Calcium	8.8 mg/dL
Alkaline phosphatase	124 mg/dL
Total bilirubin	0.8 mg/dL
Albumin	4.0 g/dL
Total protein	9.5 g/dL
WBCs	5800/µL
Hb	13.2 g/dL
Platelets	252 000/µL

Based on the elevated total protein, additional laboratory workup and bone marrow biopsy are performed to evaluate for an underlying hematologic disorder. SPEP with immunofixation demonstrates M-protein elevated at 4 g/dL, serum free κ light chain 200 mg/L, serum λ free light chain 2.5 mg/L, κ/λ ratio 80:1. Bone marrow biopsy demonstrates 15% clonal plasma cells. Bone scan demonstrates no lytic lesions.

Which of the following is the most appropriate diagnosis?

A. Amyloid light chain amyloidosis

B. Monoclonal gammopathy of unknown significance (MGUS)

C. Multiple myeloma

D. Nonsecretory multiple myeloma

E. Smoldering multiple myeloma

64. A 65-year-old man presents with new right shoulder pain for the past month. He is active and works out at the local gym five times per week, so he initially attributed the discomfort to muscle strain after lifting weights. However, the pain worsened over the subsequent days. He is referred for CT of the shoulder, which demonstrates a large destructive osseous lesion involving the upper part of the humerus with an enhancing extraosseous soft-tissue component. CT-guided biopsy of the lesion is performed, and pathology demonstrates clonal proliferation of plasma cells. Bone scan demonstrates no other bony abnormalities. Bone marrow biopsy shows normal trilineage hematopoiesis without abnormal plasma cell clonal proliferation.

Laboratory studies	
Creatinine	0.8 mg/dL
Calcium	9.0 mg/dL
Albumin	4.0 g/dL
Hb	12.9 g/dL
Platelets	198 000/µL
SPEP with immunofixation	Normal, no M spike

Which of the following is the most appropriate next step in management?

A. Combination induction chemotherapy with lenalidomide and dexamethasone (RD)
B. Combination induction chemotherapy with lenalidomide, bortezomib, and dexamethasone (RVD)
C. Observation and physical therapy referral
D. Referral to radiation oncology for radiation to the right humerus osseous lesion
E. Stem cell collection followed by high-dose melphalan and autologous stem cell transplant

65. A 62-year-old man is admitted to the hospital from clinic for management of poorly controlled bone pain. He has numerous lytic metastases throughout the lumbar and sacral spine, the bilateral femoral heads, and the pelvic bones, related to his recently diagnosed multiple myeloma. His pain is controlled with a patient-controlled analgesia (PCA), and the decision is made to proceed with treatment for his multiple myeloma during the hospitalization, in view of his pain.

Laboratory studies	
Hb	10.2 g/dL
Creatinine	1.8 mg/dL
Calcium	9.0 mg/dL (after 2 L normal saline)

Based on his age and functional status, it is determined that he would be a transplant candidate.

In addition to denosumab, which of the following would be the most appropriate initial therapy for the treatment of this patient's multiple myeloma?

A. Bortezomib/lenalidomide/dexamethasone
B. Doxorubicin/lenalidomide/dexamethasone
C. Human leukocyte antigen typing to find a match, followed by allogeneic stem cell transplant with myeloablative conditioning
D. Pomalidomide/cyclophosphamide/dexamethasone
E. Stem cell harvest, followed by high-dose melphalan conditioning and autologous stem cell transplant

66. A 35-year-old previously healthy man was found to have AML with myelomonocytic differentiation. The karyotype was normal. Leukemic cells showed a *FLT3-ITD* mutation and wild-type *NPM1*. Complete remission has been achieved following "3+7" (daunorubicin/cytarabine) induction chemotherapy. The CBC is now normal.

Which of the following treatment approaches would you recommend now?

A. 1 to 2 cycles of HiDAC, followed by myeloablative allogeneic transplant from his sibling
B. 3 to 4 cycles of HiDAC plus FLT3 inhibitor
C. 3 to 4 cycles of HiDAC, then observation
D. Myeloablative conditioning followed by allogeneic transplant from his sibling
E. Reduced intensity conditioning followed by allogeneic transplant from his sibling

67. A 34-year-old woman who, 2 weeks earlier, underwent a matched unrelated peripheral stem cell transplant for AML develops a new fever to 102°F. She had previously been breathing normally on room air, but shortly after the fever, her oxygenation falls, and she is soon on a nonrebreather at 15 L. CXR shows diffuse bilateral opacities. Physical examination reveals a diffuse erythrodermatous rash over her torso, arms, and upper thighs.

Labs are significant for a creatinine of 1.2 mg/dL (baseline 0.7), WBC 4000/µL (ANC 600/µL), Hb 7.1 g/dL, and platelets 73 000/µL. Blood and urine cultures are drawn.

What is the most appropriate approach to therapy?

A. G-CSF
B. Remove all lines and start broad-spectrum antibiotics
C. Steroids
D. Tocilizumab

68. A 76-year-old man is undergoing matched related donor allogeneic stem cell transplant for AML. He had positive CMV IgG titers in his pretransplant lab work; his donor was found to be CMV IgG negative. Today is day +21 of his transplant and his ANC is 2400/µL. You are preparing his discharge medication list.

What prophylactic medications are reasonable for him to continue after leaving the hospital?

A. Fluconazole, atovaquone, acyclovir, and ciprofloxacin
B. Fluconazole, atovaquone, letermovir, and allopurinol
C. Fluconazole, atovaquone, acyclovir, and letermovir
D. Fluconazole, atovaquone, acyclovir, valganciclovir, and ciprofloxacin
E. Fluconazole, atovaquone, valganciclovir, and ciprofloxacin

69. A 53-year-old man received mismatched related peripheral stem cell transplant two and a half months earlier for chronic myelogenous leukemia blast crisis. He was discharged from the hospital after a few posttransplant complications. He returns to clinic, however, complaining of increasing diarrhea.

Inspection of his skin reveals a maculopapular rash on both extremities. Labs are drawn and are significant for K 3.0 mEq/L, total bilirubin 2.3 mg/dL, and creatinine 1.1 mg/dL.

What is the most likely diagnosis?

A. Acute graft-versus-host disease (GVHD)
B. Chronic GVHD
C. CMV colitis
D. Engraftment syndrome

70. A 44-year-old man who underwent a matched related peripheral stem cell transplant 12 days ago begins to complain of abdominal distention. Examination reveals a new fluid wave, peripheral edema, and tenderness to right upper quadrant palpation. Cardiac examination is unremarkable. He is noted to have gained 5 lb since his last measurement 2 days earlier. He has no skin rashes, and his stool output has remained formed.

Labs are significant for aspartate transaminase (AST) 220 U/L, alanine transaminase (ALT) 330 U/L, bilirubin 6 mg/dL (direct 5.5), WBC 9000/μL, Hb 8 g/dL, platelets 70 000/μL, INR 1.3, and N-terminal pro b-type natriuretic peptide (NT-proBNP) 100 pg/mL. Right upper quadrant ultrasound is unremarkable.

What is the most likely diagnosis?

A. Acute GVHD
B. Budd-Chiari syndrome
C. Congestive heart failure
D. Sinusoidal obstruction syndrome

71. A 62-year-old woman with a 35-pack-year smoking history, COPD, and CAD is admitted with increased cough productive of bloody sputum, thought to be consistent with a COPD exacerbation. She reports that she has been feeling unwell for the past month with decreased appetite and 10-lb unintentional weight loss. On examination, she has decreased breath sounds at the right lung base and expiratory wheezing throughout the bilateral lung fields. She has temporal and supraclavicular wasting. A CT of the chest with contrast is performed and demonstrates a right middle lobe tumor measuring 6 cm. A CT-guided biopsy of the mass is performed and confirms the diagnosis of non–small cell lung cancer (NSCLC).

Which of the following are the most appropriate next steps in diagnosis and management?

A. FDG PET/CT and brain MRI; pending results, follow with mediastinal lymph node evaluation with endobronchial ultrasound and mediastinoscopy
B. Initiate chemotherapy with platinum doublet and adjuvant radiation therapy
C. Initiate concurrent pembrolizumab and radiation therapy
D. Initiate definitive chemotherapy/radiation therapy followed by adjuvant durvalumab
E. Surgical debulking followed by chemotherapy and radiation therapy

72. A 58-year-old man, nonsmoker, with no significant PMH, presents to the ED complaining of fatigue, abdominal pain, and light-headedness over the past 48 hours. On physical examination, he appears fatigued with supraclavicular and temporal wasting. His infectious disease workup is negative. A cosyntropin stimulation test demonstrates adrenal insufficiency, and the patient undergoes CT of the abdomen/pelvis, adrenal protocol, for further evaluation. The scan demonstrates adrenal metastases of unknown primary with intrahepatic and bony metastases. Further workup with CT of the chest reveals a large primary lung mass. A biopsy of the adrenal lesion confirms lung adenocarcinoma. The tumor specimen is sent for analysis for genetic mutations in epidermal growth factor receptor (EGFR), anaplastic lymphoma kinase, ROS1, and BRAF and demonstrates an exon 19 deletion in eGFR.

Which of the following is the most appropriate treatment plan for this patient?

A. Carboplatin, pemetrexed, and crizotinib
B. Carboplatin, paclitaxel, and osimertinib
C. Carboplatin, pemetrexed, and pembrolizumab
D. Osimertinib alone
E. Pembrolizumab alone

73. A 69-year-old woman with a 50-pack-year history of smoking and a diagnosis of COPD presents to establish care with a PCP for increased cough productive of sputum over the past several months. She has a friend who was recently diagnosed with lung cancer and inquires about screening chest CT. A CT of her chest is performed and demonstrates a large cavitary lung mass with bony and intra-abdominal metastases. She undergoes CT-guided biopsy and is diagnosed with squamous cell carcinoma, lung primary.

Which of the following is the most appropriate therapy for stage 4 squamous cell carcinoma with PD-L1 staining <50%?

   A. Carboplatin and paclitaxel alone
   B. Carboplatin and pemetrexed alone
   C. Carboplatin, paclitaxel, and pembrolizumab
   D. Carboplatin, pemetrexed, and pembrolizumab
   E. Pembrolizumab alone

74. A 63-year-old woman with a 30-pack-year smoking history is admitted to the hospital with shortness of breath. The admission CXR shows a large pleural effusion on her right side. She undergoes thoracentesis with improvement in her respiratory status. Pathology from her pleural fluid shows a malignant effusion. A CT scan of her lungs after drainage of the pleural effusion shows a 3.5 cm right middle lobe spiculated mass but no mediastinal lymphadenopathy. Additional imaging showed no metastatic disease in her brain or abdomen. Her lung mass is biopsied and pathology is consistent with squamous cell carcinoma.

What is the best treatment for this patient?

   A. Surgical resection of the lung mass
   B. Definitive chemoradiation
   C. Stereotactic body radiation therapy to the lung mass
   D. Systemic therapy

75. A 50-year-old woman with no smoking history presents to the oncology clinic with a new suspected diagnosis of metastatic cancer. Her only symptoms are fatigue and weight loss. On imaging, she has masses in her liver, multiple enlarged mediastinal lymph nodes, and a left lung mass. Her brain MRI showed no metastatic disease. She undergoes a CT-guided biopsy of one of her liver lesions. The pathology service notifies you a few days later that the biopsy shows adenocarcinoma consistent with a lung primary.

What is the most appropriate next step?

   A. Start chemotherapy
   B. Start immunotherapy
   C. Arrange for biopsy of the lung mass to confirm diagnosis
   D. Request molecular diagnostic testing

76. A 63-year-old woman is brought into the hospital after a generalized seizure. She has no history of neurologic illness, and this is her first seizure. Noncontrast head CT is negative for acute processes or tumors. Her sodium is measured at 111 mEq/L. She does not drink alcohol and has smoked one pack of cigarettes a day for the past 40 years.

In addition to sodium studies, what diagnostic imaging should be performed to diagnose the cause of her hyponatremia?

   A. Brain magnetic resonance angiography (MRA)
   B. Brain MRI
   C. Carotid ultrasound
   D. Chest CT

77. A 50-year-old woman presents to her PCP for her annual physical. She has high BP and a history of depression but is otherwise in good health. Her PCP refers her for her first screening colonoscopy. The patient asks if she should also be referred for lung cancer screening. She has been smoking one pack per day for the past 30 years.

When should her PCP refer her for lung cancer screening?

A. Today
B. In 5 years
C. In 10 years
D. No referral indicated

78. A 41-year-old premenopausal woman identifies a lump in her right breast. She goes to her PCP, who refers her for imaging and a subsequent biopsy. She is ultimately diagnosed with a small (0.8 mm), node-negative, low-grade estrogen receptor–positive (ER+) breast cancer with a low Oncotype DX score.

After surgery and radiation, what is the standard systemic therapy for this patient?

A. Anastrozole
B. Lapatinib
C. Tamoxifen
D. Trastuzumab

79. A 53-year-old woman with a history of hormone receptor–positive breast cancer treated 15 years ago presents to her PCP with abdominal pain. Imaging reveals multiple liver lesions, the biopsy of which identifies metastatic ER+/PR+/HER2− breast cancer.

Which of the following is NOT a therapeutic option?

A. Anastrozole
B. Everolimus
C. Lapatinib
D. Palbociclib

80. A 52-year-old woman has a suspicious mass identified on mammogram. A stereotactically guided biopsy identifies breast cancer, and further diagnostics confirm the cancer to be ER−/PR−/HER2+. She undergoes a lumpectomy and sentinel lymph node biopsy. The tumor is 3 cm, and the sentinel lymph nodes are negative.

Which is the most appropriate adjuvant therapy?

A. Docetaxel, cyclophosphamide, trastuzumab, pertuzumab
B. Letrozole plus ribociclib
C. Neratinib
D. T-DM1

81. A 40-year-old woman presents to breast clinic with a new ER+/PR+/HER2− breast cancer. Her mother was diagnosed with breast cancer at age 38, her maternal aunt developed ovarian cancer at age 63, and her maternal grandfather died of pancreatic cancer.

What is the germline mutation most likely underlying these four cancers in the same family?

A. BRCA1
B. BRCA2
C. MLH1
D. TP53

82. A 75-year-old woman presents to her PCP for her annual physical. She has been undergoing biennial mammogram screenings since she was 50 years old, and her last was at age 73. She has always had normal mammograms and is having no breast complaints.

When is her next mammogram due?

A. This year
B. 1 year
C. 5 years
D. No further mammograms indicated

83. A 53-year-old woman presents to the ER with abdominal pain and is found to have a liver mass on CT. Subsequent biopsy identifies a new triple-negative breast cancer. Mammogram identifies the primary tumor in her left breast. She presents to her oncologist to discuss treatment plans. Meanwhile, PD-L1 testing on her tumor has returned positive. She has seen advertising for immunotherapy on TV and would like to know if this is an option for her.

What will her oncologist recommend?

A. Considering a clinical trial of immunotherapy, as there is currently no approved immunotherapy agent for breast cancer
B. Considering immunotherapy in combination with chemotherapy if she fails first-line therapy
C. Starting treatment with immunotherapy alone
D. Starting treatment with immunotherapy in combination with chemotherapy first line

84. A 77-year-old man with a history of hypertension, hyperlipidemia, CAD on medical management, and mild chronic kidney disease presents to the ER with 2 to 3 months of increasing back pain, decreased appetite, and 10-lb weight loss. Examination reveals an elderly man with focal spinal tenderness on the lower back. Rectal examination reveals an enlarged, hard, and nodular right prostate lobe. His labs are significant for an Hb of 9 g/dL and a prostate-specific antigen (PSA) of 4000 ng/mL. His ECOG performance status is 2. A bone scan shows extensive metastatic disease in the entire axial skeleton, and a CT scan shows enlarged pelvic and retroperitoneal lymph nodes measuring up to 3 cm. A biopsy of the retroperitoneal lymph node shows prostatic adenocarcinoma.

What is the best up-front therapy for this patient?

A. 2 weeks of bicalutamide followed by leuprolide
B. 2 weeks of bicalutamide followed by leuprolide and docetaxel
C. Degarelix and abiraterone/prednisone
D. Docetaxel
E. Leuprolide

85. A 67-year-old very active and healthy man has a PSA checked, which returns at 6. On repeat testing 3 months later, the PSA is 6.1. He meets with a urologist to discuss these results. On rectal examination, he has a smooth but enlarged prostate without any nodules or abnormalities. The patient is quite hesitant to have invasive testing.

What is the next best step in management?

A. Likely secondary to benign prostatic hyperplasia (BPH). No further testing
B. Proceed with ultrasound-guided transrectal 12-core prostate biopsy
C. Prostate MRI
D. Repeat PSA in 6 months

86. The man in Question 85 undergoes a prostate MRI, which shows a small 4-mm lesion in the right prostatic lobe, for which he undergoes two targeted core needle biopsies. About 10% of one of the two cores shows Gleason 6 (3 + 3) prostate cancer. What is the next best step for management? Given his active lifestyle, he is very concerned about his quality of life and treatment-related toxicities.

    Which treatment is associated with the LEAST amount of morbidity?

    A. Active surveillance
    B. Brachytherapy
    C. External beam radiation therapy
    D. Robotic or laparoscopic radical prostatectomy

87. A 63-year-old man with a PSA of 10.6 and Grade Group 2 prostate cancer undergoes radical prostatectomy. He has no adverse features noted and no lymph node metastases on pathology. His PSA falls to undetectable levels 6 months after his prostatectomy, but his PSA level rises to 0.7 ng/ml after 12 months and 2.3 ng/mL after 18 months. He remains asymptomatic and continues to walk 2 miles each day. He has not yet been initiated on any androgen deprivation therapy (ADT). He undergoes a technetium-99m-methylene diphosphonate (MDP) bone scan, which is equivocal for the presence of bony disease.

    What is the most appropriate next step in management?

    A. Continued monitoring of PSA values at 6-month intervals as the PSA is not yet high enough to count as biochemical recurrence
    B. Axumin scan to assess for bone and soft-tissue metastases with subsequent ADT versus salvage radiotherapy and ADT
    C. CT chest, abdomen, and pelvis with and without contrast to assess for bone and soft-tissue metastases with subsequent salvage ADT
    D. MRI brain to assess for occult intracranial disease with plans for subsequent stereotactic radiosurgery if there are limited sites of spread

88. An 18-year-old man presents to a new PCP after transitioning away from his pediatrician. On speaking with the patient, the physician learns that he has a strong family history of cancers: his father developed pancreatic cancer at age 50, his paternal aunt developed colon cancer at age 40, and his paternal grandmother developed endometrial cancer at age 50. His germline mutation analysis reveals a MSH2 mutation.

    At what age should this patient start colon cancer screening and at what frequency?

    A. Colonoscopy at age 20, then repeat screen yearly
    B. Colonoscopy at age 20, then repeat screen every 5 years
    C. Colonoscopy at age 30, then repeat screen yearly
    D. Colonoscopy at age 30, then repeat screen every 5 years

89. A 73-year-old man with a PMH of hypertension and hyperlipidemia presents to his PCP with new fatigue. He gets winded walking upstairs and is losing his energy. He used to go to the grocery store and was able to walk the aisles, but now he is getting too tired and needs to sit on a motorized cart. Basic labs are sent, which are significant for an Hb of 7.2 g/dL (baseline 10 g/dL).

    After ruling out cardiac etiologies, he is sent for a colonoscopy, which identifies a 2-cm mass in his ascending colon. Biopsy confirms adenocarcinoma. He is referred for surgical removal but prior to this step is sent for further testing.

Which of the following are indicated at this time?

A. Carcinoembryonic antigen (CEA) level
B. CT chest/abdomen/pelvis
C. MRI brain
D. A and B
E. All of the above

90. A previously healthy and active 58-year-old man was found to have a 2-cm mass in his transverse colon on screening colonoscopy. Biopsy was consistent with adenocarcinoma of the colon. He underwent screening CT scans of the chest, abdomen, and pelvis, which revealed several metastatic lesions in the liver and a few lung nodules. He is following up with you in clinic today to review the results of the molecular testing on his tumor tissue, which was notable for high microsatellite instability (MSI-H), *KRAS*wt, and *BRAF*wt.

What do you recommend for treatment?

A. FOLFOX (folinic acid, fluorouracil [5-FU], oxaliplatin) + cetuximab (anti-EGFR mAb)
B. FOLFOX + bevacizumab (anti-VEGF mAb)
C. Pembrolizumab
D. FOLFIRI (folinic acid, 5-FU, irinotecan)
E. FOLFOXIRI (folinic acid, 5-FU, irinotecan, and oxaliplatin)

91. A 44-year-old man presents for his annual physical. He has prediabetes and hyperlipidemia. He tells you that he has recently felt easily winded with exercise and can no longer run as far as he used to. His ECG in the office is notable for frequent PVCs. You order a CBC, which reveals an Hb of 9.3 g/dL with an MCV of 78. He tells you that his father was diagnosed with colon cancer at age 60, and his mother has diabetes. He otherwise has no significant family history. He has never had a screening test for colon cancer.

What do you recommend to him for colon cancer screening?

A. Flexible sigmoidoscopy
B. Fecal occult blood testing (guaiac cards)
C. DNA fecal immunochemical testing (FIT)
D. Colonoscopy
E. None of the above. He is too young to start colon cancer screening.

92. A 45-year-old man is diagnosed with resectable pancreatic adenocarcinoma. He is treated appropriately and is seen for follow-up and survivorship. He is concerned about his two children, ages 11 and 15, because he has a strong family history of cancer, including breast cancer in his mother, breast cancer in his maternal aunt, ovarian cancer in his maternal aunt, and prostate cancer in his maternal grandfather. He inquires about genetic testing in order to better understand the risk of cancer for his children.

Which of the following is the most likely hereditary risk factor for pancreatic cancer in this family?

A. Familial atypical multiple mole melanoma (*CDKN2A*/p16)
B. Familial breast/ovarian cancer (*BRCA2*)
C. Hereditary chronic pancreatitis (mutation in cationic trypsinogen gene *PRSS1*, or *SPINK1*)
D. Hereditary nonpolyposis colorectal cancer
E. Peutz-Jeghers (*LKB1*) syndrome

93. The patient in Question 92 had *BRCA* testing performed and was found to be a carrier for a known deleterious mutation. Unfortunately, he developed metastatic disease and

was started on FOLFIRINOX (folinic acid, 5-FU, irinotecan, oxaliplatin). He had a near-complete response to this regimen and has received 6 months of therapy. However, he has developed increasing peripheral neuropathy and does not want to continue with more FOLFIRINOX. Otherwise, he still remains in good health with an ECOG performance status 0.

What is the next best option for treating this patient?

A. FOLFOX (5-FU/leucovorin + oxaliplatin)
B. Gemcitabine/abraxane
C. Hospice
D. Immunotherapy with PD-1 blocking mAb (eg, pembrolizumab)
E. Poly (ADP-ribose) polymerase (PARP) inhibitors

94. A 72-year-old man with a history of hypertension, heart failure with preserved ejection fraction, and chronic kidney disease presents with a complaint of yellowing of the eyes and 20-lb unintentional weight loss over the preceding 3 months. On physical examination, he has temporal and supraclavicular wasting, scleral icterus, and jaundice. His abdomen is distended with a positive fluid wave and tender to deep palpation at the epigastric region.

Laboratory studies	
Total bilirubin	9.0 mg/dL
Direct bilirubin	7.2 mg/dL
Alkaline phosphatase	655 U/L

Which of the following is the most appropriate next step in diagnosis?

A. Check CA 19-9 and consult gastroenterology for endoscopic retrograde cholangiopancreatography (ERCP)
B. Check CA 19-9 and pancreatic protocol CT scan or MRI with contrast
C. Check CA 19-9 and perform abdominal ultrasound
D. Pancreatic protocol CT scan or MRI with contrast followed by endoscopic ultrasound (EUS)-guided fine needle aspiration (FNA)

95. A 63-year-old man with a history of hypertension, hyperlipidemia, T2DM, and cirrhosis secondary to chronic hepatitis C presents to his PCP for a routine visit. As part of hepatocellular carcinoma (HCC) screening, he has been undergoing liver ultrasounds. A liver ultrasound done prior to the visit shows concern for a 4-cm mass lesion in the right lobe of the liver. A follow-up multiphasic liver protocol CT scan revealed a 4.5-cm mass showing arterial enhancement followed by progressive washout in the venous and delayed phase.

What is the next best step in the management of this patient?

A. Follow-up multiphasic CT in 3 months
B. Liver MRI with contrast
C. Percutaneous needle biopsy
D. Referral to multidisciplinary team for management of HCC
E. Serum α-fetoprotein (AFP) level

96. A 57-year-old woman with obesity, T2DM, hyperlipidemia, and CAD presents with increasing pain in the right upper abdomen. Investigations, including CT abdomen, reveal cirrhotic liver morphology and a 4-cm tumor in the right liver lobe. The tumor is seen invading into the portal vein, leading to its thrombotic occlusion. A biopsy of the mass reveals HCC. No other metastatic lesions are seen in the abdomen, and a CT chest is

normal. She is evaluated by a multidisciplinary oncology team and deemed not to be a candidate for surgical resection.

Which of the following therapies would NOT be appropriate for this patient?

A. Clinical trial with pembrolizumab (PD-1 mAb)
B. Sorafenib
C. Stereotactic body radiation therapy
D. Transcatheter arterial chemoembolization (TACE)

97. A 53-year-old man with a history of alcohol cirrhosis undergoes routine ultrasonography and AFP testing every 6 months. On his most recent ultrasound, he is found to have a suspicious lesion. There is no change in his AFP level.

What next step is needed to make a diagnosis of HCC?

A. Abdominal PET scan
B. Liver biopsy
C. Liver MRI
D. Repeat AFP level in 3 months

98. A 53-year-old man presents to his PCP reporting symptoms of chronic heartburn. His medical history is significant for hypertension, gastroesophageal reflux disease (GERD), a hiatal hernia, prior appendectomy, and a BMI of 31. He has no family history of malignancy, and he does not drink alcohol. He smoked one pack of cigarettes per day for 30 years until this year when he was able to quit smoking. He has been taking famotidine for many years. His medical therapy is intensified to a proton pump inhibitor (PPI).

Which of the following approaches to screen for upper GI malignancy is indicated?

A. There is no indication for screening
B. There is no indication for screening unless symptoms continue with PPI therapy
C. Upper GI endoscopy; repeat every year if Barrett esophagus present
D. Upper GI endoscopy; repeat every 3-5 years if Barrett esophagus present

99. A 36-year-old woman is seen in oncology clinic after being diagnosed with metastatic melanoma. MRI of her brain showed numerous subcentimeter intracranial metastases, and CT of her abdomen and chest showed metastases in her liver and lungs. Her pathology showed that she does not have a BRAF mutation. Other than melanoma, she has no significant PMH and is highly active, jogging three to five times per week for exercise. She does not have any symptoms from her brain metastases.

Which of the following would be the most appropriate initial therapy for this patient?

A. Ipilimumab and nivolumab
B. Pembrolizumab
C. Pembrolizumab plus stereotactic radiosurgery to intracranial metastases
D. Dabrafenib and trametinib plus stereotactic radiosurgery to intracranial metastases

100. A 52-year-old man with hypertension presents with dyspnea on exertion and bilateral lower extremity edema for the past few months. Physical examination reveals decreased breath sounds in bilateral lower lobes, massive splenomegaly at least 20 cm below the left costal margin, and 3+ pitting edema bilaterally.

Labs are notable for Cr 1.7 mg/dL (normal baseline), K 5 mEq/L, Ca 8.6 mg/dL, phosphorus 6.6 mg/dL, uric acid 14.7 mg/dL, LDH 1810 U/L, WBC 641 000/µL, hematocrit 21.5%, and platelets 71 000/µL. Peripheral smear reveals marked leukocytosis with a predominance of left-shifted myeloid cells in all stages of differentiation, including occasional blasts, as well as increased basophils and nucleated RBCs. CXR showed diffuse bilateral fine reticular nodular opacities with no pleural effusions.

Which of the following is NOT an appropriate next step?

A. Bone marrow biopsy
B. Chest/abdomen CT with contrast
C. Hydroxyurea
D. IV fluids
E. Rasburicase

101. A 29-year-old woman with AML on cytarabine and daunorubicin develops a new fever while she is neutropenic with an ANC of 0. Her nurse reports one episode of nonbloody emesis and several watery stools. Vital signs are notable for T 38.3°C, HR 105 beats/min, and BP 110/75 mmHg. Physical examination reveals right lower quadrant tenderness to palpation with minimal guarding and no rebound tenderness. Other notable labs include Cr 0.9 mg/dL, hematocrit 24%, and platelets 20 000/µL. Abdominal CT with contrast shows cecal wall thickening with no pneumatosis. Broad-spectrum antibiotics are initiated.

Which additional therapy could be considered?

A. Loperamide as needed for diarrhea
B. Morphine for pain control
C. Nasogastric suction
D. Surgical intervention

102. A 43-year-old woman presents to the ED after visiting her PCP for easy bruising and being found to have a platelet count of 27 000/µL. On arrival, her white count is noted to be 1.5 with an ANC of 330/µL. Her Hb is 9 g/dL. Her INR is 1.3. She is an otherwise healthy woman and takes only lisinopril for BP. Inspection of her peripheral blood reveals no schistocytes but rare scattered cells with high nuclear-to-cytoplasmic ratios and overall immature appearances. These are presumed to be blasts. Several of the blasts have red needle-shaped figures in the cytoplasm, suspicious for Auer rods.

What treatment should this patient receive immediately?

A. 7+3 induction
B. ATO and ATRA
C. High-dose steroids
D. Hydroxyurea

103. A 63-year-old man with a history of metastatic melanoma presents for a follow-up appointment. He is on a clinical trial medication, which he has been tolerating well. Today, however, he is reporting new lower back pain. On subsequent neuro examination, he is noted to have new right lower extremity weakness and distal numbness.

What is the next best step his providers should take?

A. Discontinue clinical trial medication
B. Lumbar puncture
C. Refer for emergency surgery
D. Stat MRI spine

104. A 72-year-old woman comes to your clinic for several months of abdominal bloating and decreased appetite. She feels full after eating a small amount, but her weight has been stable. She has noticed that her abdomen has been getting larger. She has a remote history of rectal cancer (age 40) for which she received radiation, and she has had no recurrence since. She has no family history of cancer. She has no other health conditions. She has two children, delivered vaginally. She underwent menarche at age 9 and menopause at age 56. Her screening colonoscopy last year was normal.

Examination is notable for distended abdomen with positive fluid wave. CT abdomen/pelvis demonstrates ascites and nodularity of the peritoneum, concerning for peritoneal carcinomatosis. The liver appears normal.

What is the next best step in diagnosis?

A. Obtain a CT of the chest
B. Perform a diagnostic paracentesis and send fluid for cytology
C. Send serum CA-125 testing
D. Only B and C
E. All of the above

105. The same patient from Question 104 is diagnosed with stage IV epithelial ovarian carcinoma. Germline genetic testing is negative for heritable cancer syndromes, and molecular testing of her tumor tissue is negative for *BRCA 1/2* mutations but positive for homologous recombination deficiency. She asks you what the treatment of her cancer will entail.

What do you recommend?

A. Neoadjuvant chemotherapy with carboplatin and paclitaxel, followed by cytoreductive surgery
B. Cytoreductive surgery followed by olaparib (PARP inhibitor)
C. Carboplatin and paclitaxel, no surgery
D. Gemcitabine and bevacizumab
E. Surgery alone

106. A 57-year-old previously healthy man presents to the ED after having a focal seizure at home. He noticed his right arm twitching for about 1 minute while watching TV. On further questioning, he notes that he has been waking up with headaches for the past few weeks. Examination reveals no focal neurologic deficits. An MRI of the brain is obtained, which shows a 1.5-cm-diameter mass in the left frontal lobe.

Basic labs show no abnormalities. He is up to date on his age-appropriate cancer screenings, including colonoscopy at age 55, which was negative. He smoked a few cigarettes a day over 30 years ago. His father had a heavy smoking history and died of lung cancer at age 65. He is started on levetiracetam.

What is the next best step in evaluation?

A. Consult neurosurgery to biopsy the lesion
B. Obtain CT imaging of the chest, abdomen, and pelvis
C. Forgo biopsy and start radiation therapy immediately given seizures
D. Obtain a lumbar puncture (LP) with opening pressures and send cytology on CSF

107. A 61-year-old man with no PMH was recently diagnosed with sigmoid colon adenocarcinoma and underwent laparoscopic resection with primary anastomosis. Pathology showed a T3N2a moderately differentiated adenocarcinoma, with 4/17 lymph nodes positive for malignancy—stage 3B. The tumor was microsatellite stable. His medical oncologist recommended starting adjuvant chemotherapy with FOLFOX (5-FU/leucovorin, oxaliplatin) to reduce the risk of tumor recurrence. He is brought to the ER after the first cycle with febrile neutropenia. He has been having more than seven episodes of diarrhea per day for the last 3 days, and his ANC on presentation is 250/μL.

What is the potential cause of his toxicity?

A. Dihydropyrimidine dehydrogenase deficiency
B. Error leading to incorrect dose administration
C. Expected for this chemotherapy regimen
D. Lack of G-CSF postchemotherapy
E. Oxaliplatin toxicity

108. A 53-year-old woman was recently diagnosed with metastatic melanoma (BRAF wild type) and was started on dual checkpoint blockade with ipilimumab (CTLA4 mAb) and nivolumab (PD-1 mAb). She tolerated treatment well, and the first set of restaging scans done at 4 weeks showed a partial response. Six weeks after initiating therapy, she developed abdominal pain, fevers, and profuse diarrhea up to eight times per day. Her therapy was stopped, and she was admitted to the hospital, where initial workup, including stool cultures and *Clostridiodes difficile* toxin assay, was negative. A flexible sigmoidoscopy showed diffuse severe colitis with multiple shallow ulcerations, and a biopsy confirmed an active colitis; stains for CMV were negative on the biopsy. Based on this information, she was started on treatment with IV methylprednisolone but did not show much improvement.

What treatment would you consider next in this patient?

A. Antimotility agents
B. Broad-spectrum antibiotics with gram-negative and anaerobic coverage
C. Infliximab
D. Surgical consultation

109. A 67-year-old woman with metastatic NSCLC has been treated with pembrolizumab (PD-1 mAb) for several months. She has been tolerating treatment well and continues to walk daily for exercise. She presents to clinic today for routine follow-up. On her most recent staging CT scans 2 months ago, she had metastases to the liver and adrenal glands. Routine labs today are notable for newly elevated ALT 106, AST 85, and alkaline phosphatase 190. Bilirubin is within normal limits. Examination is notable for soft, nontender abdomen without hepatomegaly.

You are concerned that her elevated liver enzymes represent hepatitis secondary to her checkpoint inhibitor therapy.

What is the most appropriate next step in management?

A. Stop pembrolizumab, start oral steroids
B. Continue pembrolizumab, recheck LFTs in 10 to 14 days
C. Obtain abdominal CT imaging and rule out viral or other etiologies of LFT abnormalities
D. Both A and C
E. Both B and C

110. A 52-year-old woman with unresectable melanoma is being actively treated with combination nivolumab and ipilimumab, which she started 2 months earlier. She is brought into the ED with profound weakness, fatigue, and headache. Her BP is found to be 70/40 mmHg.

Physical examination is notable for vitiligo skin changes on both hands and feet, a normal cardiac examination, and 1+ nonpitting edema to her midshins. Labs are notable for TSH 0.1 mU/L (normal 0.5-4.7 mU/L), free T4 0.3 (normal >0.7), and cortisol and adrenocorticotropic hormone (ACTH) levels below assay. Follicle-stimulating hormone (FSH) and luteinizing hormone (LH) levels are subsequently sent and also found to be markedly low.

The patient's immunotherapy is held, and she is given stress dose steroids, after which her BP rises to 100/70 mmHg.

What test would likely confirm her diagnosis?

A. ACTH stimulation test
B. Blood and urine cultures
C. Brain MRI
D. Thyroid ultrasound

111. A 34-year-old woman with refractory ALL undergoes a CAR-T infusion. One week later, she develops fever, chills, and tachycardia to 120 beats/min. Her baseline BP is 110/70 mmHg. Once her fevers start, her BP drops to 88/60 mmHg. She is given 2 L of fluid, and her BP recovers.

The following evening, her BP decreases again but this time does not respond to fluids. She is transferred to the ICU and started on peripheral vasopressors and broad-spectrum antibiotics.

What additional therapy should be added to the above?

A. Infliximab
B. Mycophenolate mofetil
C. Stress dose steroids
D. Tocilizumab

112. A 56-year-old woman with relapsed diffuse large B-cell lymphoma is treated with CAR-T therapy. Five days later, she becomes agitated and confused. A preliminary infectious disease and metabolic workup is negative, and ultimately she has a grand mal seizure and requires intubation and transfer to the ICU.

What therapy is indicated for this patient?

A. Levetiracetam
B. Lorazepam
C. Steroids
D. Tocilizumab
E. A, B, and C
F. All of the above

113. A 55-year-old man with pancreatic cancer is admitted to the hospital with confusion, subjective fevers, and oral discomfort 7 days after being treated with FOLFIRINOX (folinic acid, 5-FU, irinotecan, oxaliplatin) chemotherapy. His vitals are remarkable for a BP of 123/75, a HR of 97, a temperature of 38.5°C, and an oxygen saturation of 93% on room air. On physical examination, he is found to have moderate oral mucositis. He has mild left lower quadrant abdominal tenderness to palpation but no rebound or guarding. He has no skin rashes or erythema, and the implanted port for venous access within his right chest wall has no surrounding fluctuance, erythema, or tenderness. His labs show an ANC of 250. An admission CXR shows no evidence of pneumonia.

What initial therapy is the most appropriate?

A. Cefepime
B. Vancomycin and cefepime
C. Vancomycin and cefepime and micafungin
D. Vancomycin and meropenem

114. A 45-year-old woman with no major PMH other than a recent diagnosis of metastatic colon cancer presents to the ED because of intermittent shortness of breath that started yesterday. She is receiving FOLFOX (folinic acid, 5-FU, and oxaliplatin) chemotherapy for her colon cancer, which was found on staging scans to have numerous metastases to the lungs. She does not smoke. Her vital signs are notable for a BP of 133/80 and an oxygen saturation of 96% on room air. Physical examination is notable for clear lungs bilaterally and a soft systolic murmur best heard at the apex. The patient is wearing an infusion pump that she says she was told to wear at the beginning of each chemotherapy cycle. While you are interviewing the patient, she begins having worsening shortness of breath and reports substernal chest pain as well. A CT scan pulmonary embolism protocol shows no evidence of pulmonary embolism to the level of the segmental pulmonary arteries, and her ECG shows sub-millimeter ST segment depressions in leads II and III, but no ST elevations.

What is the most likely cause of her symptoms?

A. Progression of metastatic disease
B. Coronary artery plaque rupture
C. Coronary artery vasospasm
D. Occult pulmonary embolism

115. A 66-year-old man with newly diagnosed diffuse large B-cell lymphoma is admitted to the hospital with dyspnea and worsening lower extremity edema. His PMH is notable for hypertension, hyperlipidemia, COPD, T2DM, and a 30-pack-year smoking history. He says his symptoms started 2 weeks ago after he felt like he had a flu-like illness. He had initiated R-CHOP (rituximab, cyclophosphamide, hydroxydaunorubicin, oncovin, prednisone) chemotherapy the week prior to the onset of his symptoms. He says he started eating high-calorie meals after his diagnosis of cancer because of significant unintentional weight loss over the past 6 months. He is started on IV diuretics with improvement in his symptoms. A transthoracic echocardiogram shows new segmental wall abnormalities.

What is the most likely cause of this patient's new heart failure?

A. Viral myocarditis
B. Missed myocardial infarction
C. Anthracycline chemotherapy
D. Dietary indiscretion

ANSWERS

1. **The correct answer is: B. Folate deficiency.** This patient is an elderly woman with malnutrition and a diet low in leafy green vegetables and fruits. Her presentation is consistent with megaloblastic anemia from impaired DNA synthesis, resulting in ineffective erythropoiesis and macrocytosis. Her absence of neurologic symptoms and normal methylmalonic acid are consistent with folate deficiency rather than vitamin B12 deficiency. However, B12 should also be checked to make sure she is not borderline deficient. Although methylmalonic acid is very sensitive, one would not want to treat with folate and mask developing B12 deficiency.

2. **The correct answer is: D. Vitamin B12 1 mg intramuscular (IM) weekly and then monthly.** This patient has vitamin B12 deficiency, given his neurologic deficits, megaloblastic macrocytic anemia, and increased methylmalonic acid. His vegan diet likely does not include foods of animal origin rich in vitamin B12. Although less likely in light of his dietary habits, testing for pernicious anemia, including autoantibodies to parietal cells and intrinsic factor, should be performed to make sure he can absorb oral supplementation after full repletion with IM B12.

3. **The correct answer is: C. Iron/TIBC <18%, ferritin 5 ng/mL.** This patient has iron deficiency anemia based on his pica, angular cheilitis, atrophic glossitis, and guaiac positive stool. He requires a colonoscopy to screen for colon cancer and initiation of oral or IV iron.

4. **The correct answer is: A. Allogeneic stem cell transplant.** This patient most likely has a new diagnosis of aplastic anemia. For young patients, allogenic stem cell transplant offers 80% long-term survival and significantly decreased risk of malignant evolution, although it has the risk of transplant-related morbidity and mortality. Immunosuppression, such as cyclosporine or tacrolimus, is associated with a response rate of 80% to 90% and 5-year survival of 80% to 90% but is also associated with a 15% to 20% 10-year incidence of clonal disorders, including myelodysplastic syndrome, AML, and paroxysmal nocturnal hemoglobinuria. Thrombopoietin mimetics are usually reserved for refractory disease, and supportive care with transfusions, antibiotics, and growth factors is more appropriate for an elderly or treatment refractory population.

5. **The correct answer is: A. Anemia of chronic inflammation.** This patient has anemia of chronic inflammation based on her normocytic anemia and high ferritin. The best management of her anemia is treatment of her lupus, as her worsening arthralgias and new oral ulcers suggest a likely disease flare. Although iron deficiency can also co-exist with anemia of chronic inflammation, iron deficiency is unlikely in this patient given the elevated ferritin. Her normal creatinine also argues against anemia of chronic kidney disease, whereas her normal Hb last year and lack of offending exposures (ie, alcohol, isoniazid, chloramphenicol, lead) are not consistent with sideroblastic anemia.

6. **The correct answer is: A. Autoimmune hemolytic anemia.** This patient has hemolytic anemia, spherocytosis, and a positive Coombs test all consistent with warm autoimmune hemolytic anemia. The patient's lymphadenopathy and absolute lymphocytosis point to chronic lymphocytic leukemia as the underlying etiology of the autoimmune hemolytic anemia. Drug-induced hemolytic anemia from levofloxacin is less likely, given the positive Coombs test. Similarly, there is no thrombocytopenia or schistocytosis to suggest MAHA. Finally, hereditary spherocytosis would have presented at a much earlier age and is not characterized by a positive Coombs test.

7. **The correct answer is: E. Pure red cell aplasia.** This history provided suggests that the patient and her children were infected with parvovirus, which can be associated with fevers and a "slapped cheek" appearance. Her laboratory workup demonstrates a normocytic anemia without evidence of thrombocytopenia or leukopenia, making aplastic anemia less likely. Pure red cell aplasia occurs when a patient develops destructive antibodies or lymphocytes that target the bone marrow and lead to ineffective erythropoiesis. This condition can be associated with parvovirus infection, as well as with thymoma, chronic lymphocytic leukemia, autoimmune disease, and certain drugs. Bone marrow biopsy would reveal lack of erythroid precursors with normal hematopoiesis of the other cell lines. Importantly, in immunocompetent adults, parvovirus infection leads to transient anemia, so this woman is likely to recover soon without intervention. In immunocompromised patients, parvovirus can cause more prolonged anemia.

8. **The correct answer is: C. α-Thalassemia minor.** The long-standing, asymptomatic nature of the patient's anemia makes iron deficiency anemia, choice A, unlikely, despite the low MCV. The correct diagnosis based on the low MCV, the normal transferrin saturation >18%, and the Hb electrophoresis results is α-thalassemia minor. α-Thalassemia minor results from the loss of two α-chain genes. The genotype can be heterozygous for the α-thalassemia-1 trait (aa/--, more common among Asian individuals) or homozygous for the α-thalassemia-2 trait (a-/a-, more common among African individuals). Patients typically have mild anemia, hypochromia, and microcytosis, without other significant clinical manifestations, unlike α-thalassemia intermedia or major.

9. **The correct answer is: C. Exchange transfusion.** This patient has acute chest syndrome based on her new pulmonary infiltrates on CXR and her cough, fever, tachypnea, intercostal retractions, wheezing, rales, and dropping oxygen saturations. Acute chest syndrome is a leading cause of death for patients with sickle cell disease, and this patient rapidly evolves from moderate to severe acute chest syndrome. Therefore, exchange rather than simple transfusion is the most appropriate management, as exchange transfusion will allow rapid decrease in hemoglobin S (HbS) percentage while avoiding the hyperviscosity that could occur with a large-volume simple transfusion. Steroids are not standard practice for acute chest syndrome management in adults, and albuterol nebulizers will not reverse the underlying cause of her symptoms.

10. **The correct answer is: B. Plasma exchange.** This patient has thrombotic thrombocytopenic purpura leading to MAHA. He requires emergent plasma exchange to remove inhibitory autoantibodies and replace low levels of ADAMTS13 (a disintegrin-like and metalloproteinase with thrombospondin type 1 motifs 13), the enzyme required to cleave von Willebrand factor (vWF) multimers. Uncleaved ultrahigh-molecular-weight vWF multimers lead to platelet thrombi and hemolytic anemia. Fresh frozen plasma will replace ADAMTS13 but will not remove inhibitory autoantibodies. Thus, it can be used to temporize but will not provide a durable improvement. RBC and platelet transfusions will similarly not reverse the underlying disorder.

11. **The correct answer is: B. Glucose-6-phosphate dehydrogenase (G6PD) testing.** G6PD testing is required, as G6PD deficiency is more common in African Americans and patients of Mediterranean descent. TMP-SMX is a frequent cause of hemolytic anemia in patients with G6PD deficiency. If anemia is severe or the patient is symptomatic, RBC transfusion should be given. Patients should be advised to avoid oxidizing agents in the future. Note that G6PD levels may be normal in the setting of an acute crisis if the patient has developed a significant reticulocytosis, because these younger cells have a higher G6PD content.

12. **The correct answer is: A. Administer 4-factor prothrombin complex concentrate (4F-PCC).** Warfarin-associated intracranial hemorrhage with prolonged PT-INR should be treated with 4F-PCC, rather than fresh frozen plasma. The rationale for this is that the 4F-PCC is administered in a smaller volume and will lead to more rapid INR reversal. 4F-PCC contains the vitamin K–dependent coagulation factors, which include II, VII, IX, and X. Although vitamin K should also be administered, it should be given as 10 mg of an IV infusion. There is no indication to transfuse platelets in this patient with a normal platelet count and no evidence of platelet dysfunction. With regard to RBC transfusion, this is reserved for large-volume blood loss. In this patient, although the intracranial hemorrhage produces a significant clinical effect, the true blood loss is likely relatively small.

13. **The correct answer is: A. Acquired platelet disorder; DDAVP (desmopressin acetate).** Bleeding in the setting of uremia is often multifactorial but includes platelet dysfunction and abnormal platelet-endothelial interactions. This is considered an acquired platelet disorder, given that there is a normal platelet count, but decreased platelet function, in a patient without a known congenital etiology for platelet dysfunction and with an identifiable acquired trigger. The factors thought to contribute to platelet dysfunction in the setting of uremia include uremic toxins, anemia, and increased nitric oxide production by endothelial cells (inhibit platelet aggregation). Administration of DDAVP acts by increasing the release of large factor VIII: vWF multimers from endothelial cells and is a rapid-acting, low-risk intervention for the management of uremic bleeding. It may also potentiate platelet activation and granule release. The other accepted initial intervention is dialysis to correct the uremia. Platelet transfusion will not be effective, because the platelets will become dysfunctional in the uremic plasma. Insulin does not contribute to bleeding.

14. **The correct answer is: E. Skin biopsy with direct immunofluorescence microscopy.** Palpable purpura is a common manifestation of small vessel vasculitis. The erythematous papules and plaques will eventually progress to raised, nonblanchable lesions. In this young patient with palpable purpura, abdominal pain, and new renal failure, the most likely diagnosis is immunoglobulin A (IgA) vasculitis. In patients with IgA vasculitis, skin biopsy will show leukocytoclastic vasculitis on histopathologic evaluation and IgA on direct immunofluorescence. The first step in the diagnosis of patients with defined skin lesions is a skin biopsy. Renal biopsy presents increased risk of bleeding because of the invasive nature of the procedure, although it would also demonstrate IgA deposits. Anti–glomerular basement membrane antibody disease presents with rapidly progressive glomerulonephritis and, in some cases, pulmonary alveolar hemorrhage, but would not be expected to present with abdominal pain or palpable purpura. Although ANCA vasculitis may produce a similar rash, affected patients are typically older (age 60s) and do not present with abdominal pain.

15. **The correct answer is: E. Thrombotic thrombocytopenic purpura.** This patient is a young woman who has MAHA (Coombs negative), thrombocytopenia, schistocytes on peripheral smear (indicative of MAHA), elevated LDH, and elevated indirect bilirubin, all consistent with thrombotic thrombocytopenic purpura because of an acquired autoantibody. Thrombotic thrombocytopenic purpura is more common in women and Black patients. Given this patient's history of hypothyroidism, most likely from chronic autoimmune hypothyroidism, also known as Hashimoto thyroiditis, this patient may be at a higher risk for autoimmune disorders. It is important to recognize the diagnosis of thrombotic thrombocytopenic purpura early, because the treatment is emergent plasma exchange therapy. HUS also presents with MAHA, but renal failure is a hallmark, which

was not seen in this patient and is only variably seen in TTP. HUS is also more common in children and after a diarrheal illness. Primary immune thrombocytopenia is less likely in this case because the patient also has hemolytic anemia, and Evans syndrome (immune thrombocytopenia plus hemolytic anemia) is also less likely because of the negative Coombs test. Drug-induced thrombocytopenia is not likely with concurrent hemolytic anemia. Potential drug culprits for thrombocytopenia include quinine, antimicrobials, quetiapine, and chemotherapy agents. The patient would not have required antimicrobial prophylaxis for her trip to Europe.

16. **The correct answer is: C. Stop heparin, send PF4-heparin ELISA, start bivalirudin.** This patient most likely has immune (antibody)-mediated HIT, which typically occurs after 4 to 10 days of heparin exposure but can occur earlier if the patient has been exposed to heparin within the preceding 100 days because of persistent antibodies. Thrombotic events can occur in up to 50% of patients. The 4T score can be used clinically to assess the pretest probability of HIT and thrombosis in this patient. This patient has a very high 4T score based on the degree of platelet drop (>50% with nadir above 20 000), timing of the thrombocytopenia (within 1 day given prior heparin exposure in the last month), associated DVT, and no other clear explanation of her thrombocytopenia. Immediate discontinuation of heparin and initiation of alternative anticoagulation (parenteral agents include argatroban, bivalirudin, danaparoid, or fondaparinux; oral agents include the direct-acting oral anticoagulants) is indicated if there is a high probability of antibody-mediated HIT. Warfarin is not an accepted therapy for initial management of thrombosis in HIT, because there will be an initial depletion of the anticoagulant factors protein C and S prior to depletion of the vitamin K–dependent clotting factors, which can exacerbate thrombosis and lead to peripheral gangrene. In contrast, type I HIT can occur after 1 to 4 days of heparin therapy without prior heparin exposure and is mediated by the direct effect of heparin (nonimmune). Patients typically are without thrombosis, have platelet count >100 000/µL, and can safely continue on heparin with close observation.

    For diagnosis of HIT, the PF4-heparin ELISA should be sent first. If the ELISA is highly positive and the 4T score is high, then HIT is confirmed. If the result is indeterminate or mildly positive with a low-intermediate 4T score, a functional HIT assay, such as the serotonin release assay, is indicated. If the ELISA is negative, HIT is extremely unlikely, and other causes of thrombocytopenia should be investigated.

17. **The correct answer is: D. Immune thrombocytopenic purpura.** This is a classic presentation of immune thrombocytopenia that has a bimodal age distribution for disease onset. In children and younger adults, the disease typically presents following a viral syndrome with sequelae from severe thrombocytopenia. The large morphology of platelets is also classic for immune thrombocytopenia. Although an aleukemic leukemia is a possibility, the lack of constitutional symptoms, preserved Hb, WBC, and absence of any abnormal leukocytes in the peripheral blood all point against it. Tick-borne diseases such as ehrlichiosis often have associated thrombocytopenia, but the lack of a clinical syndrome including constitutional symptoms, fevers, associated leukopenia, and LFT abnormalities is not consistent with ehrlichiosis. Lastly, although drug-associated thrombocytopenia has to be considered, this clinical syndrome is more consistent with immune thrombocytopenia.

18. **The correct answer is: B. Intravenous immunoglobulin (IVIG) + steroids.** The patient has spontaneous bleeding and a platelet count <10 000/µL, which requires urgent treatment with the goal of increasing his platelet count into a safe range (generally >30 000/µL). In particular, the presence of blood blisters on mucosal surfaces can be indicative of higher chances of spontaneous bleeding such as in intracranial or visceral

locations. Steroids form the backbone of immune thrombocytopenia treatment and are considered first-line therapy in the acute setting and generally lead to a response in platelet count in 4 to 7 days after therapy is initiated. In cases of severe thrombocytopenia and high risk of CNS bleed, IVIG can also be added. Platelet count response to IVIG is typically seen within 1 to 2 days. Given the immune nature of platelet clearance in immune thrombocytopenia, there is generally no role for platelet transfusion. Splenectomy or thrombopoietin agonist therapies are effective treatment strategies for the management of immune thrombocytopenia in the chronic phase.

19. **The correct answer is: D. Platelet transfusion with a platelet goal >50 000/μL.** In general, platelet goal >50 000/μL is recommended for most surgical procedures. This patient likely has multifactorial thrombocytopenia from hepatitis C, chronic liver disease, and splenomegaly. Hence, platelet transfusion is the most effective strategy to rapidly bring the platelet count to goal. Romiplostim is often used in the preprocedural setting for elective procedures where there is time to titrate the medicine and allow for a platelet response, which may take up to 1 to 2 weeks. Romiplostim is advised for patients with immune thrombocytopenia in the case where platelet transfusions are not an effective therapy. This patient has a mildly deranged INR, likely secondary to hepatic dysfunction, which does not reflect a true coagulopathy.

20. **The correct answer is: D. Type 3 vWD.** DDAVP is a synthetic analog of vasopressin that causes a transient release of vWF from storage granules in the vascular endothelium, leading to an increase in serum concentrations. Hence, it is a reasonable strategy for prophylaxis and treatment of minor bleeding in patients with mild type 1 vWD and mild hemophilia A (factor VIII deficiency), because vWF increases the circulating half-life of factor VIII from approximately 30 minutes to 24 hours. It has also been seen to be effective in platelet dysfunction of end-stage renal disease. Type 3 vWD is a rare variant of vWD characterized by a severe deficiency or near absence of any vWF, leading to a severe bleeding diathesis. DDAVP is ineffective in type 3 vWD because there is no vWF present in storage granules (which are Weibel-Palade bodies).

21. **The correct answer is: D. Type 2 HIT.** Type 2 HIT is an immune-mediated disorder with generation of platelets against the heparin-PF4 complex, which leads to microvascular platelet thrombi and a massively procoagulant state. However, the generation of antibodies against heparin-PF4 needs at least 5 days of exposure to IV unfractionated heparin. In patients with prior exposure to heparin type 2, HIT may occur sooner than 5 days, but this patient has no prior PMH and is on no medications. Type 1 HIT is a non–immune thrombocytopenia caused by direct effects of heparin binding to platelets and causing clearance from the circulation and is seen within the first 2 days of IV unfractionated heparin initiation. This phenomenon is not prothrombotic and improves over time even with continuation of therapy with heparin. Intra-aortic balloon pump use is associated with thrombocytopenia, which is thought to be mechanical in etiology.

22. **The correct answer is: B. IV vitamin K.** This woman is presenting with a peripheral smear concerning for acute PML, which is associated with DIC, often leading to life-threatening bleeding. However, she is not actively bleeding, and her labs are consistent with mild DIC. Platelets should be administered for a platelet count <10 000/μL (in the absence of active bleeding). Patients with serious bleeding and a significantly prolonged PT or activated PTT or a low fibrinogen level should receive coagulation factor replacement, such as fresh frozen plasma or cryoprecipitate, the latter of which provides fibrinogen with less volume than fresh frozen plasma. Therefore, she currently has no indication for platelets, cryoprecipitate, or fresh frozen plasma. Vitamin K is the most

appropriate therapy at this time, particularly in the setting of antibiotic therapy that may suppress vitamin K–producing intestinal flora. PCCs are usually contraindicated in DIC, given the risk of thrombosis.

23. **The correct answer is: D. Idarucizumab.** Dabigatran is a direct thrombin inhibitor. The patient last took dabigatran 3 hours prior to presentation, and the half-life is around 12 hours without renal insufficiency. Because he has a major potentially life-threatening bleed, reversal of dabigatran with idarucizumab is indicated. If idarucizumab is not available, an activated PCC, such as FEIBA, could be administered instead, although this carries a significant prothrombotic risk. Fresh frozen plasma is generally avoided in bleeding associated with direct oral anticoagulants, given associated risks, including transfusion reactions, thrombosis, and volume overload, and the absence of data supporting its use except in the case of a coexisting coagulopathy. Andexanet-alfa is indicated for the reversal of factor Xa inhibitors in patients with life-threatening bleeds associated with factor Xa inhibitors, such as rivaroxaban, apixaban, and edoxaban.

24. **The correct answer is: B. Emicizumab.** Emicizumab is a recombinant humanized bispecific mAb that bridges activated factors IX and X and hence replaces the function of factor VIII. It is not inhibited by antibodies that bind to factor VIII and is now approved for primary prophylaxis in patients with hemophilia A and high titer of inhibitors. Given the high titers of inhibitors (alloantibodies produced in response to frequent and long-term recombinant factor VIII infusion), a higher dose of factor VIII would not work. Hemophilia A is a deficiency in factor VIII, and levels of factor IX are normal in these patients; hence, recombinant factor IX therapy would be of no benefit. Recombinant factor VIIa activates the extrinsic coagulation pathway, which does not need factor VIII, and has been used in the past for patients with hemophilia and high titer of inhibitors in the setting of acute bleeding events. However, this is associated with a high risk of thrombotic complications and is not used for prophylaxis. In the context of efficacy and approval for emicizumab, the utility of factor VIIa in patients with inhibitors and acute bleeding is less clear. Please note that emicizumab does not work immediately: it requires about a month of loading dose treatment.

25. **The correct answer is: C. Flow cytometry for CD55 and CD59.** This patient has hemolytic anemia, pancytopenia, and mesenteric venous thrombosis, which together suggest a diagnosis of paroxysmal nocturnal hemoglobinuria, a rare, acquired hematopoietic stem cell disorder resulting from a somatic mutation in a gene on the X chromosome. The diagnostic test of choice is flow cytometry for the glycophosphatidylinositol-linked proteins CD55 and CD59, which are characteristically decreased on RBCs and granulocytes. Protein C and S and antithrombin III levels are affected by acute thrombosis and anticoagulation and are therefore best assessed more than 2 weeks after completing anticoagulation. A positive activated protein C resistance assay is consistent with factor V Leiden. These other inherited thrombophilias would not explain this patient's hemolytic anemia or pancytopenia.

26. **The correct answer is: D. Warfarin.** This patient presents with arterial thrombosis and elevated antiphospholipid antibodies on two occasions, confirming the diagnosis of antiphospholipid syndrome. Long-term anticoagulation with warfarin has been shown to be more effective for secondary thrombosis prevention in patients with antiphospholipid syndrome than direct oral anticoagulants, especially for those patients with a history of arterial thrombosis. Lifelong use of enoxaparin imposes significant costs and burden on patients and is therefore usually reserved for patients with antiphospholipid syndrome who are or become pregnant.

27. **The correct answer is: D. No anticoagulation.** Although factor V Leiden does carry a slightly increased risk of venous thromboembolism, in the absence of a history of a clot or a high-risk circumstance (eg, major surgery), there is no indication for anticoagulation in these patients, although use of venous thromboembolism prophylaxis at times of surgery should be considered.

28. **The correct answer is: B. No treatment.** This patient has stage 0 chronic lymphocytic leukemia, where the only abnormality is an elevated WBC count. Stage 1 is diagnosed when lymph nodes are enlarged, stage 2 when spleen is enlarged, stage 3 when the patient becomes anemic, and stage 4 when thrombocytopenic. Treatment typically does not begin until stage 3, or if symptomatic from lymphadenopathy and/or splenomegaly.

29. **The correct answer is: C. Microscopic cholesterol emboli.** Eosinophilia that develops during a hospitalization is typically secondary to a drug exposure or procedure. Typical drugs are antibiotics, and the eosinophilia will resolve after discontinuation. Post-catheterization cholesterol emboli may also cause secondary eosinophilia. The vasculature of the kidneys is most vulnerable when this occurs.

30. **The correct answer is: C. Drug reaction.** This patient is on two medications that have been associated with drug-induced neutropenia: phenytoin and TMP-SMX. CMV infection (option A) can also cause neutropenia; however, this patient has no concerning signs or symptoms for CMV and drug reaction is more likely. Myelodysplastic syndrome (option B) is uncommonly seen in patients this young, and is characteristically associated with cytopenia in more than one cell line (ie, leukopenia *and* anemia, etc). Finally, cyclic neutropenia (option D) is a rare congenital neutropenia syndrome characterized by recurrent neutropenia (often every 3 weeks) and associated fevers, malaise, and mucosal ulceration, which this patient does not have.

31. **The correct answer is: A. Tissue necrosis.** Though neutrophilia is commonly seen as a marker of infection, it can also arise as a reaction to inflammation such as in patients with burns and tissue necrosis. The exact cause can sometimes be difficult to tease out, as many different inflammatory conditions and medications can cause an increase in the ANC. This patient has had a broad infectious disease workup that has been negative for bacterial infection (option B). Given his critical state, it would not be inappropriate to maintain a high index of suspicion and start empiric antibiotic therapy; however, tissue necrosis is the most likely cause of neutrophilia here. Fungal infection (option D) is often seen in patients with immunocompromise and long-term neutropenia. Congenital neutrophilia is associated with dextrocardia and would be unlikely in this previously healthy patient (option C).

32. **The correct answer is: B. Chronic myelogenous leukemia.** Basophilia is not typically an isolated finding but rather needs to be put into context. It may be seen in any of the preceding conditions; hence clinical context is critical for distinguishing etiology. The presentation with elevated WBC count with excess mature granulocytes and preserved differentiation, without symptoms of leukostasis or tumor lysis, is classic for chronic myelogenous leukemia.

33. **The correct answer is: D. Order washed blood products only.** Patients can have allergic reactions including hives and rarely anaphylaxis to transfused proteins within blood products. This is especially pronounced in patients with IgA deficiency because of anti-IgA antibodies that develop after exposure to IgA, and subsequently react against donor IgA. Although diphenhydramine is the correct therapy to administer for urticaria,

washed blood products will reduce the risk of further allergic reactions in future transfusions. Irradiation of blood products is performed to reduce T-cell number and reduce the risk of transfusion-associated GVHD. Running the transfusion more slowly would be unlikely to prevent reoccurrence of hives as the same antigens would still be exposed to the patient's immune system.

34. **The correct answer is: A. CMV-negative.** This patient requires CMV-negative RBCs because he is a solid organ transplant recipient on immunosuppression at risk for CMV infection. Leukoreduction dramatically reduces the risk of febrile nonhemolytic transfusion reactions, human leukocyte antigen alloimmunization, and CMV transmission. However, CMV and other viruses may be transmitted in plasma, so CMV-negative is preferred for renal transplant patients. Furthermore, a few viable lymphocytes remain after leukoreduction, so patients at risk for transfusion-associated GVHD, such as recipients of hematopoietic stem cell transplants (HSCTs), require irradiated RBC.

35. **The correct answer is: A. Consult the blood bank.** This patient is experiencing a delayed hemolytic transfusion reaction, which usually occurs 1 or 2 weeks after a blood transfusion. Most delayed hemolytic transfusion reactions are characterized by extravascular hemolysis and are clinically silent. However, patients with sickle cell disease are more likely to be symptomatic because of mild intravascular hemolysis. Consulting the blood bank will prompt an antibody screen to identify the specific RBC antigen to which the patient has become sensitized, so future reactions can be prevented. Transfusing another unit of packed RBCs before the antigen is identified could result in another hemolytic transfusion reaction and so should be avoided. Infection is a less likely cause of fever and jaundice in this patient given the positive Coombs test, so blood cultures are not necessary. Finally, discharge home would be premature, because the patient requires serial blood checks to confirm that the hemolysis is not worsening.

36. **The correct answer is: C. Transfusion-associated circulatory overload.** This patient has transfusion-associated circulatory overload, for which she has many risk factors, including a history of heart failure and COPD, as well as age >85 years, female sex, and small body habitus. This could have been prevented by a slower transfusion rate, reduced transfusion volume, and diuretic administration prior to transfusion. The other transfusion reactions listed as answer options occur during or soon after a transfusion rather than hours later and are more likely to cause hypotension rather than hypertension.

37. **The correct answer is: A. Allogeneic stem cell transplant.** This patient has myelodysplastic syndrome with symptomatic anemia and neutropenia with recurrent cellulitis. However, she has very good cytogenetics with a low blast count, so she has a very low revised International Prognostic Scoring System (IPSS-R) score of 1.5, which corresponds to a median overall survival approaching 9 years. She should therefore be treated with supportive care measures, including antibiotics and erythropoietin-stimulating agents, as well as low-intensity therapies, such as azacitidine and decitabine. Allogeneic stem cell transplant is reserved for patients with high or very high IPSS-R scores with a good performance status.

38. **The correct answer is: C. Pneumococcal vaccine every 5 years.** Patients with myelodysplastic syndrome should receive age-appropriate vaccinations, including yearly influenza vaccines and every 5-year pneumococcal vaccines. However, they should not receive live vaccines. Similarly, prophylactic antibiotics and G-CSFs have not been shown to provide benefit and are therefore not recommended by National Comprehensive Cancer Network (NCCN) guidelines.

39. **The correct answer is: A. Allogeneic stem cell transplant.** This patient has my-elodysplastic syndrome with symptomatic anemia and thrombocytopenia. He has poor cytogenetics and a very high IPSS-R score of 8, which corresponds to a median overall survival of under 1 year. He is medically fit with good performance status, so he is a good candidate for allogeneic stem cell transplant, which offers the only hope of a cure. Hypomethylating agents are more appropriate for patients with poor performance status. His disease does not have an IDH1 or IDH2 mutation that could be targeted with ivosidenib or enasidenib, respectively. Based on his adverse cytogenetics, intensive chemotherapy is unlikely to achieve long-term benefit and is associated with a high toxicity rate.

40. **The correct answer is: B. Clopidogrel.** The patient most likely has polycythemia vera, and although all patients should be started on low-dose aspirin, he also meets criteria for phlebotomy and hydroxyurea. Polycythemia vera is diagnosed in men with Hb >16.5 g/dL or hematocrit >49%, and in women with Hb >16 g/dL or hematocrit >48% who do not have other explanations (eg, hypoxemia, erythropoietin-producing syndromes, dehydration). Roughly 95% of patients will have the activating JAK2 V617F mutation. Patients should also have erythropoietin levels measured, because low erythropoietin levels make polycythemia vera more likely. Treatment entails phlebotomy to goal hematocrit <45%, low-dose aspirin, and hydroxyurea if high risk, which includes age ≥60 or prior thrombus.

    Of note, protein C and S levels are often low after a clotting event, so measuring these levels at that time is not indicative of a deficiency. Repeat testing would have to be performed after the DVT, although in this case, the patient has a better explanation for his presentation.

41. **The correct answer is: D. RBC transfusion.** The patient has myelofibrosis (MF), likely secondary to lupus. Secondary MF may also arise from polycythemia vera, ET, other hematologic and solid cancers, and toxins. By contrast, primary MF arises de novo, similar to other myeloproliferative neoplasms. Symptoms of MF are typically secondary to anemia and subsequent splenomegaly. If the patient has no symptoms and is not anemic, there is no indication for treatment. If the patient were younger and had a poor prognosis, she may attempt more aggressive treatment with an allogeneic stem cell transplant, the only potential cure. For an elderly symptomatic patient like this one, however, supportive care, including blood transfusions, is standard.

42. **The correct answer is: D. Observation.** The patient is <60 years old, has no history of thrombosis, and his platelet count is <1 500 000/μL, so he has no indication for aspirin or hydroxyurea.

43. **The correct answer is: E. Start hydroxyurea and aspirin 81 mg daily.** Patients over 60 years old with a history of thrombosis (stroke) are at high risk of recurrent thrombosis, regardless of JAK2 mutational status (International Prognostic Score for Essential Thrombocythemia (IPSET) thrombosis score; Blood. 2012;120:5128). He should be started on aspirin 81 mg daily and receive cytoreductive treatment with hydroxyurea. There is no role for anticoagulation (options C and D). Observation is no longer appropriate now that he has had a thrombotic event (option F).

44. **The correct answer is: D. Cytogenetics: t(8;21), NPM1+.** In addition to CBC with differential, the diagnostic evaluation for acute leukemia includes peripheral smear and bone marrow biopsy with flow cytometry and cytogenetics. The peripheral smear will demonstrate anemia, thrombocytopenia, and circulating blasts, the origin of which can be determined by flow cytometry (ALL vs AML). In addition, the presence of specific

cytogenetic abnormalities, including t(15;17), t(8;21), inv(16), or t(16;16), is sufficient for a diagnosis of AML regardless of the blast count. This patient has AML based on blasts showing myeloid markers, including myeloperoxidase, CD13, and CD33.

Cytogenetics and molecular abnormalities are key in helping determine the risk of relapse in AML. In the question, only translocation (8;21) and NPM1 gene mutation positivity confer a favorable prognosis. Other markers of favorable prognosis include inv(16), t(16;16), and biallelic CEBPA mutations. t(15;17) leads to a fusion PML-retinoic acid receptor α (PML-RARA) oncoprotein and is diagnostic of acute PML, a unique subset of AML that is associated with a very high cure rate on modern therapies including ATRA and ATO. Deletions 5 and 7, 3q26 aberrations, t(6;9); 11q23 aberrations, and complex karyotype confer an unfavorable prognosis, as do the gene mutations FLT3-ITD, MLL-PTD, TP53, and RUNX1. t(9;22) signifies the presence of BCR-ABL fusion transcript, which is not found in AML but identifies a high relapse risk subset of ALL.

45. **The correct answer is: A. Liposomal cytarabine and daunorubicin on days 1, 3, and 5.** This patient has most likely developed cytotoxic therapy–related AML based on her history of breast cancer requiring chemotherapy. Therefore, the most appropriate induction therapy for this patient is liposomal cytarabine and daunorubicin on days 1, 3, and 5. Standard induction therapy would be indicated for patients who are under the age of 60 years, or who are over the age of 60 years but eligible for intensive chemotherapy, and who do not have targetable mutations. Choice E, with the addition of midostaurin, describes the appropriate induction therapy for patients with FLT3-mutated AML. Choice D, with the addition of gemtuzumab ozogamicin, describes the appropriate induction therapy for patients with CD33-positive AML. The reduced intensity therapy is indicated for patients who are over the age of 60 years and require nonintensive chemotherapy because of medical comorbidities or functional status. For patients under the age of 45 years, induction therapy includes standard therapy or HiDAC for 6 days followed by idarubicin or daunorubicin for 3 days.

46. **The correct answer is: D. Differentiation syndrome; treat with dexamethasone 10 mg twice daily and supportive care.** The most likely explanation for the patient's acute presentation is differentiation syndrome, which occurs in approximately 25% of patients who are treated with ATRA for acute PML. Differentiation syndrome is a life-threatening complication of therapy with differentiating agents while leukemic blasts are present. Signs and symptoms of differentiation syndrome include fever, pulmonary infiltrates, shortness of breath, edema, hypotension, and acute kidney injury. Although acute respiratory distress syndrome may also be characterized by shortness of breath, hypoxemia, and bilateral pulmonary infiltrates, the diagnosis of differentiation syndrome is more likely in this patient, who is undergoing induction therapy for acute PML with ATRA.

The treatment for differentiation syndrome includes both dexamethasone 10 mg twice daily and supportive care with diuresis, vasopressors, oxygen support, and dialysis as needed. Supportive care alone is not sufficient for this life-threatening condition. Treatment with additional chemotherapy agents, such as daunorubicin, is not indicated, because this syndrome indicates a response to therapy, rather than resistance to therapy or worsening disease. Antibiotics are indicated if an infectious source is identified, but the differentiation syndrome alone does not require treatment with antibiotics.

47. **The correct answer is: B. If she discontinues the imatinib, she will have a 60% chance of recurrence in 24 months.** This patient has achieved a complete molecular remission with imatinib-based chemotherapy, which occurs in about one-fourth of patients. The official recommendation is to remain on imatinib indefinitely, but she will not

be able to conceive, as imatinib is teratogenic. There are many tyrosine kinase inhibitor discontinuation trials that all show an approximate 40% freedom from molecular relapse rate at 2 years. Should she decide to discontinue imatinib, she will require an intensive monitoring strategy for the next 24 months (*Lancet Oncol.* 2010;11:1029).

48. **The correct answer is: A. Blinatumomab.** Blinatumomab is approved for patients with CD19-positive relapsed or refractory B-cell ALL and was shown to be superior to standard chemotherapy options with respect to remission rates as well as improvement in overall survival (*NEJM.* 2017;376:836).

    Inotuzumab and CAR-T are also new options for patients with relapsed or refractory ALL. Inotuzumab is only approved for patients with CD22+ lymphoblasts, but only a subset of the lymphoblasts are CD22 positive. There are two CAR-T products that are approved for relapsed B-ALL: brexucabtagene autoleucel and tisagenlecleucel. Brexu-cabtagene autoleucel is approved for adults with relapsed/refractory B-ALL (like our patient), but tisagenlecleucel is only approved for patients up to 26 years of age. In any case, blinatumomab would still be preferred for her.

49. **The correct answer is: A. AML.** This patient has acute leukemia based on the presence of >20% circulating blasts in the peripheral blood. Chronic myelogenous leukemia leads to increase in myeloid cells all along the differentiation spectrum of the myeloid lineage and does not have high blast counts (unless it is accelerated phase or blast crisis). Assignment of lineage is critical to expedient management of these patients and is done by flow cytometry on peripheral blood (if there is evidence of circulating blasts) or bone marrow. Myeloid blasts express markers myeloperoxidase, CD13, CD33, and CD117. Lymphoid blasts can be either B or T cells and are identified by respective markers. B-cell blasts: CD19, CD20, CD22. T-cell blasts: CD3, CD4, CD8.

50. **The correct answer is: D. All of the above.** This case demonstrates that patients with acute leukemia may present with several complications from their disease or related sequelae. In particular, high burden of disease with a very high blast count increases the risk of leukostasis because of visceral microvascular sludging and occlusion, leading to end organ dysfunction. This classically presents with respiratory and CNS-related symptoms, and its treatment includes urgent initiation of cytoreductive therapy, leukapheresis, and intensive critical care. This patient also shows lab evidence of spontaneous tumor lysis with hyperkalemia, renal dysfunction, and elevated LDH. This often occurs in patients with high disease burden and rapidly proliferative disease, leading to spontaneous tumor cell lysis. Given the replacement of the normal immune system by the leukemic clone, patients with acute leukemia are at a very high risk for infection, and all fevers should be urgently investigated and patients should receive empiric broad-spectrum antibiotic therapy.

51. **The correct answer is: A. <50.** Primary CNS lymphoma typically occurs when a patient's CD4 count drops below 50/mm^3. Non-Hodgkin lymphoma (NHL) is an AIDS-defining malignancy. Patients are also typically infected with Epstein-Barr virus. Treatment involves intrathecal methotrexate, steroids, and possible radiation and/or temozolomide. The regimen may necessitate significant myeloablation, to the point of considering an autologous HSCT.

52. **The correct answer is: C. Observation.** This patient has asymptomatic chronic lymphocytic leukemia, which does not warrant treatment. Chronic lymphocytic leukemia is not treated unless patients have disease-related symptoms (eg, pain from lymphadenopathy or hepatosplenomegaly) or have developed cytopenias. First-line therapy would often be ibrutinib, but other regimens such as venetoclax + rituximab can be considered, as well as venetoclax and/or obinutuzumab depending on cytogenetics.

53. **The correct answer is: C. Diffuse large B-cell lymphoma (DLBCL).** The patient has undergone a Richter transformation, a progression of chronic lymphocytic leukemia to DLBCL. This occurs in roughly 5% of chronic lymphocytic leukemia patients and carries a poor prognosis. Patients are then treated for DLBCL, rather than for the initial chronic lymphocytic leukemia. DLBCL treatment often includes R-CHOP (rituximab, cyclophosphamide, doxorubicin = hydroxydaunorubicin, vincristine = oncovin, prednisone) with or without radiation.

54. **The correct answer is: C. Positron emission tomography (PET)-CT scan; bone marrow biopsy.** The most important next step in diagnostic workup is excisional lymph node biopsy (not FNA because this will not reveal the surrounding architecture) with immunophenotyping and cytogenetics to confirm the diagnosis. Because staging requires identification of the number of lymph node regions involved, the presence of disease on one or both sides of the diaphragm, and the presence or absence of involvement of extralymphatic organs, full-body imaging is needed. PET-CT scan is preferred, because CT alone will not reliably detect spleen and liver involvement. In addition, PET response to treatment can be prognostic and can at times guide treatment. Bone marrow biopsy is indicated, as this would be a site of extranodal disease. Head CT and/or MRI is not indicated in the absence of symptoms.

55. **The correct answer is: A. ABVD (doxorubicin, bleomycin, vinblastine, dacarbazine) and repeat PET-CT after 2 cycles.** This patient has classical Hodgkin lymphoma, stage 2, nonbulky. The first-line therapy for stage 1-2 Hodgkin lymphoma is ABVD with or without radiation therapy. Although she would, in theory, be considered for involved-site radiation based on the disease being confined to only two sites, the potential risk of secondary malignancy in the breast and/or cardiomyopathy as a consequence of mediastinal radiation outweighs the potential benefit, particularly because chemotherapy alone is curative in more than half of the patients. PET-CT after the first two cycles is recommended for restaging. Patients with progressive disease at this time might be considered for escalation of therapy to a more aggressive regimen such as BEACOPP, whereas those with remarkable response to the first two cycles would be candidates for elimination of bleomycin for the remaining four cycles in order to reduce pulmonary toxicity. It would not be appropriate to plan for escalated BEACOPP prior to reimaging in early-stage disease, making choice C incorrect. Both Brentuximab-vedotin and pembrolizumab are active agents for Hodgkin's disease, but are currently only approved for more advanced stage (brentuximab-vedotin) or relapsed/refractory disease (both). Combination chemotherapy with ABVD is standard up-front therapy for Hodgkin lymphoma, and there is no role for radiation therapy alone (choice D) in this patient.

56. **The correct answer is: A. CXR, echocardiogram, pulmonary function tests.** The late effects after treatment for Hodgkin lymphoma include increased risk for second cancers (approximately 4.6× risk for up to 40 years), particularly breast (if received radiation therapy), lung, and hematologic malignancies. Because this patient did not undergo chest or neck radiation, her risk of breast cancer is relatively closer to average, while her risk of lung cancer, acute leukemia, myelodysplastic syndrome, and NHL remains elevated. CBC with differential is done to evaluate for hematologic malignancy. CXR should be performed to evaluate for lung cancer given her symptoms. As she is at increased risk for cardiac and pulmonary disease because she received 6 cycles of both doxorubicin (cardiotoxic) and bleomycin (pulmonary toxicity), she should therefore undergo echocardiogram and pulmonary function testing. TSH, T4 and cortisol testing do not need to be part of the initial workup for this patient. Although hypothyroidism or hypophysitis could contribute to fatigue and shortness of breath in some cases, the risk of thyroid or pituitary disease in this patient is similar to that of the general population, because the increased risk among patients with Hodgkin lymphoma applies only to those who receive neck radiation.

57. **The correct answer is: A. R-CHOP (rituximab, cyclophosphamide, doxorubicin, vincristine, prednisone).** This patient without double- or triple-hit diffuse large B-cell lymphoma (DLBCL) should be treated with standard R-CHOP chemotherapy; DA-R-EPOCH can be considered for double or triple-hit DLBCL. Treatment with CAR-T is typically reserved for relapsed or refractory DLBCL after two or more prior therapies, although it is also considered in patients with early first relapse (within 12 months from first treatment). ABVD is the chemotherapy regimen used in Hodgkin lymphoma, not DLBCL.

58. **The correct answer is: A. Quadruple therapy for treatment of the _H. pylori_ (bismuth, metronidazole, tetracycline, omeprazole).** This patient has a type of mucosa-associated lymphoid tissue (MALT) lymphoma, in this case, _H. pylori_ associated. More than 75% of patients with _H. pylori_–associated early-stage gastric MALT lymphoma will have regression of their disease and a durable long-term response with treatment of the _H. pylori_ alone. If the patient had persistent disease after eradication of _H. pylori_, radiation therapy or rituximab monotherapy would be appropriate. Similarly, if the patient had no evidence of _H. pylori_ at diagnosis, it would be appropriate to proceed with radiation or rituximab as first-line therapy.

59. **The correct answer is: B. Bone marrow biopsy with cytogenetics and gene mutation analysis; skeletal survey.** This patient's initial presentation with hypercalcemia, renal disease, anemia, and bone pain along with a large monoclonal IgG-κ is consistent with a diagnosis of multiple myeloma. The criteria for diagnosing multiple myeloma include clonal bone marrow plasma cells ≥10% and at least one myeloma-defining event, which can include either myeloma-related organ or tissue impairment (lytic bone lesions, calcium >11 mg/dL, creatinine >2 mg/dL, or Hb <10 g/dL), or any one of several biomarkers, including bone marrow plasma cells ≥60%, serum free light chain ratio ≥100:1, or more than one focal lesion on MRI studies. This patient has already undergone serum testing consistent with multiple myeloma but requires a bone marrow biopsy with cytogenetics and gene mutation analysis to help guide treatment and stratify risk. In addition, his complaint of hip pain is concerning for lytic bone lesion that may be at risk for pathologic fracture, and therefore a skeletal survey is indicated for further workup. PET-CT alone without bone marrow biopsy would be inappropriate. Furthermore, although PET-CT is more sensitive than plain films for detecting myelomatous bony lesions, starting with plain films or CT myeloma survey is the typical recommended practice at most centers. β_2-Microglobulin level and serum albumin should also be sent for staging purposes. In this patient, who meets several diagnostic criteria for multiple myeloma, it would not be appropriate to defer further workup and repeat testing in 6 weeks or 6 months.

60. **The correct answer is: B. 1% per year; 25% lifetime risk.** This patient has a diagnosis of κ light chain MGUS. This diagnosis requires an abnormal free light chain ratio in the absence of lytic bone lesions, renal failure, or hypercalcemia. This patient should undergo a skeletal survey to confirm that there are no bony lesions. The prevalence of MGUS in the population is about 3% in patients over age 50, 5% in patients over age 70, and 7.5% in patients over age 85. The prognosis is favorable for most patients with MGUS, because there is a 1% per year risk of progression to multiple myeloma, Waldenström macroglobulinemia, or a malignant lymphoproliferative disease and a 25% lifetime risk. Patients should be followed closely after diagnosis with repeat SPEP in 6 months and then yearly thereafter if stable.

61. **The correct answer is: D. Hyperviscosity syndrome.** This patient's overall clinical presentation with anemia, elevated monoclonal IgM spike, and cryoglobulinemia is most consistent with a diagnosis of Waldenström macroglobulinemia, which is a B-cell

neoplasm (lymphoplasmacytic lymphoma) that secretes monoclonal IgM. Approximately 90% of these patients will have MYD88 L265P mutations. In addition, patients with Waldenström macroglobulinemia should not have lytic bone lesions. Clinical manifestations can include amyloidosis and glomerulopathy because of IgM deposition in the skin, intestines, and kidney, although this patient does not have any signs consistent with this. Patients can also have chronic autoimmune hemolytic anemia and peripheral neuropathy because of autoantibody activity of IgM, although also not present in this patient. Type I cryoglobulinemia, leading to Raynaud phenomenon and vasculitis, is also present in this patient, but does not explain the neurologic and pulmonary symptoms. This patient's symptoms are most consistent with hyperviscosity syndrome, which occurs in about 15% of patients with Waldenström macroglobulinemia. Symptoms will typically present when the relative serum viscosity is >5 or 6. The symptoms include blurred vision, headache, dizziness, change in mental status, congestive heart failure, and pulmonary infiltrates. The management is plasmapheresis.

62. **The correct answer is: B. Start bendamustine + rituximab.** Indications for treatment in patients with Waldenström macroglobulinemia include hyperviscosity, neuropathy, organomegaly, amyloidosis, cold agglutinin disease, cryoglobulinemia, cytopenias related to the disease, and bulky adenopathy. For asymptomatic patients with incidentally diagnosed Waldenström macroglobulinemia, observation with close laboratory and clinical follow-up is appropriate. However, this patient has symptoms of peripheral neuropathy, most likely IgM related, and requires treatment. Patients with Waldenström macroglobulinemia and peripheral neuropathy can have antibodies to myelin-associated glycoprotein or others that contribute to the development of neuropathy, unrelated to serum viscosity. This patient does not have symptoms or laboratory evidence of hyperviscosity, and therefore plasmapheresis, choice E, is not indicated. There are several preferred regimens for the initial treatment of Waldenström macroglobulinemia, including bendamustine/rituximab, bortezomib/dexamethasone/rituximab, and zanubrutinib. Bortezomib would be an inappropriate choice for this patient, because it can worsen symptoms of neuropathy. Autologous stem cell transplant is recommended frequently for patients with multiple myeloma but is not indicated as first-line treatment for Waldenström macroglobulinemia.

63. **The correct answer is: E. Smoldering multiple myeloma.** This patient has smoldering multiple myeloma, which is diagnosed in patients with M-protein >3 g/dL and/or 10% to 60% bone marrow clonal plasma cell infiltrate, without myeloma-related organ or tissue impairment or amyloidosis. The workup for this patient demonstrates an elevated M-protein and >10% bone marrow plasma cell infiltration but absence of lytic lesions, anemia, hypercalcemia, and renal insufficiency. However, if the serum free light chain ratio was >100, this would qualify as multiple myeloma. The findings are inconsistent with MGUS, which requires M-protein <3 g/dL and marrow plasmacytosis <10%. Nonsecretory multiple myeloma is diagnosed in patients with no M-protein, but marrow plasmacytosis and myeloma-related organ or tissue impairment. The patient does not have clinical features or pathologic findings consistent with amyloidosis.

64. **The correct answer is: D. Referral to radiation oncology for radiation to the right humerus osseous lesion.** This patient has a solitary bone plasmacytoma, which is defined as a lytic lesion without plasmacytosis or other myeloma-related organ or tissue impairment, including other bone lesions, calcium >11 mg/dL, creatinine >2 mg/dL, or Hb <10 mg/dL, with SPEP negative for M spike. Because the disease is localized, the most appropriate next step in management would be either radiation or surgical reconstruction. In this case, radiation would be appropriate. Observation and referral to physical

therapy would be inappropriate, because the patient would be at risk for worsening pain and possibly pathologic fracture. Although choices A, B, and E are appropriate systemic therapies to consider in multiple myeloma, they are not indicated in the case of a solitary plasmacytoma.

65. **The correct answer is: A. Bortezomib/lenalidomide/dexamethasone.** Induction regimens with the best response rate for multiple myeloma combine proteasome inhibitors (bortezomib, carfilzomib) with immunomodulators (lenalidomide). Other active drugs include prednisone, dexamethasone, melphalan, and cyclophosphamide. A patient's candidacy for transplant is important to establish prior to induction, as the preferred regimens differ for patients who may go on to receive a transplant. However, stem cell transplant is not recommended as initial induction therapy for patients with multiple myeloma. Autologous stem cell transplant is recommended for some patients, after they undergo induction, in order to allow for high-dose consolidative therapy. Allogeneic stem cell transplant is rarely used for patients with multiple myeloma. Common induction regimens for transplant candidates include triplets, such as bortezomib/lenalidomide/dexamethasone, bortezomib/cyclophosphamide/dexamethasone, or carfilzomib/lenalidomide/dexamethasone, most of which combine proteasome inhibitors with immunomodulators. Pomalidomide/cyclophosphamide/dexamethasone, choice D, is indicated only for patients with previously treated, relapsed, or refractory multiple myeloma.

66. **The correct answer is: D. Myeloablative conditioning followed by allogeneic transplant from his sibling.** The patient has a high risk of relapse based on the presence of the *FLT3-ITD* mutation, in the setting of wild-type *NPM1*. Given the elevated risk of disease relapse (ie, adverse risk group) an allogeneic transplant is the best treatment strategy for him; that the patient has a fully matched donor is a plus. In a young patient with adverse risk AML without any comorbidities, myeloablative conditioning is tolerable and reduces the risk of leukemia recurrence in addition to the antileukemic effects from graft versus leukemia effect of the allogeneic transplant itself. Option C could be a reasonable approach for consolidation therapy for patients with favorable-risk AML (such as *NPM1* mutated without *FLT3* mutation or with low fraction of leukemic cells having the *FLT3* mutation [low VAF]). FLT3 inhibitors (option B) have shown improvement in overall survival when added to standard induction chemotherapy followed by maintenance dosing; however, this would only be preferred in patients who are unable to undergo allogeneic transplant because of age or comorbidities. Given this patient's age, availability of fully matched sibling donor, and high risk of disease recurrence, an allogeneic transplant would be the best choice for consolidation therapy.

67. **The correct answer is: C. Steroids.** This patient has developed engraftment syndrome, which occurs typically 1 to 4 days after ANC >500. Major characteristics are fever, noncardiogenic pulmonary edema, and erythrodermatous rash. If only two of the prior criteria are present, diagnosis can be supported by renal dysfunction, hepatic dysfunction, encephalopathy, or unexplained weight gain. Treatment of engraftment syndrome entails steroids 1 mg/kg, rapidly tapered over 3 to 4 days.

68. **The correct answer is: C. Fluconazole, atovaquone, acyclovir, and letermovir.** Patients undergoing allogeneic HSCT are at risk of bacterial, fungal, and viral infections, both because of initial pancytopenia from chemotherapy and immunosuppressive medications used to prevent GVHD. Fluconazole or posaconazole for prophylaxis against candidal infections is often given through day 75, though some centers no longer require fungal prophylaxis. TMP-SMX or atovaquone is started for *Pneumocystis carinii* pneumonia/*Pneumocystis jirovecii* pneumonia (PJP) prophylaxis after engraftment (because

of concerns for marrow suppression) and continued for 365 days or until immunosuppression is stopped. Acyclovir or valacyclovir may be used for herpes simplex virus (HSV) and varicella zoster virus (VZV) prophylaxis through 365 days. Patients who have positive CMV antibody titers, meaning they have been exposed to CMV in the past, are at risk of CMV reactivation, and over the first 100 days after transplant should receive CMV viral load monitoring and/or prophylaxis against reactivation (prophylaxis especially for high-risk patients—like those with CMV seronegative donors, HLA-mismatched donors, or receiving T-cell-depleting therapies or high-dose immunosuppression for GVHD). Valganciclovir, ganciclovir, or letermovir are all approved for prophylaxis, and choice can be influenced by complications (valganciclovir and ganciclovir can be myelosuppressive) and formulation (ganciclovir is given IV). This patient is at high risk for CMV reactivation as their donor is CMV-negative (so the graft will not include CMV targeted memory T cells to suppress CMV reactivation) and letermovir is a good choice, which reduces the risk of clinically significant CMV reactivation and is associated with lower mortality and good tolerability (*NEJM.* 2017;377:2433-2444). Fluoroquinolones are used for prophylaxis against bacterial infections while patients are neutropenic (options A, D, and E); however, this patient is no longer neutropenic. Finally, allopurinol is used to protect against hyperuricemia in the days leading up to transplant, while patients are receiving conditioning chemotherapy (option B), which no longer applies to this patient.

69. **The correct answer is: A. Acute graft-versus-host disease (GVHD).** The combination of diarrhea, maculopapular rash, and liver dysfunction makes acute GVHD the most likely diagnosis. Acute GVHD occurs typically within 6 months of transplant and is characterized by involvement of these three systems. Severity is graded based on percentage of body area involved by rash, level of bilirubin elevation, and volume of diarrhea. The mismatched related peripheral stem cell transplant increased the patient's risk for GVHD. This patient's symptoms and labs are all mild (grade 1), but he will likely need a biopsy to support the GI GVHD diagnosis, which will then be managed with increased immunosuppression. (Of note, if <25% of his skin were involved, he could be initially managed with topical steroids alone.)

70. **The correct answer is: D. Sinusoidal obstruction syndrome.** This patient is presenting with hepatic sinusoidal obstruction syndrome. The diagnosis is typically made based on a clinical syndrome of serum bilirubin >2 mg/dL, hepatomegaly or right upper quadrant pain, and sudden weight gain >2% baseline body weight. Although several conditions predispose patients to the risk of sinusoidal obstruction syndrome, patients who have undergone hematopoietic cell transplants are at increased risk, particularly within the first 3 weeks. Diagnosis must also exclude other causes of hepatic failure, including infection, GVHD, Budd-Chiari syndrome, and ischemia.

71. **The correct answer is: A. FDG PET/CT and brain MRI; pending results, follow with mediastinal lymph node evaluation with endobronchial ultrasound, mediastinoscopy.** The key information required to make a treatment determination here is the stage of the cancer. Hence, the initial workup focuses on evaluation of distant metastatic disease with a PET/CT and brain MRI and, if negative, to fully evaluate local extent of tumor within the mediastinum. The latter is critical in helping decide the approach to treating locally advanced tumors, including the role of radiation and feasibility of surgical approaches.

72. **The correct answer is: D. Osimertinib alone.** Deletions in EGFR exon 19 are activating mutations and these are predominantly found in nonsmokers with lung cancer. Presence of EGFR mutations is predictive of response to EGFR inhibitors, which are

more efficacious and less toxic than standard cytotoxic chemotherapy. In this patient, with stage 4 NSCLC with EGFR-positive mutation analysis, the most appropriate first-line therapy is osimertinib, a third-generation EGFR tyrosine kinase inhibitor. Osimertinib has shown more efficacy than earlier generation inhibitors (erlotinib, gefitinib) in the up-front setting, and this is thought to be related to its activity against both canonical EGFR mutations found in treatment-naïve patients (L858R and exon 19 deletions) and T790M resistance mutations found in almost 50% of patients who progress on early generation EGFR inhibitors. Additionally, osimertinib has better brain penetration than earlier generation EGFR inhibitors. Osimertinib should not be combined with carboplatin and paclitaxel as first-line therapy. Crizotinib is also a tyrosine kinase inhibitor, but targets ROS1 and should be used in patients with ROS1 mutation. Pembrolizumab alone and carboplatin/pemetrexed/pembrolizumab can be used for patients with PD-L1 staining >50% without other targetable mutations.

73. **The correct answer is: C. Carboplatin, paclitaxel, and pembrolizumab.** For patients with metastatic squamous cell carcinoma, PD-L1 staining is recommended. For those with >50% staining, pembrolizumab alone or chemotherapy + pembrolizumab can be considered as first-line therapy. For those with PD-L1 <50%, the first-line therapy is carboplatin/paclitaxel plus pembrolizumab. For patients with metastatic squamous non-small cell lung cancer, adding pembrolizumab to chemotherapy was shown to have a survival benefit for at all levels of PD-L1 expression.

74. **The correct answer is: D. Systemic therapy.** Regional spread involving a pleural effusion or pleural metastases are classified as stage IV disease. Unfortunately, the presence of malignant cells in this patient's pleural fluid cytology necessitates the use of systemic, rather than curative, treatment options. Had the patient not had a malignant pleural effusion, and if a brain MRI was also negative for metastatic disease, then this patient could have been considered for local therapies such as surgery (the gold standard) or stereotactic body radiotherapy. Definitive chemoradiation is typically used in unresectable stage III disease.

75. **The correct answer is: D. Request molecular diagnostic testing.** All patients with metastatic lung adenocarcinoma should have molecular testing performed for at least *EGFR*, *ALK*, and *ROS1*, as well as consideration of molecular testing for *KRAS*, *BRAF*, *NTRK1/2/3*, *METex14* skipping, and *RET* and immunohistochemical staining for PD-L1 (there is debate whether to simply check all at once or to test if *EGFR*, *ALK*, and *ROS1* are negative). Metastatic squamous cell carcinoma should be tested for PD-L1 expression, and testing for the aforementioned other genes should be considered (but is not yet recommended for all cases). The patient's biopsy is sufficient evidence of a metastatic lung cancer and so a confirmatory biopsy of the primary lung mass is not indicated, as it would not change management. A general principle in oncology is (whenever feasible) to biopsy presumed metastatic sites, as this approach provides diagnostic information on both the metastasis and the primary through pathology, whereas biopsy of a primary site leaves open the question of what disease process the presumed metastatic sites actually represent. The correct initial systemic therapy for metastatic lung adenocarcinoma will depend on the mutational profile.

76. **The correct answer is: D. Chest CT.** This patient has a smoking history and significant hyponatremia. Although sodium studies are indicated, this patient also has a concerning story for a paraneoplastic syndrome secondary to a small cell lung carcinoma, so a chest CT is warranted.

77. **The correct answer is: A. Today.** The U.S. Preventive Services Task Force (USPSTF) has updated their recommendations for annual low-dose CT for individuals aged 50 (rather than 55) to 80 with a 20-pack-year (rather than 30) smoking history who currently smoke or quit within the past 15 years.

78. **The correct answer is: C. Tamoxifen.** Tamoxifen is the standard systemic therapy for low-risk, early-stage ER+ breast cancer in premenopausal women. An aromatase inhibitor such as anastrozole would be first-line therapy for postmenopausal women. In premenopausal women, however, aromatase inhibitors do not block ovarian production of estrogen and so can only be used with concurrent medical or surgical ovarian suppression. Combined aromatase inhibition and ovarian suppression is more effective than tamoxifen alone in younger women with high risk of disease (ie, involved lymph nodes, high tumor grade, large tumor size, high Oncotype DX score). Adjuvant endocrine therapy for 10 years is generally superior to treatment for 5 years. However, the disease-free and overall survival benefits of extended therapy are small for patients, such as this woman, with low-risk disease, so therapy could be stopped before 10 years if she experiences adverse effects, such as intolerable hot flashes or thrombosis.

79. **The correct answer is: C. Lapatinib.** Options for metastatic hormone receptor–positive, HER2-negative breast cancer include aromatase inhibitors (eg, anastrozole), CDK 4/6 inhibitors (eg, palbociclib), and mammalian target of rapamycin (mTOR) inhibitors (eg, everolimus) added to aromatase inhibitors (eg, exemestane). Lapatinib is a reversible HER2 inhibitor, which is not indicated in HER2-negative disease.

80. **The correct answer is: A. Docetaxel, cyclophosphamide, trastuzumab, pertuzumab.** HER2+ breast cancer is treated with HER2-targeted therapy. These agents include the mAbs trastuzumab and pertuzumab, tyrosine kinase inhibitors, including lapatinib and neratinib, and the antibody-drug conjugate trastuzumab emtansine (T-DM1). In the adjuvant setting, docetaxel (Taxotere), cyclophosphamide, trastuzumab (Herceptin), pertuzumab (TCHP) is now considered standard therapy based on the Adjuvant Pertuzumab and Herceptin in Initial Therapy of Breast Cancer (APHINITY) trial (*N Engl J Med.* 2017;377:122-131). Letrozole, an aromatase inhibitor, plus ribociclib, a CDK4/6 inhibitor, is an appropriate first-line therapy for metastatic hormone receptor–positive, HER2-negative breast cancer.

81. **The correct answer is: B. BRCA2.** Although both BRCA1 and BRCA2 increase the risk of breast and ovarian cancer, there is a greater association of pancreatic cancer with BRCA2 mutations. Of note, BRCA mutated cancers are often more sensitive to therapies that target the homologous recombination repair pathway, including platinum therapy and PARP inhibitors. PARP inhibitors are approved for metastatic breast cancer with germline BRCA1/2 mutations.

82. **The correct answer is: D. No further mammograms indicated.** The USPSTF recommends biennial mammogram screening for women aged 50 to 74. In the absence of prior abnormal mammograms and no current breast complaints, there is no indication for this patient to continue regular mammogram screening.

83. **The correct answer is: D. Starting treatment with immunotherapy in combination with chemotherapy first line.** In March 2019, the Food and Drug Administration (FDA) granted accelerated approval for first-line atezolizumab in combination with chemotherapy for PD-L1-positive patients with triple-negative breast cancer. Pembrolizumab in combination with chemotherapy is now also approved for treatment of triple-negative breast cancer in patients with a PD-L1 combined positive score (CPS) of 10 or more.

84. **The correct answer is: C. Degarelix and abiraterone/prednisone.** This patient has newly diagnosed hormone-sensitive metastatic prostate cancer. The backbone of therapy for hormone-sensitive metastatic prostate cancer is ADT, either with a long-acting LH-releasing hormone (LHRH) agonist (eg, leuprolide) or LHRH antagonist

(eg, degarelix). The choice of ADT is variable between experts. However, leuprolide alone is associated with a transient androgen burst, given its agonist activity on the LHRH receptor, and can hence worsen symptoms or precipitate crises in patients with high-volume disease. Hence, either it is phased into treatment after pretreating with an androgen receptor blocker (bicalutamide) for a couple of weeks or treatment is initiated with a direct antagonist of the LHRH receptor, which is not associated with the androgen surge. Several would favor the latter approach, particularly in patients with a high volume of disease such as this patient, although this is a more expensive therapy.

We have recently learned from several clinical trials that the addition of newer generation antiandrogen abiraterone (CYP17 lyase inhibitor) or chemotherapy in the form of docetaxel to ADT improves overall survival in patients with hormone-sensitive metastatic prostate cancer (especially those with high disease burden). Given this patient's age, multiple comorbidities, and poor performance status, he is not a good candidate for docetaxel chemotherapy. Hence, degarelix with abiraterone/prednisone is the best option among those listed.

85. **The correct answer is: C. Prostate MRI.** The patient has a persistently elevated PSA, which could be secondary to prostate cancer. He is 67 years and, without any major medical issues, has a long life expectancy. In such patients, diagnosing early prostate cancer can help prevent future cancer-related mortality. A few years ago, the only way to investigate this PSA further was a transrectal ultrasound (TRUS)-guided 12-core biopsy. Recent advances in prostate imaging with MRI now allow visual identification of any potential pathologic lesions. In a recent study (*NEJM.* 2018;378:1767) prostate MRI was compared head-to-head with standard TRUS-guided prostate biopsy in patients with a similar epidemiologic profile as our patient. Approximately 30% of patients in the study were able to forgo a prostate biopsy because the MRI revealed no concerning lesions. Patients with visualized lesions on the MRI underwent a more focused biopsy rather than the blind 12-core biopsy. Not surprisingly, a higher percentage of patients undergoing prostate MRI were diagnosed with clinically significant prostate cancer (Gleason grade ≥7) compared with standard biopsy given the targeted approach.

86. **The correct answer is: A. Active surveillance.** Active surveillance is a strategy to avoid or delay treating patients with low-risk prostate cancer that is unlikely to pose a health issue for many years, and that patients may die with rather than die of. Active surveillance is, as the name suggests, an active strategy with close follow-up and testing, including repeat PSA measurements, prostate biopsies, and/or MRI, to identify patients with early progression for treatment and hence not reduce the chance of cure while avoiding therapy in patients with truly low-risk disease. Choices C and D are standard of care for localized clinically significant prostate cancer but have associated toxicities. In a patient with low-risk Gleason 6 prostate cancer from a targeted MRI-guided biopsy, active surveillance is a reasonable approach as long as he understands that if the disease is seen to be progressing (elevation in PSA, change to higher Gleason grade), then treatment with choices C or D would be appropriate.

87. **The correct answer is: B. Axumin scan to assess for bone and soft-tissue metastases with subsequent ADT versus salvage radiotherapy and ADT.** Indications for salvage radiotherapy include an undetectable PSA that becomes subsequently detectable and increases on two measurements or a PSA that remains persistently detectable after radical prostatectomy. The patient falls in the former category. Next-generation imaging such as an Axumin scan is generally preferred over conventional imaging (ie, CT scan) in such patients who are candidates for local salvage therapy,

particularly if the PSA is 0.5 to 2.0 ng/mL, given the Axumin scan's greater sensitivity to detect disease both locoregionally and at distant sites. Depending on if recurrence is found at the resection bed or at distant sites, RT + ADT versus ADT alone can be considered. If, however, local therapy would not be feasible when considering what imaging to obtain, conventional imaging with a CT scan would be reasonable (and salvage ADT alone could be considered) although disease may not be found until the PSA is >10. In men who have undergone radical prostatectomy, a PSA recurrence is defined as a serum PSA of 0.2 ng/mL or higher, confirmed by a repeat test. By contrast, in men who have undergone definitive radiotherapy, a recurrence is defined as a rise of 2 ng/mL or more above the nadir PSA, confirmed by a repeat test.

88. **The correct answer is: A. Colonoscopy at age 20, then repeat screen yearly.** This patient likely has hereditary nonpolyposis colorectal cancer (HNPCC) based on his family history: ≥3 family members with HNPCC-associated cancers, two generations affected, and at least one diagnosis before age 50. This was confirmed by germline mutation testing, which showed a mutation in PMS2, one of the components of the mismatch repair pathway. Other components of the mismatch repair pathway that can be mutated in HNPCC include MLH1, MSH6, and PMS2. Patients with this familial syndrome should undergo genetic counseling, begin screening at age 20 to 25 years, and continue with screening colonoscopies every 1 to 2 years.

89. **The correct answer is: D. A and B.** In patients with a known colon cancer diagnosis, CEA is measured in order to subsequently measure response to therapy. Of note, CEA is not a screening tool. Patients then undergo CT chest/abdomen/pelvis to look for metastatic disease. This disease preferentially metastasizes to the liver, lungs, and peritoneum in that order. Brain metastases are less common, so head imaging is not indicated unless neurologic symptoms are present.

90. **The correct answer is: C. Pembrolizumab.** This patient's tumor has MSI-H. Pembrolizumab has been shown to be superior to chemotherapy (+/- bevacizumab or cetuximab) in terms of progression-free survival in patients with metastatic colon cancer that is MSI-H or deficient in mismatch repair proteins (dMMR) (*NEJM.* 2020;383:2207). Thus, pembrolizumab is now recommended as first-line therapy for these patients.

91. **The correct answer is: D. Colonoscopy.** This patient has a positive history of colon cancer in a first-degree relative, which means he should start routine colon cancer screening at age 40 or 10 years before his father's age of diagnosis, whichever is earlier. All of the options listed are appropriate screening tests for routine screening of asymptomatic individuals per the USPSTF guidelines. However, this patient is presenting with symptomatic microcytic anemia concerning for iron deficiency. In an adult male, iron deficiency anemia is highly suspicious for colon cancer and requires diagnostic workup with colonoscopy. When there is suspicion for malignancy, the purpose of testing is no longer for screening but for diagnosis. Colonoscopy is far more sensitive and specific than the other modalities listed and is the most appropriate diagnostic test.

92. **The correct answer is: B. Familial breast/ovarian cancer BRCA2.** Although all syndromes listed can lead to a hereditary form of pancreatic cancer, this particular pattern of cancers of the breast, ovary, and prostate points toward BRCA2 mutations. The penetrance for developing pancreatic cancer in patients with BRCA2 inherited mutations is lower than that for breast and ovarian cancers.

93. **The correct answer is: E. Poly (ADP-ribose) polymerase (PARP) inhibitors.** PARP inhibitors target poly (ADP-ribose) polymerase. BRCA2 functions in the homologous

recombination DNA repair pathway and tumors that have lost BRCA2 (and hence homol-ogous recombination deficient tumors) are exquisitely sensitive to loss of PARP, which is normally involved in repairing single-strand breaks. This exquisite sensitivity of BRCA-null tumor cells to PARP inhibition is known as synthetic lethality, a phenomenon where a defect in either of two genes has little effect on the cell or organism but a combination of defects in both genes results in death. Hence, nontumor cells in the patient (which have not lost the second copy of BRCA2) do not suffer the same toxicity to PARP inhibition as tumor cells. Recently, maintenance PARP inhibitor therapy with olaparib was shown to prolong disease progression in metastatic pancreatic cancer patients who had a genomic BRCA2 mutation. Because this patient's main toxicity is neuropathy (which is secondary to oxaliplatin), continuing chemotherapy with FOLFOX (5-FU/leucovorin + oxaliplatin) or a regimen consisting of abraxane (also causes neurotoxicity) would likely worsen these symptoms. Regarding option D, immunotherapy, specifically checkpoint blockade with PD-1 inhibitors, has not shown efficacy in pancreatic cancers except for a very small sub-set of patients (~1% or less) who have pancreatic cancer secondary to Lynch syndrome, leading to MSI-H (microsatellite unstable). Because the patient has a good performance status and an excellent response to up-front FOLFIRINOX, the option for therapy hospice (option C) at this point would not be appropriate.

94. **The correct answer is: D. Pancreatic protocol CT scan or MRI with contrast followed by endoscopic ultrasound (EUS)-guided fine needle aspiration (FNA).** Pancreatic protocol CT scan with IV contrast, including arterial and venous phase imaging or MRI with contrast, is the most important next step in diagnosis. If no lesion is seen, the next step would be EUS, or magnetic resonance cholangiopancreatography (MRCP). Following imaging to define the lesion size and location, EUS-guided FNA is the preferred modality to obtain tissue diagnosis. Although it is useful to check CA 19-9 preoperatively and trend postoperatively to assess for recurrence, this is not an essential test in diagno-sis. Abdominal ultrasound is useful for assessing the liver, gallbladder, and kidneys but less sensitive for pancreatic lesions.

95. **The correct answer is: D. Referral to multidisciplinary team for manage-ment of HCC.** HCC is one of the rare tumors that can be diagnosed without a biopsy in patients with liver cirrhosis and characteristic findings on multiphasic liver CT scan or contrast-enhanced liver MRI. The American College of Radiology has established LI-RADS (Liver Imaging Reporting and Data System) to standardize the interpretation of surveillance liver imaging for HCC. LI-RADS category 5 implies definitive HCC, and these patients do not need a biopsy for confirmation. LI-RADS 5 criteria for masses >2 cm include arterial phase hyperenhancement and one of the following: (1) washout appearance (nonperipheral); (2) enhancing capsule; (3) threshold growth = size increase of a mass by ≥50% in ≤6 months.

96. **The correct answer is: D. Transcatheter arterial chemoembolization (TACE).** TACE is a minimally invasive technique of locally delivering chemotherapy (coated on gel beads) into the hepatic artery branches feeding the tumor and represents a reasonable approach to palliate unresectable locally advanced nonmetastatic HCC. However, TACE is generally contraindicated in patients with portal vein thrombosis of the main vein or first-order right or left branches because of high risk of hepatic insufficiency from post-TACE ischemic liver injury. Patients with HCC and associated portal vein thrombosis have a worse overall prognosis and, in general, are not considered candidates for liver transplantation, surgical resection, and TACE. Stereotactic body radiation therapy, a type of highly focused radiation therapy, can still be used in such cases.

97. **The correct answer is: C. Liver MRI.** A diagnosis of HCC can be made via a three-phase contrast-enhanced abdominal CT or MRI. CT or MRI is indicated if either a mass is found on ultrasound or if AFP levels are found to be increasing.

98. **The correct answer is: D. Upper GI endoscopy, repeat every 3-5 years if Barrett esophagus present.** Screening with esophagogastroduodenoscopy (EGD) is recommended to assess for Barrett esophagus given the presence of multiple risk factors (chronic GERD, male, age ≥50, obesity, smoking, hiatal hernia). A family history of esophageal cancer is also a risk factor, although the patient does not have this. If dysplasia is found, repeat screening should be performed every 3-5 years to reassess any potential progression. The patient should also have their medical therapy intensified and efforts made to reduce the chronic stress of reflux onto the squamous epithelium of the distal esophagus (eg, weight loss, stop smoking).

99. **The correct answer is: A. Ipilimumab and nivolumab.** Checkpoint inhibitor therapy is a cornerstone of therapy for metastatic melanoma. BRAF/MEK inhibitors such as dabrafenib/trametinib can also be considered in first-line therapy, but only if activating BRAF V600E mutations are present. Dual checkpoint inhibitor therapy is associated with an improved response rate, particularly for intracranial metastases. Although dual therapy is also associated with more checkpoint inhibitor–related toxicities than monotherapy, in this young and fit patient with intracranial disease, the benefits of dual therapy likely outweigh the risks. Furthermore, this patient has small and asymptomatic brain lesions that can be treated with systemic dual checkpoint inhibitor therapy. If she had large or symptomatic lesions, then surgery or stereotactic radiosurgery might be considered for local therapy as well.

100. **The correct answer is: B. Chest/abdomen CT with contrast.** This patient has a new diagnosis of chronic myelogenous leukemia with increased creatinine, phosphorous, and uric acid, as well as borderline high potassium, all consistent with impending tumor lysis syndrome. A chest/abdomen CT will not help diagnose chronic myelogenous leukemia, and contrast should be avoided in the setting of renal dysfunction associated with tumor lysis syndrome. Instead, a bone marrow biopsy is necessary to confirm the diagnosis of chronic myelogenous leukemia. Rasburicase is appropriate to treat this patient's elevated uric acid, and although there is a risk of hemolysis without having first checked G6PD deficiency status, in this patient with an extremely elevated uric acid and evidence of renal injury, the benefits likely outweigh the risks. Hydroxyurea is helpful for cytoreduction while awaiting diagnostic confirmation, although it requires close monitoring for worsening tumor lysis syndrome. IV fluids are helpful for tumor lysis syndrome prevention.

101. **The correct answer is: C. Nasogastric suction.** This patient has neutropenic enterocolitis, in which microbial infection in the setting of severe neutropenia has led to necrosis of various layers of the bowel wall. Nasogastric suction should be considered as a supportive therapy, as well as bowel rest, IV fluids, and nutritional support. Morphine and loperamide are opioid and antidiarrheal agents, respectively, that may aggravate ileus and so should be avoided. Although a surgery consult may be appropriate, surgical intervention should similarly be avoided in this neutropenic and thrombocytopenic patient, unless she clinically deteriorates or develops perforation with free air or persistent GI bleeding despite medication interventions. Of note, neutropenic patients should have no anorectal manipulation (medications, exams, rectal tubes), but placement of nasogastric tubes is acceptable.

102. **The correct answer is: B. ATO and ATRA.** This patient has a presentation concerning for acute PML, given the easy bruising and the Auer rods. Such patients have a very high cure rate, but mortality typically occurs early if the condition is not identified. Roughly 90% of these patients will present with DIC with evidence of bleeding, and the primary cause of death is intracranial hemorrhage. This patient should receive ATO and ATRA, and her labs should be monitored closely to keep her platelets >10 000/µL, fibrinogen >100 mg/dL, and normal PT/PTT/INR.

103. **The correct answer is: D. Stat MRI spine.** The patient is exhibiting signs of spinal cord compression, an oncologic emergency. Although surgery may ultimately be indicated, this cannot be performed before imaging confirmation. The patient must thus undergo immediate spine MRI. He may also receive high-dose steroids to manage sequelae.

104. **The correct answer is: E. All of the above.** This patient is presenting with new likely malignant ascites and evidence of peritoneal carcinomatosis. With her history of pelvic radiation, ovarian carcinoma should be high on the differential. Ovarian cancer often presents insidiously with nonspecific history of bloating, abdominal pain, and urinary or bowel symptoms. Prompt diagnosis is essential so that treatment can be initiated, and peritoneal sampling and tumor markers (CA-125) are often pursued in tandem. Positive cytology on ascitic fluid can be diagnostic. If it is not, then biopsy of an identified lesion would be indicated. An elevated CA-125 is not diagnostic on its own, but is a helpful adjunctive piece of information. CT chest should also be obtained to complete staging.

105. **The correct answer is: A. Neoadjuvant chemotherapy with carboplatin and paclitaxel, followed by cytoreductive surgery.** The mainstay of treatment of ovarian carcinoma is cytoreductive surgery and chemotherapy. Even with metastatic disease, cytoreductive surgery has been shown to improve survival. First-line preferred chemotherapy is carboplatin and paclitaxel, which can be either prior to (neoadjuvant—usually 3 of 6 total cycles prior) or following (adjuvant) surgery. Neoadjuvant chemotherapy can increase the likelihood of maximal surgical cytoreduction and reduces surgical complications; survival is equivalent. PARP inhibitors such as olaparib (option B) are not recommended for adjuvant therapy. They are approved as maintenance therapy following first-line chemotherapy and surgical cytoreduction, for women with tumors that are *BRCA* mutant (germline or somatic), homologous recombination deficient, or have responded to platinum therapy. The greatest benefit is seen in patients with tumors that are *BRCA* mutant or homologous recombination deficient positive. Gemcitabine with or without bevacizumab (option D) is used in patients with platinum-resistant disease, meaning those who have recurrence within 6 months after their last treatment with platinum doublet (eg, carboplatin and paclitaxel) but do not meet the standard of care for first-line adjuvant therapy.

106. **The correct answer is: B. Obtain CT imaging of the chest, abdomen, and pelvis.** A new isolated brain lesion is highly suspicious for malignancy. Among CNS tumors, metastatic lesions are more common than primary CNS tumors, and their discovery should prompt a workup for systemic malignancy (most commonly lung, breast, melanoma, and renal cell carcinoma) with total body imaging. Biopsy of the CNS lesion (option A) may be necessary, but in this stable patient, full staging should be done first to strategize where to biopsy. If body imaging reveals other lesions suspicious for malignancy, biopsy of those lesions may be more feasible and is often preferred. However, in choosing a place to biopsy, a guiding principle is to biopsy a location that can reveal both diagnosis AND stage (eg, it is generally preferred to biopsy lesions distant from the suspected primary lesion). Seizures are a common presenting symptom of CNS tumors and the mainstay of management is antiepileptic medication. Radiation would not be warranted at this time (option C). Finally, LP for cytology (option D) can be considered if there is specific concern for CNS lymphoma after further imaging.

107. **The correct answer is: A. Dihydropyrimidine dehydrogenase deficiency.** Up to 80% of 5-FU (and its oral prodrug capecitabine) is degraded by liver enzyme dihydropyrimidine dehydrogenase into inactive metabolites. Polymorphisms in dihydropyrimidine dehydrogenase that lead to partial or complete deficiency of enzyme activity are associated with increased exposure to 5-FU and its active metabolites and can present with serious hematologic, GI, CNS, and dermatologic toxicity. Uridine triacetate, a pyrimidine derivative, competitively inhibits incorporation of 5-FU in RNA and is an approved agent to be given within 96 hours of completion of treatment with either 5-FU or capecitabine in cases of severe and unexpected toxicity. Symptoms present are not routinely seen after FOLFOX, which is given on an outpatient basis without G-CSF support in most cases. Although option B is possible, dihydropyrimidine dehydrogenase deficiency needs to be considered first.

108. **The correct answer is: C. Infliximab.** This patient has severe checkpoint inhibitor–induced colitis, which is refractory to steroids. Checkpoint inhibitors derepress the immune system to generate antitumor effect. However, autoimmune side effects can occur with these agents. In particular, use of dual checkpoint inhibitors targeting both the CTLA4 and the PD-1 axis can have more severe toxicities and more unusual toxicities not seen with monotherapy. In this case, the timing of the diarrhea in relation to the treatment duration fits well with occurrence of checkpoint inhibitor–induced colitis. Infection is the most important differential diagnosis and has been ruled out with stool cultures and *C. difficile* toxin. CMV colitis can often occur in these patients who tend to be immunocompromised and can often be missed. CMV colitis was also evaluated on the colonic biopsy specimen and was negative. Hence, given the timing of the symptoms, and findings on sigmoidoscopy and active colitis on biopsy, there is very little doubt as to this being checkpoint inhibitor–induced colitis. The first-line treatment for severe checkpoint-induced colitis is parenteral steroids. A subset of patients can be refractory to steroids and are treated with anti–tumor necrosis factor (TNF)-α antibody such as infliximab.

109. **The correct answer is: E. Both B and C.** This patient has elevations in her liver enzymes while on pembrolizumab, an immune checkpoint inhibitor, concerning for an immune-related adverse event (IRAE). The AST and ALT elevations are <3× the upper limit of normal and alkaline phosphatase is <2.5× the upper limit of normal, consistent with a grade 1 IRAE. She feels overall well and has no signs or symptoms to suggest other types of immune-related inflammation. Management of grade 1 IRAEs generally consists of supportive care and continuation of treatment. There is no need for steroids (option A). It is important, however, not to anchor on a diagnosis of treatment-related hepatitis and to rule out other etiologies such as viral infection and progression of known liver metastases (option C).

110. **The correct answer is: C. Brain MRI.** Although there are many infectious and autoimmune causes of hypotension in a patient on immunotherapy, the combination of thyroid, adrenal, and gonadal abnormalities suggests a problem high in their respective axes. Hypophysitis is a rare but serious side effect of ipilimumab and nivolumab, the chances of which are increased with combination therapy. The clinical syndrome raises suspicion, which can be confirmed with MRI. Meanwhile, immunotherapy agents should be held, and, given the severe hemodynamic risk, the patient should also receive steroids.

111. **The correct answer is: D. Tocilizumab.** When the patient's BP first dropped but was fluid responsive, she had developed grade 2 cytokine release syndrome. When she was no longer fluid responsive, this became grade 3 cytokine release syndrome. Currently, the interleukin-6 inhibitor tocilizumab is indicated at grade 3 cytokine release syndrome, although practices are moving toward grade 2. Steroids are avoided if possible, given they have not been definitely shown to not interfere with the efficacy of CAR-T. TNF-α inhibitors like infliximab are sometimes given for colitis, and mycophenolate mofetil is sometimes given for hepatitis.

112. **The correct answer is: E. A, B, and C.** The patient has developed immune effector cell–associated neurotoxicity syndrome (ICANS), which is characterized by cerebral edema, delirium, aphasia, seizures, and, potentially, death. If patients progress to the severity of seizure and intubation, they should be treated with antiepileptics and steroids. Tocilizumab is indicated for cytokine release syndrome but not for ICANS.

113. **The correct answer is: A. Cefepime.** Febrile neutropenia requires up-front broad-spectrum antibiotic coverage with an agent that has antipseudomonal activity. However, monotherapy is preferred, and vancomycin is only added if hypotension, pneumonia, clinically apparent soft-tissue or catheter infection, mucositis plus quinolone antibiotic prophylaxis, or gram-positive organisms in blood cultures are present. The presence of an indwelling line or mucositis in and of themselves does not warrant addition of vancomycin therapy in febrile neutropenia. Antifungal coverage such as micafungin should be added if fevers continue despite 4 or more days of appropriate antibiotics and the ANC has not yet recovered. Meropenem is not indicated unless the patient has a history of multidrug-resistant organisms (eg, extended-spectrum β-lactamase-producing bacteria).

114. **The correct answer is: C. Coronary artery vasospasm.** FOLFOX includes 5-FU, which is often administered through a chemotherapy infusion pump, and can cause coronary vasospasm. In this young patient without risk factors for CAD, chemotherapy toxicity is more likely than an acute coronary syndrome, despite the thrombogenic potential of cytotoxic chemotherapy. Pulmonary metastases would be unlikely to cause acute worsening of shortness of breath and chest pain as the patient is experiencing. An occult pulmonary embolism should always be considered in patients with active malignancy and shortness of breath, but substernal chest pain would be less typical of pulmonary embolism and chemotherapy-related toxicity is more likely in this scenario.

115. **The correct answer is: B. Missed myocardial infarction.** The patient had a flu-like illness 2 weeks ago, which was likely a missed myocardial infarction rather than a true viral infection given the evidence of new segmental wall motion abnormalities plus new-onset heart failure in a patient with significant risk factors for CAD (eg, hypertension, hyperlipidemia, type 2 diabetes, smoking). Anthracycline chemotherapy such as hydroxydaunorubicin can cause a dilated cardiomyopathy, but this is generally a dose-dependent toxicity that becomes more likely with higher cumulative lifetime doses. Anthracycline-related cardiomyopathy causing heart failure would be less likely after the patient has only received one cycle of R-CHOP. Dietary indiscretion would be more likely to cause heart failure symptoms in a person with a preexisting history of heart failure. It certainly could lead to initial presentations of heart failure, but the patient's segmental wall motion abnormalities and history of symptom onset make missed myocardial infarction more likely.

INFECTIOUS DISEASES

QUESTIONS

1. A 78-year-old woman with a history of chronic obstructive pulmonary disease (COPD), hypertension, and gastroesophageal reflux disease presents with 4 days of productive cough, fever, and malaise. She feels short of breath when she walks. Her granddaughter recently had a cold, but she cannot recall any other sick contacts in the assisted living facility where she resides. She has not received any antibiotics in the last 3 months. On physical examination, her temperature is 37.6°C, pulse 90/min, respirations 32 breaths/min, and blood pressure (BP) 150/87 mmHg. Her examination is notable for diminished lung sounds and crackles in the right lower base, without egophony or wheezing. Her laboratory findings demonstrate a white blood cell (WBC) count of 16 800/μL with 89% neutrophils, 1.2% bands, 8% lymphocytes, erythrocyte sedimentation rate (ESR) 48 mm/h, C-reactive protein 33 mg/L, platelets 90 000/μL, and creatinine 0.6 mg/dL. Chest x-ray (CXR) has stable emphysematous changes and evidence of right lower lobe and right middle lobe opacification.

   What is the most likely diagnosis?

   A. Acute exacerbation of bronchiectasis
   B. Aspiration pneumonitis
   C. COPD exacerbation
   D. Severe community-acquired pneumonia

2. If the patient in Question 1 were immunocompromised, which of the following tests should NOT be used?

   A. Blood cultures
   B. Procalcitonin
   C. Sputum Gram stain and culture
   D. Viral respiratory testing

3. What would be the appropriate empiric therapy for the patient in Question 1?

   A. Ceftriaxone plus azithromycin
   B. Doxycycline
   C. No antibiotics; provide supportive care
   D. Vancomycin plus cefepime

4. Which vaccines should you ensure the patient in Question 1 has received as part of normal health maintenance?

   A. Influenza vaccine
   B. Pneumococcal 20-valent conjugate vaccine
   C. Zoster recombinant vaccine
   D. All of the above

5. If the patient in Question 1 had been in the hospital within the last 1 month for treatment of a urinary tract infection (UTI), what would be the most appropriate empiric treatment for her pneumonia?

   A. Cefepime and vancomycin
   B. Ceftriaxone and metronidazole
   C. Ceftriaxone and vancomycin
   D. Ciprofloxacin

6. If influenza testing was positive in the patient in Question 1, what would be the appropriate treatment?

   A. Zanamivir 10 mg twice daily for 5 days
   B. Oseltamivir 75 mg once daily for 5 days
   C. Oseltamivir 75 mg twice daily for 5 days
   D. Supportive measures only

7. A 54-year-old woman with a history of ischemic cardiomyopathy who is status post heart transplant 12 days ago has developed new fevers. She has evidence of waxing and waning delirium, but otherwise denies any localizing infectious symptoms such as headache, neck stiffness, photophobia, cough, shortness of breath, abdominal pain, dysuria, or diarrhea. She has a stage 1 pressure ulcer on her sacrum and one peripherally inserted central catheter line in her right upper extremity. She has an external pacemaker with a clean, dry incision site. On physical examination, her temperature has peaked to 39.4°C, pulse 115/min, respirations 18 breaths/min, and BP 126/82 mmHg. Her examination is notable for decreased alertness with orientation to person, place, but not time. She has decreased lung sounds bilaterally. Cardiac examination reveals S1, S2, and S4 heart sounds with no murmurs, rubs, or gallops. Her abdomen has positive bowel sounds and is nontender. Her extremities are symmetrically edematous. She has no rashes. Her labs are notable for creatinine 1.8 mg/dL and WBC count 19 300/μL with 93% neutrophils. A CXR demonstrates atelectasis at the bases and mild pulmonary edema. Urinalysis has 1+ glucose mg/dL, 1+ protein mg/dL, and specific gravity 1.016 (reference range 1.001-1.035), with 0 to 2 WBCs/high-power field (hpf). Two sets of blood cultures result in the growth of yeast in two out of four bottles at 72 hours; 1,3-β-D-glucan and galactomannan serum tests are pending.

   Which of the following factors does NOT increase the risk for invasive fungal infection?

   A. Central venous catheters
   B. Foley catheter
   C. Hematologic malignancy
   D. Total parenteral nutrition
   E. Tumor necrosis factor (TNF)-α inhibitors

8. All of the following may result in a positive 1,3-β-D-glucan serum test EXCEPT for which?

   A. Hemodialysis with cellulose membranes
   B. Invasive aspergillosis
   C. Invasive mucormycosis
   D. Recent administration of albumin
   E. Recent administration of intravenous immunoglobulins (IVIGs)

9. Which species of fungi can be detected by galactomannan serum testing?

   A. *Aspergillus* species
   B. *Histoplasma* species
   C. *Penicillium* (*Talaromyces*) species
   D. A and C
   E. All of the above

10. Which diagnostic test is necessary in the patient in Question 7?

    A. Ophthalmology consult

    B. Repeat blood cultures

    C. Transthoracic echocardiogram

    D. All of the above

11. What is your empiric management for the patient in Question 7?

    A. Initiate an echinocandin

    B. Initiate fluconazole

    C. Remove all central venous catheters

    D. A and C

    E. B and C

12. A 56-year-old man presents 8 months after an allogeneic stem cell transplant with increased cough and shortness of breath. He has been on a prolonged course of steroids for complications of graft-versus-host disease of the skin. He is on trimethoprim-sulfamethoxazole (TMP-SMX) for *Pneumocystis* prophylaxis. On examination, he is afebrile, pulse 92/min, respirations 22 breaths/min, BP 122/85 mmHg, and O_2 saturation 90% on room air. A computerized tomography (CT) scan of the chest is notable for multiple scattered pulmonary nodules with nodular consolidations and surrounding ground glass opacities ("halo sign"). Serum galactomannan is elevated.

What is the most likely diagnosis?

    A. Bronchiolitis obliterans

    B. Invasive pulmonary aspergillosis

    C. Methicillin-resistant *Staphylococcus aureus* (MRSA) pneumonia

    D. Respiratory syncytial virus (RSV)

13. The patient in Question 12 develops an allergic reaction to TMP-SMX.

What alternative antimicrobial can be used for *Pneumocystis* prophylaxis?

    A. Atovaquone

    B. Acyclovir

    C. Ertapenem

    D. Amoxicillin/clavulanic acid

14. A 36-year-old woman with a history of recurrent nephrolithiasis and poorly controlled diabetes presents with urinary burning, frequency, and suprapubic tenderness. The patient is sexually active with one male partner and does not use condoms. On physical examination, her temperature is 37.4°C, pulse 70/min, respirations 16 breaths/min, and BP 118/79 mmHg. Her examination is notable for a nontoxic appearance, normal cardiovascular evaluation, and suprapubic tenderness. She does not have costovertebral tenderness.

What is the most likely diagnosis?

    A. Acute pyelonephritis

    B. Acute uncomplicated cystitis

    C. Neurogenic bladder from diabetes

    D. None of the above

15. Which of the following should NOT be considered for workup of the patient in Question 14?

    A. Complete blood count (CBC)

    B. CT abdomen and pelvis

    C. *Neisseria gonorrhoeae* and *Chlamydia trachomatis* testing

    D. Urinalysis and urine culture

16. Which of the following could be considered for empiric treatment in the patient in Question 14?

A. Fosfomycin
B. Nitrofurantoin
C. TMP-SMX
D. All of the above

17. A 36-year-old man with a remote history of renal transplant presents with burning, frequency, and foul-smelling urine for several days. He received TMP-SMX last month for an extended β-lactamase *Escherichia coli* UTI. His symptoms resolved for a few weeks and now have returned. He is sexually active and does not use condoms. On physical examination, his temperature is 38°C, pulse 80/min, respirations 16 breaths/min, and BP 118/79 mmHg. His examination is notable for a nontoxic appearance, normal cardiovascular evaluation, and suprapubic tenderness. No urethral discharge or genital lesions are noted. He does not have costovertebral tenderness.

What is the most likely diagnosis?

A. Complicated UTI
B. Transplant rejection
C. Uncomplicated UTI
D. None of the above

18. What is the appropriate workup for the patient in Question 17?

A. CT abdomen and pelvis
B. *N. gonorrhoeae* and *C. trachomatis* testing
C. Prostate examination
D. Urinalysis and urine culture
E. All of the above

19. What is the empiric treatment for the patient in Question 17?

A. Ciprofloxacin
B. IV carbapenem
C. Nitrofurantoin
D. TMP-SMX

20. A 73-year-old man with a history of gout, hypertension, diabetes, and alcohol use disorder presents with a right plantar foot wound of 1-year duration that has become acutely painful. One week prior to admission, at an urgent care clinic, the patient received a dose of IV antibiotics and had a foot radiograph, which was not suggestive of osteomyelitis. He has received ongoing wound care with a local podiatrist. His home medications include allopurinol, indomethacin, and lisinopril. He recently completed a prednisone taper for a gout flare. On physical examination, his temperature is 37.6°C, pulse 72/min, respirations 16 breaths/min, and BP 160/92 mmHg. His extremities are notable for a 4 × 3 cm ulcerated lesion on the right plantar foot at the base of the great toe. There is a black necrosis at the center of the lesion, with erythematous, well-defined edges. The erythema extends beyond the edges by 4 cm. With a probe, the subcutaneous tissue is identified; however, the probe does not reach the bone.

What is the most likely diagnosis?

A. Chronic osteomyelitis
B. Diabetic foot infection
C. Gout flare
D. Necrotizing fasciitis

21. Which of the below characteristics would support a diagnosis of acute osteomyelitis in the patient in Question 20?

   A. ESR >70 mm/h

   B. Probing to bone or grossly visible bone

   C. Ulcer duration longer than 1 to 2 weeks

   D. Ulcer size >2 cm^2

   E. All of the above

22. What is the optimal empiric treatment for the patient in Question 20?

   A. Ciprofloxacin and metronidazole

   B. Piperacillin-tazobactam

   C. Vancomycin and ertapenem

   D. Vancomycin and levofloxacin

   E. Vancomycin, cefepime, and metronidazole

23. A 39-year-old woman with active IV drug use and untreated hepatitis C presents with acute-onset fevers and chills. She last injected IV heroin into her arm 12 hours before arrival. On examination, she is in acute distress, febrile to 40.3°C, pulse 118/min, BP 97/70 mmHg, respirations 18 breaths/min, and oxygen saturation 99% on room air. She is alert and oriented ×3; however, she is unable to turn her neck or lift her right arm. Brudzinski and Kernig testing are both positive. The remainder of the examination is notable for injection site marks along the bilateral antecubital fossa. Labs are notable for WBC count of 20 000/μL with 87% neutrophils. Blood cultures result in methicillin-sensitive *Staphylococcus aureus* (MSSA), and she is initiated on oxacillin. A transthoracic echocardiogram was negative for endocarditis. Despite appropriate antistaphylococcal antibiotics, the patient has persistent bacteremia with neck pain and focal neurologic symptoms.

What is the most likely diagnosis?

   A. Aortic root abscess not observed on a transthoracic echocardiogram

   B. Epidural abscess

   C. MSSA meningitis

   D. Recurrent IV drug use while hospitalized

   E. None of the above

24. For the patient in Question 23, what is the appropriate duration of antimicrobial therapy?

   A. 2 weeks from initiation of oxacillin

   B. 6 weeks from initiation of oxacillin

   C. 2 weeks from surgical debridement

   D. 6 weeks from surgical debridement

   E. Oxacillin can be discontinued 48 hours after clearance of cultures

25. A 22-year-old healthy woman presents after cutting her left foot on a boat propeller while swimming in a lake. The accident occurred 24 hours ago, with only a small abrasion along the dorsum of her foot. The site became increasingly painful; therefore, she presented to the hospital. Her examination is notable for a young woman in acute distress, diaphoretic, with an edematous, erythematous right foot. Erythema reaches her ankle, and the tissue appears boggy. There is no drainage, no crepitus on examination. She is febrile at 40.1°C, pulse 112/min, respirations 16 breaths/min, and BP 100/62 mmHg. Labs are notable for Cr 1.7 mg/dL, WBC count 22 400/μL with 98% neutrophils, 6% bands, and lactate 3.4.

What is the most likely diagnosis?

   A. Necrotizing fasciitis

   B. Pyoderma gangrenosum

   C. Pyomyositis

   D. Severe cellulitis

   E. Shark bite

26. For the patient in Question 25, in addition to initiating IV antibiotics, which team should be urgently consulted?

  A. Ophthalmology
  B. Surgery
  C. Neurology
  D. Physical therapy

27. A 52-year-old man, who has been training for his first marathon, presents with 1 week of left-sided facial numbness, left facial paralysis, left ear tinnitus, and painful tongue lesions. He presented to the emergency department (ED) 4 days prior and was told he has viral-associated Bell palsy and should take 60 mg of prednisone daily. He did as instructed and his symptoms progressed. Patient re-presented to the ED when he developed new severe left-sided headaches and hearing loss. On physical examination, he is afebrile, pulse 70/min, respirations 12 breaths/min, and BP 115/78 mmHg. He has obvious left-sided facial paralysis without evidence of rash. Inspection of his mouth reveals white coating along his tongue and vesicles lining his palate. He is oriented but has decreased arousal. Serum laboratory findings are unremarkable.

  What is the most likely diagnosis?

  A. Acute human immunodeficiency virus (HIV) infection
  B. Facial nerve paresis secondary to Lyme disease
  C. Herpes zoster ophthalmicus
  D. Melkersson-Rosenthal syndrome
  E. Ramsay Hunt syndrome

28. Of the studies you may send on the patient in Question 27, which has the LOWEST sensitivity for diagnosing active infection?

  A. Direct fluorescent antibody testing on scrapings from vesicular skin lesions
  B. Varicella zoster virus polymerase chain reaction (PCR) from lesion
  C. Varicella zoster virus viral culture

29. The patient in Question 27 became increasingly delirious over the next 12 hours. Lumbar puncture (LP) is performed, which shows WBC 320/mm^3 with 70% polymorphonuclear cells (PMNs), glucose 110 mg/dL, and total protein 100 mg/dL.

  What is the most likely etiology given his history and these results?

  A. Bacterial superinfection meningitis
  B. Herpes simplex virus (HSV)-1 encephalitis
  C. Stroke
  D. Varicella zoster encephalitis

30. A 68-year-old man with a history of hypertension, gout, obesity, cervical stenosis status post recent cervical laminectomy, and spinal fixation 5 days ago is brought in by his wife for confusion. There were no complications with the surgery and the patient was discharged on postoperative day 3 with oxycodone. At home, his pain steadily escalated; therefore, the patient increased his doses of oxycodone, gabapentin, and ibuprofen. On physical examination, his temperature is 39.6°C, pulse 106/min, respirations 24 breaths/min, and BP 170/96 mmHg. He is oriented and able to hold a conversation but appears lethargic. Pupils are equally round and reactive. Cervical collar is in place. The incision site appears clean, dry, and intact without induration or tenderness. He is able to move all four limbs without focal deficits. Cardiac pulmonary evaluation is normal. Laboratory findings demonstrate Cr 1.9 mg/dL, K 5.4 mEq/L, WBC count 20 800/µL with 87% neutrophils, 3.2% bands, and platelets 306 000/µL; urinalysis with 1+ protein, 1+ urobilinogen, and 10 to 20 WBC/hpf.

What is the most likely diagnosis?

A. Bacterial meningitis
B. Cerebral vascular event
C. Medication-induced altered mental status
D. Viral encephalitis

31. Which of the following scenarios does NOT require head imaging prior to LP?

A. Patient with known epilepsy
B. Focal neurologic findings
C. New-onset seizure
D. Papilledema
E. Primary central nervous system (CNS) lymphoma

32. The LP of the patient in Question 30 shows WBC 1200/mm³ with 80% PMNs, glucose 25 mg/dL, and total protein 600 mg/dL.

What is the most likely etiology given his history and these results?

A. Bacterial meningitis
B. Drug-induced aseptic meningitis
C. HSV encephalitis
D. Tuberculous (TB) meningitis

33. What is the most appropriate empiric treatment regimen for the patient in Question 30?

A. Hold on antibiotics until further culture data are obtained
B. IV acyclovir
C. Liposomal amphotericin B
D. Vancomycin and cefepime

34. A 34-year-old woman with a history of IV drug use presents to ED with 5 days of fever, shaking chills, and malaise. She has no other significant past medical history and takes no medications. She endorses daily use of IV heroin. On examination, she is febrile at 39.2°C, pulse 107/min, BP 105/67 mmHg, respirations 16 breaths/min, and oxygen saturation 97% on room air. Examination is notable for a 2/6 systolic murmur heard best in the left lower sternal border and scattered crackles on pulmonary examination. She has multiple injection site marks noted on her arms and legs, as well as a few erythematous macules on her bilateral palms. Labs are notable for a WBC count of 18 000/μL with 92% neutrophils. Her basic metabolic panel and liver function tests (LFTs) are within normal limits. A CXR is notable for diffuse bilateral nodular densities.

What are the next steps in the workup and management of this patient?

A. Initiate empiric broad-spectrum antibiotics
B. Obtain an echocardiogram
C. Obtain an electrocardiogram (ECG)
D. Obtain blood cultures
E. All of the above

35. The blood cultures of the patient in Question 34 return with four out of four bottles growing MSSA. Transthoracic echocardiogram is notable for an 8-mm mobile vegetation on the tricuspid valve and a transesophageal echocardiogram (TEE) is ordered for better assessment.

What additional steps should be taken at this time?

A. Narrow antibiotics to a β-lactam (ie, nafcillin or cefazolin)
B. Obtain CT chest to assess for pulmonary emboli
C. Screen for HIV and hepatitis C
D. B and C
E. A, B, and C

36. The patient in Questions 34 and 35 clears her blood cultures after 48 hours of antibiotic therapy. TEE is negative for any significant valvular abscess or perforation, and cardiac surgery is not felt to be indicated. Chest CT is notable for several subpleural nodular lesions and a few wedge-shaped densities without necrosis caused by septic infarcts.

    What are the next steps for management?

    A. Continue antibiotics for 2 weeks from date of first negative blood cultures and follow along with weekly labs
    B. Continue antibiotics for 6 weeks from date of first negative blood cultures and check weekly labs
    C. Continue antibiotics for 2 weeks from date of first negative blood cultures; no indication to check weekly labs
    D. Continue antibiotics for 6 weeks from date of first negative blood cultures; no indication to check weekly labs

37. Which of the following are indications for antimicrobial prophylaxis for dental procedures?

    A. History of infective endocarditis
    B. History of ventricular septal defect repaired as a child
    C. Presence of a bioprosthetic aortic valve
    D. A and C
    E. A, B, and C

38. A 45-year-old man presents to establish primary care. He moved to the United States from Eastern Europe 6 months ago and reports that he has no prior medical issues and takes no medication. He received the bacillus Calmette-Guérin (BCG) vaccine as a child. On physical examination, he is afebrile and his vital signs are within normal limits. He is well appearing with clear lung sounds bilaterally and no lymphadenopathy. You decide to screen him for TB.

    Which test should you proceed with?

    A. CXR
    B. Induced sputum for mycobacterial culture and smear for acid-fast bacilli (AFB)
    C. Interferon-γ release assay
    D. Tuberculin skin test

39. If the TB interferon-γ release assay of the patient in Question 38 returns indeterminate, what do you do next?

    A. Order a tuberculin skin test for comparison
    B. Reassure—this is expected with the BCG vaccine
    C. Repeat interferon-γ release assay
    D. Treat empirically for latent TB infection

40. The TB interferon-γ release assay of the patient in Question 38 returns positive. He denies any recent fever, chills, night sweats, or weight loss. He has no pulmonary symptoms. He has no known history of contacts who had TB. His HIV testing is negative. He undergoes a CXR, which is clear.

What is the next best step in the management and treatment of this patient?

A. Initiate isoniazid daily (with vitamin B6) for 9 months
B. Initiate rifampin daily for 4 months
C. Initiate rifampin, isoniazid, pyrazinamide, and ethambutol for 2 months followed by rifampin with isoniazid for 4 months
D. Either A or B

41. Suppose instead the patient in Question 38 endorses several months of intermittent fever and cough. His CXR was normal.

What would be your next steps?

A. Monitor and recheck interferon-γ release assay in 1 year
B. Obtain CT chest imaging
C. Send three induced sputum cultures for AFB smear and mycobacterial culture
D. B and C

42. A 37-year-old man presents to clinic requesting an HIV test. He reports that a former sexual partner of his recently notified him that he was diagnosed with HIV. The patient reports that he has been sexually active with multiple male partners in the past and reports that he does not always use condoms. Medical history is notable for one prior episode of gonococcal urethritis 2 years ago and an episode of primary syphilis 5 years ago. He reports that he had a negative HIV test about 10 years ago. On examination, he is afebrile, heart rate (HR) 87 beats/min, and BP 124/85 mmHg. He is anxious appearing. Head and neck examination are normal. He has a regular rate and rhythm and lungs are clear. His abdominal examination is benign, and he has no rashes. A HIV screen test for HIV-1/2 antibody/antigen is sent and returns positive. The HIV-1/2 differentiation assay is positive for HIV-1.

In addition to CD4 cell count, HIV viral load and genotype, CBC with differential, basic metabolic panel, and LFTs, of the laboratory workup listed below, which is NOT recommended in those with a new HIV diagnosis?

A. Fasting lipids
B. Glucan and galactomannan
C. Hemoglobin A_{1c} (HbA$_{1c}$)
D. Hepatitis A, B, C serologies
E. Interferon-γ release assay

43. The CD4 cell count of the patient in Question 42 returns at 172 cells/μL and his HIV-1 viral load is 364 000 copies/mL. His CBC, basic metabolic panel, and liver enzymes are all within normal limits. Further history and examination are unrevealing for any evidence of opportunistic infection.

When should antiviral treatment be started?

A. At this visit, if patient is agreeable to start
B. Begin with *Pneumocystis jiroveci* prophylaxis and, if tolerated, start antiretroviral therapy 1 week later
C. Once the results of his genotype return
D. When CD4 cell count is <100 cells/μL
E. When the patient develops signs/symptoms of an opportunistic infection

44. The patient in Questions 42 and 43 is started on antiretroviral treatment as well as TMP-SMX for *P. jiroveci* pneumonia prophylaxis. At a follow-up visit 6 months later, he is feeling well, has maintained a CD4 cell count of over 300 cells/μL on monthly checks over the past several months, and HIV viral load is now nondetectable.

Which of the following is correct?

A. He can stop TMP-SMX at this time

B. He should continue on TMP-SMX until CD4 cell count remains above 200 cells/μL for 12 months

C. He should continue on TMP-SMX until he has been on antiretroviral therapy for 12 months

D. He will need to remain on lifelong TMP-SMX

45. A 24-year-old man presents to you seeking consideration for HIV preexposure prophylaxis (PrEP). He reports that he has multiple male sex partners but always uses condoms. He has a history of rectal gonorrhea 1 year ago. Routine sexually transmitted infection screening, including HIV screening, is done and negative. Additional laboratory workup shows a normal CBC and a comprehensive metabolic panel.

What would you offer this patient, at this time, for HIV PrEP?

A. No indication for PrEP because patient is using condoms regularly

B. Start tenofovir/emtricitabine (TDF/FTC) as needed after unprotected sex

C. Start TDF/FTC daily

D. Start TDF/FTC and dolutegravir daily

46. A 62-year-old nurse in the intensive care unit presents after having had a needlestick exposure a few hours ago. The patient she was drawing labs on has a history of IV drug use, untreated hepatitis C virus (HCV, with a detectable viral load), and HIV infection. His most recent HIV viral load is unknown and viral load result on this admission is pending.

What would you offer the nurse at this time, for HIV postexposure prophylaxis (PEP)?

A. Await results of the patient's HIV viral load and hold off on treatment unless it is detectable

B. Await results of the patient's HIV viral load and only start PEP if detectable and once the genotype can be confirmed

C. Start TDF/FTC daily for 4 weeks

D. Start TDF/FTC with an integrase inhibitor (dolutegravir or raltegravir) daily for 4 weeks

47. What would you do for the nurse in Question 46 at this time regarding her HCV exposure?

A. Start glecaprevir/pibrentasvir for 8 weeks

B. Start sofosbuvir/velpatasvir for 12 weeks

C. Obtain testing for HCV RNA now. If negative, no further testing is required

D. Obtain testing for anti-HCV now and HCV RNA 3 weeks later

E. Not undergo any further testing or treatment

48. A 23-year-old man from Massachusetts presents after passing out on the football field during practice. On examination, he is afebrile, HR 48 beats/min, and BP 110/83 mmHg. His ECG is notable for a new third-degree heart block. The patient denies any significant family history of cardiac issues, takes no medications, and denies any known tick bites. On further review of systems, he does report that he had a nonpainful, nonpruritic rash on his right side a few weeks ago that resolved on its own.

Which of the following is true regarding management?

A. Blood cultures would be useful to confirm the diagnosis

B. The condition is reversible with administration of antibiotics

C. The patient will need a permanent cardiac pacer

D. The patient will need lifelong suppressive antibiotics

E. The underlying infection can be sexually transmitted

49. The mother of the patient in Question 48 also notes a target-shaped lesion on her popliteal fossa. She is otherwise asymptomatic with a normal screening ECG. She is initiated on appropriate treatment.

What side effects of the treatment should you counsel her on?

A. Esophagitis
B. Photosensitivity
C. Diarrhea
D. All of the above

50. A 65-year-old man with a remote history of splenectomy presents with 1 week of progressive fatigue and weakness, followed by 2 days of fever, malaise, and dark-colored urine. He lives in Cape Cod, Massachusetts, and enjoys spending time outdoors. He denies any known tick bites though he does report that he had a circular red rash with central clearing on the back of his leg, about 1 week ago, that has since resolved. On examination, his temperature is 38.6°C, HR 118 beats/min, and BP 116/62 mmHg. He appears jaundiced. Labs are notable for WBC 4000/μL, Hb 8.6 g/dL, platelets 110 000/μL, total bilirubin 7.2 mg/dL, alanine aminotransferase (ALT) 68 U/L, and aspartate aminotransferase (AST) 72 U/L.

Given his presentation and risk factors, what would be the next best step?

A. Check Lyme ELISA (enzyme-linked immunosorbent assay) screen, blood parasite smear, human granulocytic anaplasmosis PCR
B. Check Lyme ELISA screen, blood parasite smear, human monocytic ehrlichiosis PCR
C. No testing indicated; start empiric azithromycin
D. No testing indicated; start empiric doxycycline

51. Blood parasite smear for the patient in Question 50 shows intraerythrocytic forms and it is estimated that he has 8% parasitemia. His other lab tests are pending.

What treatment should be initiated?

A. Azithromycin and atovaquone
B. Azithromycin, atovaquone, and doxycycline
C. Ceftriaxone and azithromycin
D. Doxycycline alone
E. Vancomycin and cefepime

52. For the patient in Question 50 what other pathogens may he have been exposed to by this disease vector?

A. Rocky Mountain spotted fever
B. West Nile virus
C. Bartonellosis
D. Powassan virus
E. All of the above

53. A 28-year-old man presents with intermittent fevers for the last week. Patient reports that every few days he develops chills, headaches, and muscle pain. He has no past medical history and takes no medications. He is sexually active with one partner, denies IV drug use, and drinks alcohol on occasion. He works for the Peace Corps, but his last trip out of the country was 1 month ago to Ethiopia. On examination, his temperature is 37.1°C, HR 80 beats/min, and BP 128/62 mmHg. He appears fatigued, but in no acute distress. Labs are notable for WBC count 12 600/μL, Hb 10.4 g/dL, platelets 106 000/μL, ALT 72 U/L, AST 65 U/L, international normalized ratio (INR) 1.3 (reference range 0.9-1.1), and creatinine 1.4 mg/dL.

Given his risk factors and presentation, which condition could he have that would be a medical emergency that must be presumed until proven otherwise?

A. Acute HIV infection
B. Dengue
C. Epstein-Barr virus
D. Malaria
E. Typhoid fever

54. What would be the next step in the diagnostic workup of the condition of the patient in Question 53?

A. PCR study
B. Blood smear with staining
C. Blood culture
D. Abdominal ultrasound

55. A 72-year-old woman presents with 2 weeks of headache and fever. The headache is mostly on the left side of her face and worsened with chewing. She reports no known sick contacts or recent travel. On examination, her temperature is 38.4°C, HR 92 beats/min, and BP 128/67 mmHg. Cranial nerves, including visual acuity, are intact, and she has no focal neurologic deficits and no meningeal signs. Labs, including CBC, basic metabolic panel, and LFTs, are all within normal limits. Her ESR is elevated to 82 mm/h.

Which of the following is the next best step in management?

A. Obtain brain magnetic resonance imaging (MRI)
B. Obtain LP
C. Obtain temporal artery biopsy
D. Start high-dose prednisone

56. A 63-year-old man with a recent hospitalization for bacterial pneumonia is now presenting with 2 days of fever, abdominal cramping, and watery diarrhea. On examination, HR is 102 bpm, BP 120/72 mmHg. He is noted to have dry mucous membranes and diffuse mild abdominal tenderness. He is placed on contact precautions because of concern for *Clostridiodes difficile* colitis.

What is the most appropriate therapy to initiate?

A. IV vancomycin
B. PO vancomycin
C. PO fidaxomicin
D. PO clindamycin
E. IV ceftriaxone and metronidazole

ANSWERS

1. **The correct answer is: D. Severe community-acquired pneumonia.** This patient likely has community-acquired pneumonia. The potential etiologies include a bacterial infection, such as *S. pneumoniae*, *Haemophilus influenzae*, or *Moraxella catarrhalis*, or viral causes, such as influenza, rhinovirus, or RSV. Infectious Diseases Society of America (IDSA) 2019 guidelines for community-acquired pneumonia define severe community-acquired pneumonia as having septic shock or respiratory failure and one of the following minor criteria: a respiratory rate >30 breaths/min, PaO_2/FiO_2 (P/F) ratio of <250, multilobular infiltrates, confusion, uremia, leukopenia, thrombocytopenia, hypothermia, or hypotension. Having three or more of these criteria alone also qualifies as severe community-acquired pneumonia. This patient has a respiratory rate of 32 breaths/min, thrombocytopenia, and multilobular infiltrates, classifying her as severe community-acquired pneumonia.

2. **The correct answer is: B. Procalcitonin.** Additional information that is useful for patients presenting with community-acquired pneumonia includes sputum Gram stain and culture (adequate sample if >25 PMNs/low-power field [lpf] and <10 squamous cells/lpf), blood cultures, viral testing, and procalcitonin. Procalcitonin is a biomarker that is upregulated in acute respiratory infections caused by bacterial, but not viral, etiologies. The use of procalcitonin varies across hospital systems and could be considered to help direct the use of antibiotics at some institutions; however, it is NOT validated in immunocompromised hosts and therefore would not be advised.

3. **The correct answer is: A. Ceftriaxone plus azithromycin.** For community-acquired pneumonia, the local *S. pneumoniae* resistance patterns should be considered. Monotherapy with azithromycin or doxycycline should not be used if prevalence of resistance is >25%. Additionally, for patients with comorbidities, such as chronic heart, lung, liver, or renal disease, diabetes mellitus, alcoholism, malignancy, or asplenia, guidelines suggest either combination therapy (cephalosporin + macrolide/doxycycline) or monotherapy (levofloxacin). Of the choices listed, ceftriaxone and azithromycin would be appropriate in this patient. Oral monotherapy with levofloxacin (not listed as an option here) could also be considered. Living in an assisted living facility does not qualify her to be treated for resistant organisms encountered with hospital-acquired infections. She also has not received antibiotics in the last 3 months, which lowers her risk for resistant organisms; therefore, vancomycin and cefepime would not be indicated. Duration of therapy for community-acquired pneumonia is 5 to 7 days with clinical improvement.

4. **The correct answer is: D. All of the above.** After 65 years of age, all immunocompetent adults should receive one dose of pneumococcal conjugate vaccine (PCV) 15 or 20. If patients aged 19 through 64 years have chronic medical conditions (chronic heart, lung, liver disease, diabetes, alcoholism, cigarette smoking), then one dose of PCV 15 or 20 should be administered. If PCV15 is used, patients should receive one dose of PPSV23 1 year later. Every person should receive the influenza vaccine annually. For those with an egg allergy, with respiratory distress or angioedema, the influenza vaccine should still be administered under the supervision of a health care provider in a medical setting. Zoster recombinant vaccine (Shingrix) is recommended in all adults 50 years or older. It is a 2-dose series administered at least 2 to 6 months apart, regardless of a previous episodes of herpes zoster or previously received zoster vaccination. In this case, all of the vaccines listed would be indicated for this patient if she has not received them already.

5. **The correct answer is: A. Cefepime and vancomycin.** Empiric treatment for hospital-acquired pneumonia depends on the presence or absence of risk factors for multidrug-resistant pathogens, knowledge of predominant pathogens within the health care setting, and the individual's prior microbiology data. The most important predictive factor that places an individual at risk for multidrug-resistant organisms is if they have received IV antibiotics within the past 90 days. Two organisms that are necessary to consider in hospital-acquired pneumonia are *Pseudomonas aeruginosa* and MRSA. For this reason, the only antibiotic option that would treat both of those organisms would be a combination of cefepime (for *Pseudomonas*) and vancomycin (for MRSA).

6. **The correct answer is: C. Oseltamivir 75 mg twice daily for 5 days.** Antiviral therapy should be initiated as soon as possible and is most likely to provide benefit when initiated within the first 48 hours of illness. Treatment should NOT be held in patients with indications for therapy who present >48 hours after the onset of symptoms, especially those requiring hospitalization. Oseltamivir 75 mg twice daily for 5 days would be recommended in this patient if she were diagnosed with influenza as the etiology of her community-acquired pneumonia. The once-daily dose of oseltamivir is recommended for influenza chemoprophylaxis or if patients have renal dysfunction. Zanamivir is an inhaled antiviral agent used for influenza treatment and prophylaxis that is contraindicated in patients with asthma or COPD and should not be used in severe influenza. Baloxavir is a single dose treatment for influenza that is also an acceptable alternative.

7. **The correct answer is: B. Foley catheter.** This patient is immunosuppressed given her recent heart transplant, and this puts her at increased risk for invasive fungal infections. Other risk factors for fungemia include administration of total parenteral nutrition, hematologic malignancy, solid organ transplant, biologic therapies (including TNF-α inhibitors), and IV drug use. In this case, the source was likely her peripherally inserted central catheter line, which should be removed immediately. The Foley catheter is unlikely to be a source of her candidemia.

8. **The correct answer is: C. Invasive mucormycosis.** The 1,3-β-D-glucan assay detects a cell wall component in many fungi, including *Aspergillus* species, *Candida* species, and *P. jiroveci*; however, it is typically negative in patients with mucormycosis or cryptococcosis. The 1,3-β-D-glucan assay can be falsely positive with: IVIG or albumin, surgical gauze, certain types of dialysis membranes, and infections with certain bacteria that contain cellular β-glucans (*P. aeruginosa*).

9. **The correct answer is: E. All of the above.** Galactomannan is a major constituent of *Aspergillus* cell walls. An enzyme immunoassay that detects the galactomannan antigen is available for use in blood and bronchoalveolar lavage fluid as an adjuvant test for the diagnosis of aspergillosis. Serum galactomannan assay is helpful in the setting of suspected invasive aspergillosis in patients with hematologic malignancies. The test can be positive in the setting of infections with *Fusarium* spp, *Penicillium* spp, and *Histoplasma capsulatum* because of cross-reactivity, and there can be false positives in the setting of IVIG, and historically with piperacillin-tazobactam (rarely the case now with new preparation of piperacillin-tazobactam).

10. **The correct answer is: D. All of the above.** Blood cultures with yeast are NEVER to be considered contaminants. It is important to collect daily blood cultures until they are negative. Other important diagnostic tests for fungemia include an ophthalmology consult to evaluate for endophthalmitis and a transthoracic echocardiogram to evaluate for endocarditis, particularly in cases of persistent fungemia or if any evidence of embolic phenomena is present.

11. **The correct answer is: D. A and C.** The most likely cause of yeast in this patient's blood is *Candida* species. The first step is to remove any potential sources of infection (in this case, the peripherally inserted central catheter line) and to obtain an Infectious Disease consult. There is high mortality associated with candidemia in immunocompromised hosts. Empiric treatment for *Candida* species is an echinocandin, such as micafungin, because *Candida glabrata* and *Candida krusei* can have resistance against azole antifungals. For *Candida albicans*, there is little resistance in the absence of prior exposure to azoles; therefore, this patient could be transitioned to fluconazole after susceptibility is confirmed.

12. **The correct answer is: B. Invasive pulmonary aspergillosis.** This patient most likely has invasive pulmonary aspergillosis. Risk factors for this include prolonged and profound neutropenia or immunosuppression. In this case, the patient has a history of stem cell transplant and also was recently on steroids. The presence of a positive serum galactomannan and CT findings make aspergillosis most likely.

13. **The correct answer is: A. Atovaquone.** Oral atovaquone (1500 mg orally once daily with food), dapsone (100 mg daily, need to check glucose-6-phosphate dehydrogenase status), and aerosolized pentamidine (300 mg monthly) are alternative regimens for *Pneumocystis* pneumonia (PCP) prophylaxis. TMP-SMX is considered first line, however, because of its cost, coverage, side effects, and efficacy. Therefore, an alternative drug should only be used if TMP-SMX is not an option for the patient.

14. **The correct answer is: B. Acute uncomplicated cystitis.** This is most likely acute uncomplicated cystitis. Her symptoms are confined to the bladder without evidence of upper tract involvement or systemic signs. It is important to note that a history of nephrolithiasis, poorly controlled diabetes, HIV, urinary strictures with stents, and immunocompromised patients are not automatically considered complicated UTIs; however, there should be a lower threshold to treat these individuals as complicated infections.

15. **The correct answer is: B. CT abdomen and pelvis.** Further workup includes a urinalysis, urine culture, and CBC. Pyuria on urinalysis is suggestive of infection. In sexually active patients with UTI symptoms and "sterile pyuria," you should also test for sexually transmitted diseases such as *N. gonorrhoeae* and *C. trachomatis*. Consider CT imaging only when the patient is severely ill, symptoms persist for 72 hours despite antibiotics, and there is suspicion for obstruction from stone, renal abscess, or recurrent symptoms within a few weeks of treatment.

16. **The correct answer is: D. All of the above.** If a patient has uncomplicated acute cystitis and no prior UTIs with multidrug-resistant organisms, empiric treatment options include nitrofurantoin monohydrate/macrocrystals 100 mg twice daily for 5 days, TMP-SMX 1 DS tablet orally twice per day for 3 to 5 days, or fosfomycin 3 g orally for one single dose. For complicated cystitis, a longer course of 7 to 14 days with either a fluoroquinolone or TMP-SMX may be given.

17. **The correct answer is: A. Complicated UTI.** This is a complicated UTI. Individuals with renal transplants and pregnant women are treated as complicated UTIs regardless of whether the infection extends beyond the bladder.

18. **The correct answer is: E. All of the above.** All men with UTIs should have a prostate examination to test for prostatitis. The diagnostic studies include urinalysis, urine culture, and CBC. Pyuria on urinalysis indicates infection. CT imaging would be appropriate in this patient given his recurrent symptoms within a few weeks of completing treatment. In sexually active patients with UTI symptoms, consider also testing for sexually transmitted infections such as *N. gonorrhoeae* and *C. trachomatis*.

19. **The correct answer is: B. IV carbapenem.** For a complicated UTI, the treatment strategy depends on the patient's risk for multidrug-resistant organisms. If, in the last 3 months, the patient had a multidrug-resistant gram-negative bacilli infection, an inpatient stay, and used a fluoroquinolone, TMP-SMX, or a broad-spectrum β-lactam, then cefepime or a carbapenem is the correct first-line medication for a complicated UTI while awaiting results of susceptibility testing. This patient has recently received TMP-SMX for a UTI and has a history of drug-resistant organisms, qualifying him for a carbapenem as empiric therapy. If there are no multidrug-resistant risk factors, then the drug of choice is a fluoroquinolone, TMP-SMX, or a β-lactam. Subsequent treatment should be tailored according to culture results.

20. **The correct answer is: B. Diabetic foot infection.** This patient likely has a diabetic foot infection. The risk factors for diabetic foot infections include peripheral neuropathy, which leads to decreased awareness of injury; peripheral vascular disease, which impairs necessary blood flow for healing; and poor glycemic control, which impairs neutrophil function. If the patient had chronic osteomyelitis, you would expect to see findings on the foot radiograph, which can typically demonstrate abnormalities by 2 weeks after infection.

21. **The correct answer is: E. All of the above.** Clinical findings that help support osteomyelitis include (1) probing to bone or grossly visible bone; (2) ulcer size >2 cm; (3) ulcer duration longer than 1 to 2 weeks. Ultimately, MRI is the most sensitive imaging study to detect osteomyelitis if the plain radiograph is negative.

22. **The correct answer is: E. Vancomycin, cefepime, and metronidazole.** This is a moderately severe diabetic foot infection. Antibiotic treatment should target gram-positive organisms (vancomycin, linezolid, daptomycin), gram-negative bacilli (fluoroquinolones, advanced-spectrum β-lactams), and anaerobic organisms (metronidazole, unless a carbapenem, piperacillin-tazobactam, or ampicillin-sulbactam is included in the regimen). *P. aeruginosa* is a common pathogen with diabetic foot infections; therefore, ertapenem would not be an appropriate agent for empiric therapy. Other treatments including limb elevation, non–weight-bearing status, wound care, tight glycemic control, and venous insufficiency are critical for wound healing. Surgical consultation is necessary for debridement and revascularization (or, if these measures are unsuccessful, amputation).

23. **The correct answer is: B. Epidural abscess.** Patients who present with bacteremia, fevers, and back pain should raise concern for an epidural abscess. Classic symptoms include focal back pain, electric shock–like pain, motor and/or sensory weakness, and paralysis. It is important to recognize this clinical presentation, obtain prompt imaging, and involve neurosurgery as necessary for early decompression. Blood cultures can help identify the pathogen in 60% of cases. LP for examination of cerebrospinal fluid (CSF) is often not performed because diagnostic yield is low.

24. **The correct answer is: D. 6 weeks from surgical debridement.** Epidural abscesses often require both surgical debridement to achieve source control and long-term antimicrobial therapy. The duration of antimicrobial therapy is typically 4 to 6 weeks. If surgical debridement is pursued, the date of surgery or the date of clearance of blood cultures (whichever occurs later) is counted as the start time for an antibiotic course, rather than the first day that the patient received antibiotics.

25. **The correct answer is: A. Necrotizing fasciitis.** Necrotizing fasciitis involves deep soft tissues and results in rapid destruction of several fascial planes. It has a high mortality if not recognized early. The infection should be suspected in patients with soft tissue infection (edema, erythema) that progresses rapidly (hours), and if any signs of systemic illness are present (fever, hemodynamically unstable). Other skin manifestations include crepitus

or severe pain out of proportion to examination. Treatment includes early and aggressive surgical exploration with debridement of necrotic tissue as well as broad-spectrum antibiotic therapy. This patient's presentation is more consistent with β-hemolytic strep infection instead of polymicrobial necrotizing fasciitis, but regardless, empiric treatment should target gram-positive, gram-negative, and anaerobic organisms, and in addition, add the antitoxin antibiotic clindamycin. In this patient, who has had water exposure, it is important to consider *Aeromonas* and *Pseudomonas* species.

26. The correct answer is: B. Surgery. Necrotizing fasciitis is both an infectious disease and a surgical emergency. To prevent further deterioration of the patient both broad-spectrum antibiotics as discussed earlier and surgical debridement should be urgently pursued.

27. The correct answer is: E. Ramsay Hunt syndrome. Ramsay Hunt syndrome, otherwise known as herpes zoster oticus, is varicella zoster virus reactivation within the eighth cranial nerve that involves ipsilateral facial paralysis, hearing abnormalities (ear pain, decreased hearing, tinnitus, hyperacusis), and often vesicles within the auditory canal. Patients can also experience altered taste perception, tongue lesions, and lacrimation.

28. The correct answer is: C. Varicella zoster virus viral culture. Viral PCR yields the highest sensitivity for diagnosing varicella zoster virus reactivation, with direct fluorescent antigen testing from scrapings of an active vesicular lesion the second-best diagnostic study. Isolating the virus and culture takes 1 week for results and yields only 50% to 75% compared with PCR-positive samples. Varicella zoster virus immunoglobulin G (IgG) would have no utility in diagnosing active infection in this patient.

29. The correct answer is: D. Varicella zoster encephalitis. The LP results, along with delirium, are consistent with viral encephalitis. Herpes zoster–associated encephalitis typically presents with delirium within days following vesicular abruption but may occur prior to the onset of rash. Varicella zoster virus encephalitis is more common in immunocompromised patients, but it is also seen in a healthy host, like this patient. When cranial or cervical dermatomes are involved with the varicella zoster virus reactivation or patients develop disseminated herpes zoster, they are at a higher risk for developing encephalitis.

30. The correct answer is: A. Bacterial meningitis. Given the patient's confusion, fever, and recent neurosurgery, there is a high likelihood his presentation is due to post–neurosurgical bacterial meningitis. Infections from gram-positive skin flora are the most likely organisms in the setting of CSF shunts, recent neurosurgery, or penetrating head trauma and should be considered in this case. Patients with meningitis commonly present with fever, headache, and meningeal signs. Although they may appear lethargic, they will have a normal sensorium. This is different from patients with encephalitis, who have mental status changes consistent with delirium. Patients can have features of both diseases; however, in this patient, it would be unusual for him to develop viral encephalitis following neurosurgery. Additionally, his examination is not consistent with encephalitis.

31. The correct answer is: A. Patient with known epilepsy. Head imaging prior to an LP is considered if the patient has a history of CNS disease (primary CNS lymphoma), new-onset seizure, focal neurologic findings, or papilledema; therefore, patients with a known diagnosis of epilepsy do not require head imaging before the procedure.

This patient does not meet the criteria for head imaging. When approaching bacterial meningitis as a possible diagnosis, you should first and foremost obtain blood cultures and then initiate appropriate antibiotics. Steroids may also be given when pneumococcal meningitis is suspected and, if done, should be given before or with the first dose of antibiotics. LP should also be performed as soon as possible but should not delay initiation of antibiotics and/or steroids. Note the yield of CSF culture is unlikely to be changed if the LP is obtained within 4 hours of antibiotic initiation. Additional CSF studies that can be ordered on the basis of clinical suspicion include AFB smear and culture, fungal culture and stain, cryptococcal antigen, Venereal Disease Research Laboratory (VDRL) test, HSV/ varicella zoster virus/enteroviral PCR, and cytology.

32. **The correct answer is: A. Bacterial meningitis.** Given the markedly elevated CSF WBC count with a neutrophil predominance elevated WBC count, very low glucose, and very high total protein, bacterial meningitis would be most likely. Given his recent neurosurgical procedure, this patient is at risk for *Staphylococcus aureus*, coagulase-negative staphylococci, and gram-negative bacilli (including Pseudomonas aeruginosa).

33. **The correct answer is: D. Vancomycin and cefepime.** This patient likely has bacterial meningitis and should be initiated on vancomycin and cefepime empirically while awaiting Gram stain and culture results from the CSF.

34. **The correct answer is: E. All of the above.** This patient's presentation and examination are highly concerning for infectious endocarditis, especially given her risk from IV drug use. She has murmur on examination and evidence of vascular phenomena with palmar Janeway lesions and possible septic pulmonary emboli on CXR. This patient should have blood cultures drawn immediately, prior to the initiation of antibiotics. At least two sets of blood cultures should be drawn with two bottles per set. After blood cultures are drawn, she should be started on empiric broad-spectrum antibiotics, including coverage of MRSA. IV vancomycin and cefepime would be a good empiric option. An ECG should be obtained to assess for any conduction abnormalities that may raise concern for a perivalvular abscess, and an echocardiogram should be obtained to assess for valvular vegetations. It would be reasonable to start with a transthoracic echocardiogram, although she may also need a TEE, depending on the transthoracic echocardiogram quality and findings.

35. **The correct answer is: E. A, B, and C.** This patient has MSSA bacteremia with tricuspid valve endocarditis. Infectious diseases should be consulted immediately. A CT scan of the chest can be done, given the abnormal CXR, to assess for septic pulmonary emboli and rule out any sites of abscess or empyema that could require drainage. She should be narrowed from empiric MRSA coverage (ie, vancomycin) to a β-lactam (cefazolin, oxacillin, or nafcillin), which is superior to vancomycin for the treatment of MSSA infections. Blood cultures should be checked every 24 to 48 hours until negative. She should be screened for hepatitis C and HIV.

36. **The correct answer is: B. Continue antibiotics for 6 weeks from date of first negative blood cultures and check weekly labs.** She should continue IV antibiotics treatment with oxacillin, nafcillin, or cefazolin for 6 weeks from date of first negative blood cultures given that this is right-sided endocarditis complicated by septic emboli. During this time, she should be monitored with weekly labs (basic metabolic panel, LFTs, and CBC with differential) for possible side effects from long-term antibiotics (ie, acute renal failure, liver injury, eosinophilia, neutropenia).

37. **The correct answer is: D. A and C.** Antibiotic prophylaxis is recommended prior to dental procedures (which is defined by any manipulation of gingival tissue or periapical region of teeth or perforation of oral mucosa) in patients with a history of infective endocarditis, prosthetic heart valves, prosthetic valve repair material, cardiac transplants with valvulopathy, and unrepaired or incompletely repaired congenital heart disease. Additionally, it is indicated for patients with repaired congenital heart disease if within 6 months of the initial surgery. It would not be indicated for someone with a remote ventricular septal defect repaired as a child. The prophylactic regimen is typically amoxicillin 2 g orally 30 to

60 minutes before the procedure. Alternatively, clindamycin can be used in patients with a penicillin allergy.

38. **The correct answer is: C. Interferon-γ release assay.** A blood interferon-γ release assay should be checked as the next step for this patient. Prior receipt of the BCG vaccine, particularly later than infancy, can result in a reactive tuberculin skin test. The interferon-γ release assays do not cross-react with BCG and therefore have better specificity in BCG recipients. Induced sputum and CXR would not be done prior to TB screening if the patient does not have any symptoms concerning for active TB.

39. **The correct answer is: C. Repeat interferon-γ release assay.** The two most common interferon-γ release assay tests include QuantiFERON and T-SPOT. If the interferon-γ release assay results are indeterminate, from either a strong negative control response or a weak response to positive control, then the interferon-γ release assay should be repeated. If the repeat interferon-γ release assay results are indeterminate, then you can proceed with the tuberculin skin test. This is not an expected result from the BCG vaccine and reassurance would be incorrect in this scenario.

40. **The correct answer is: D. Either A or B.** This patient does not have any signs or symptoms concerning for active pulmonary TB (fever, cough, night sweats, weight loss), is not immunocompromised, and has a clear CXR. He likely has a latent TB and has no evidence of active TB. He also has no known or suspected contacts with multidrug-resistant TB; therefore, treatment options for latent TB in this case would include rifampin daily for 4 months daily isoniazid and rifampin for 3 months, or isoniazid daily (with vitamin B6) for 9 months. Isoniazid and rifapentine weekly for 12 weeks is also an option. Treatment for active TB (answer choice C) would not be indicated in this scenario.

41. **The correct answer is: D. B and C.** In this case, the patient requires further evaluation for active TB. Airborne infection isolation should be instituted. He should have three sputum samples, induced if necessary, for AFB stain and mycobacterial culture. TB PCR, which is more sensitive than AFB smear, should be checked on one of the samples. Negative sputum testing does not necessarily exclude the diagnosis of active pulmonary TB. The patient should also undergo chest CT imaging because his CXR was negative. Patients who are diagnosed with pulmonary TB (and are not suspected to have multidrug-resistant TB) should be initiated on four-drug therapy with rifampin, isoniazid, pyrazinamide, and ethambutol while awaiting susceptibility testing.

42. **The correct answer is: B. Glucan and galactomannan.** All patients with a newly diagnosed HIV infection should have the following baseline labs checked: CD4 cell count, HIV viral load and genotype (of the reverse transcriptase and protease genes, to assess for drug resistance), CBC with differential, basic metabolic panel, LFTs, fasting lipids, HbA$_{1c}$, syphilis screen, hepatitis (A, B, and C) serologies, and routine gonorrhea and chlamydia screening. Depending on the patient's CD4 cell count, toxoplasmosis IgG may be done, as this informs options for opportunistic infection prophylaxis in patients with CD4 cell count <200/μL and, if negative, provides the opportunity on counseling for prevention of infection. In patients with profound immunocompromise, cytomegalovirus IgG is also useful to detect those at risk for cytomegalovirus retinitis and primary infection. Patients should also have a tuberculin skin test or an interferon-γ release assay, with an appropriate review of symptoms, to assess for TB infection. Neither glucan nor galactomannan is advised in the routine workup for new diagnosis of HIV.

43. **The correct answer is: A. At this visit, if patient is agreeable to start.** In the absence of certain severe opportunistic infections (e.g. CNS infection with tuberculosis or cryptococcus), patients should be counseled and started on antiretroviral therapy

immediately. This can even be done the same day as or prior to his full set of labs or geno-type returning. First-line regimens include two nucleoside reverse transcriptase inhibitors with either an integrase inhibitor or a protease inhibitor boosted with ritonavir or cobici-stat. Additionally, he should be started on *P. jiroveci* pneumonia prophylaxis with TMP-SMX because his CD4 cell count is below 200 cells/µL. If he is unable to take TMP-SMX, other options include atovaquone, dapsone (need to check glucose-6-phosphate dehydrogenase status), or aerosolized pentamidine.

44. **The correct answer is: A. He can stop TMP-SMX at this time.** *P. jiroveci* pneu-monia prophylaxis can be stopped once a patient's CD4 cell count is >200 cells/µL for 3 to 6 months while on suppressive antiretroviral therapy. This patient can therefore stop TMP-SMX at this time.

45. **The correct answer is: C. Start TDF/FTC daily.** PrEP is highly effective at prevent-ing HIV transmission in HIV serodiscordant couples and consists of the HIV-uninfected partner taking TDF-FTC daily. Some studies have also suggested on-demand use may be effective, in which the person takes two tablets of TDF-FTC prior to the sex act and one tab every 24 hours after for two doses (thus four tablets total per sex act), however this regimen is not recommended as first-line therapy. Taking PrEP only after a sexual encoun-ter is not currently advised. Even though the patient reports using condoms, he is at high risk of acquiring HIV infection and PrEP should be advised.

46. **The correct answer is: D. Start TDF/FTC with an integrase inhibitor (dolute-gravir or raltegravir) daily for 4 weeks.** A needlestick exposure from a patient with known HIV warrants PEP. Triple-drug therapy, typically consisting of tenofovir and em-tricitabine with an integrase inhibitor (dolutegravir or raltegravir), should be started ASAP (<2 hours), but at most within 72 hours of possible exposure. You should not await the results of the source patient's viral load or genotype to initiate treatment. If the source pa-tient has known HIV resistance, then a different regimen might be considered with the help of an Infectious Disease specialist, but treatment should never be delayed for a genotype or viral load testing.

47. **The correct answer is: D. Obtain testing for anti-HCV now and HCV RNA 3 weeks later.** Following a needlestick exposure from a patient with untreated HCV, there is no available postexposure prophylactic regimen. Rather, a screening strategy is employed where the employee will be screened for HCV antibodies upon exposure and, if negative, then screened for HCV RNA at 3 weeks, then HCV antibodies again 4 months after the initial exposure. Glecaprevir/pibrentasvir and sofosbuvir/velpatasvir are both reg-imens for treatment of known HCV.

48. **The correct answer is: B. The condition is reversible with administration of antibiotics.** This patient has Lyme carditis, a manifestation of early disseminated infec-tion from the spirochete *Borrelia burgdorferi*. This is transmitted from the deer tick *Ixodes scapularis*, common throughout New England, the mid-Atlantic states, and the Midwest. It is not sexually transmitted. Lyme carditis can result in first-, second-, or third-degree heart block. Although patients may sometimes need a temporary pacer, the condition is revers-ible with antibiotic treatment. A permanent cardiac pacer is usually unnecessary. Lyme will not grow readily in culture, so blood cultures would not be useful to confirm the diagnosis. This patient should be initiated on IV ceftriaxone and can be switched to an oral agent (ie, doxycycline) upon clinical improvement. Treatment is typically for 14 to 21 days. He will not need lifelong antibiotics for this condition.

49. **The correct answer is: D. All of the above.** Doxycycline is first-line treatment for primary Lyme disease as evidenced by the classic targetoid rash of erythema migrans. Unlike the patient's son who will require IV ceftriaxone, this patient will only require PO doxycycline for 10 days. Common side effects of doxycycline include pill esophagitis, photosensitivity, and diarrhea. Patients should be counseled on sun protection as well as taking the pill with sufficient liquid and remaining upright for 30 minutes following ingestion.

50. **The correct answer is: A. Check Lyme ELISA (enzyme-linked immunosorbent assay) screen, blood parasite smear, human granulocytic anaplasmosis PCR.** There is a high concern for tick-borne illness, especially given his geographic location. His recent rash is typical for erythema migrans, which occurs in up to 80% of patients with early Lyme infection and can be seen 1 to 2 weeks after a tick bite. His other lab abnormalities, however, raise concern for potential coinfection with another tick-borne infection. Specifically, his anemia with evidence of hemolysis raises concern for infection with *Babesia microti*, the primary agent of human babesiosis in the United States. An older patient with asplenia is at high risk for severe infection and should be hospitalized. A blood smear should be sent to examine for intracellular parasites and, if present, to measure parasitemia. He should also be tested for coinfection with other tick-borne diseases that may also cause pancytopenia (without hemolysis) and transaminitis, particularly anaplasmosis (*Anaplasma phagocytophilum*). Ehrlichiosis (*Ehrlichia chaffeensis*) is relatively uncommon in Massachusetts, and although testing is considered, it would be more useful to test for coinfection with anaplasmosis of the options listed. Although empiric treatment is indicated, testing should be done, and none of the regimens listed above would provide adequate coverage.

51. **The correct answer is: B. Azithromycin, atovaquone, and doxycycline.** He should be started on treatment for babesiosis with IV azithromycin and atovaquone. Given that he also likely had primary Lyme infection based on his history of erythema migrans, he should receive treatment with doxycycline as well. Evidence of erythema migrans is sufficient to clinically diagnose early Lyme disease even without further testing. Note that doxycycline would also treat empirically for ehrlichiosis and anaplasmosis while tests are pending. Infectious Diseases should also be consulted in patients who have severe symptoms, who are asplenic or otherwise immunocompromised, or if the parasitemia burden is 4% or higher.

52. **The correct answer is: D. Powassan virus.** Lyme and babesia are most commonly spread by the *I. scapularis* tick found primarily in the Northeast United States. The *I. scapularis* tick is also known to be a vector for Powassan virus, a rare but increasingly prevalent cause of encephalitis. The vectors for Rocky Mountain spotted fever, West Nile virus, and bartonellosis are the dog tick, mosquito, and cat/flea respectively.

53. **The correct answer is: D. Malaria.** The epidemiology of fever among returned travelers is highly dependent on geography. In a recent traveler to sub-Saharan Africa, malaria should be of the highest concern, even if afebrile at the time of the evaluation. Fevers in malaria wax and wane and physical examination may be normal. Notably, the incubation time for malaria is usually 7 to 30 days and can be longer.

A thorough history and physical should always guide diagnostic workup. In this scenario, laboratory testing should include basic metabolic panel, CBC and differential, LFTs, blood cultures, and immediate performance of rapid diagnostic testing (RDT) for malaria. Although the other conditions are also possible, the patient should be presumed to have malaria until proven otherwise, and an Infectious Disease consult should be obtained. Malaria is a medical emergency with high risk or rapid deterioration and death, particularly with falciparum malaria. Prompt initiation of treatment is essential.

54. **The correct answer is: B. Blood smear with staining.** Malaria is diagnosed with a thin and thick peripheral blood smear with a Giemsa stain. Under microscopy, ring forms can be identified. The smears may also aid in identification of the malaria species, as the malaria species morphology is variable depending on the stage of infection. If malaria is suspected and the initial smear is negative, additional smears should be prepared and examined over the subsequent 48 to 72 hours. RDTs for detection of malaria parasite antigens are commonly used in endemic regions and at many medical centers in the United States. Positive results should be followed up by blood smear examination.

55. **The correct answer is: D. Start high-dose prednisone.** The majority of cases of fever of unknown origin are from a noninfectious etiology. In this case, the patient's symptoms of temporal headache with jaw pain and elevated ESR are most concerning for giant cell arteritis. Although temporal artery biopsy is helpful for diagnosis, steroids should be started immediately when this condition is suspected because if left untreated, this patient is at risk of loss of vision. Neither brain MRI nor LP would be indicated as the next best step.

56. **The correct answer is: C. PO fidaxomicin.** Fidaxomicin is considered first-line treatment for nonfulminant *C. difficile* colitis. PO vancomycin is a less expensive alternative agent with similar rates of clinical response, but with higher rates of recurrence compared with fidaxomicin. IV vancomycin and PO clindamycin are not effective agents against *C. difficile* colitis. Fulminant *C. difficile* colitis, characterized by shock and evidence of ileus or toxic mega colon, is treated with PO vancomycin and IV metronidazole with consideration of fecal transplantation and colectomy as a last resort.

ENDOCRINOLOGY

QUESTIONS

1. A 28-year-old woman presents to the emergency department (ED) with severe headache and visual field disturbances. A computed tomography (CT) scan of the head is performed, which identifies a 3-cm sellar mass as well as intralesional hyperdensities concerning for hemorrhage. On examination, the patient is in moderate distress because of pain, with temperature (T) 37.5°C, heart rate (HR) 100 beats/min, blood pressure (BP) 90/60 mmHg, and respiratory rate (RR) 22 breaths/min. She is alert and oriented, and extraocular movements are intact with no diplopia. The following labs are acquired:

   - Sodium: 132 mEq/L
   - Potassium: 4.2 mEq/L
   - Creatinine: 0.8 mg/dL

   What is the next best step in her management?

   A. Administer intravenous (IV) hydrocortisone 50 mg
   B. Assess thyroid function and antidiuretic hormone (ADH)
   C. Refer for brain magnetic resonance imaging (MRI) pituitary protocol
   D. Refer for neurosurgical consultation

2. The patient in Question 1 receives IV hydrocortisone and is evaluated by neurosurgery for emergent surgery. She undergoes transsphenoidal surgery in the evening with preliminary pathology of the lesion showing pituitary adenoma with necrosis. The patient is feeling well the following day.

   What is the expected result of the cosyntropin stimulation test the morning following the surgery, assuming she received stress dose dexamethasone prior to and after the surgery?

   Cortisol levels (μg/mL) with cosyntropin stimulation test:

   A. Baseline: 0.2; 30 min: 1.3; 60 min: 2.2
   B. Baseline: 0.5; 30 min: 15.3; 60 min: 20.5
   C. Baseline: 2.5; 30 min: 4.5; 60 min: 12.2
   D. Baseline: 6.3; 30 min: 17.1; 60 min: 22.3

3. A 45-year-old woman presents to endocrinology clinic for evaluation of weight gain. The patient reports sudden-onset 40-lb weight gain 6 months ago. She has also noted easy bruising and mild leg swelling. On examination, the patient has a BP of 145/90 mmHg, HR 80 beats/min, and RR 15 breaths/min. There is evidence of facial rounding and plethora. She exhibits central adiposity with adipose collections on the back of her neck. She has 1+ pitting edema in her legs bilaterally. Hemoglobin A_{1c} (HbA_{1c}) was recently noted as 6.4%, increased from 5.3% a year prior. The patient denies snoring, headache, or visual field changes.

   What would be the next best step in her management?

   A. Order a low-dose dexamethasone suppression test (DST)
   B. Order fasting insulin-like growth factor-1 (IGF-1) level
   C. Order morning cortisol with adrenocorticotropic hormone (ACTH)
   D. Refer for pituitary MRI

4. A dexamethasone suppression test (DST) is performed in the patient in Question 3, which shows a morning cortisol of 9.5 µg/mL. Concomitant ACTH level was 15 µg/mL. The patient performed two separate 24-hour urine cortisol collections, both of which were three times the upper limit of normal. The patient received a pituitary protocol MRI, which showed a 4-mm pituitary lesion concerning for microadenoma.

What is the next best step in her management?

A. Initiate ketoconazole 200 mg twice daily
B. Perform late-night salivary cortisol measurements two times
C. Refer to neurosurgery for microadenoma resection
D. Refer to radiology for inferior petrosal sinus sampling

5. A 40-year-old man presents to his primary care physician (PCP) office because of joint pain. He reports increasing stiffness in his knees and shoulders over the past 2 years. He also has noted increasing swelling in his hands and feet. The swelling has required him to purchase new shoes, as the old ones no longer fit. He also reports that his wife states that his snoring has gotten worse. On examination, the patient exhibits thickened digits on his hands and feet. He has multiple skin tags on his chest. He has an enlarged jaw and brow when compared to his ID photo taken 4 years ago. His oral and nasal examinations show no lesions or malformations.

Which of the following would be the next best step in his diagnosis?

A. Checking growth hormone after an oral glucose load
B. Fasting morning growth hormone level
C. Glucagon stimulation test
D. Measurement of serum IGF-1

6. The IGF-1 level of the patient in Question 5 is noted to be 1034 ng/mL (normal: 125-320 ng/mL). He receives an oral glucose tolerance test with 75 g glucose, and post-glucose growth hormone level is 2.1 ng/mL (normal: <1.0 ng/mL). A pituitary MRI shows a 9-mm lesion within the pituitary. No invasion of the cavernous sinus or compression of the optic chiasm is noted.

What is the next best step in his management?

A. Initiate lanreotide 30 mg monthly
B. Initiate pegvisomant 10 mg daily
C. Refer to neurosurgery for resection
D. Refer to radiation oncology for radiosurgery

7. A 27-year-old male with no significant past medical history was an unrestrained passenger in a motor vehicle accident (MVA). He sustained a traumatic head injury. He was admitted to the neurosurgical service where he required decompressive craniotomy. During his post-operative course, he was noticed to have significant urinary output from his Foley catheter. Laboratory values reveal serum sodium 151 mEq/L and urine osmolality 95 mOsm/kg.

What is the next best step in his management?

A. Initiate continuous normal saline infusion
B. Initiate desmopressin
C. Initiate continuous D5W infusion
D. Strict NPO diet

8. A 30-year-old woman, who is otherwise healthy, presents for secondary amenorrhea. Six months ago, she noted a lack of menses. Pregnancy test was negative at that time and

1 month ago. She has also noted occasional breast tenderness and milky discharge from both breasts. She has developed an intermittent headache over the past 2 weeks that improves with Tylenol. She denies dizziness or changes in her vision.

What is the most likely source of her symptoms?

A. Adrenal hyperplasia
B. Ovarian tumor
C. Pituitary mass
D. Surreptitious medication use

9. A prolactin level is checked in the patient in Question 8, which is elevated to 120 ng/mL (normal: <22 ng/mL). Thyroid-stimulating hormone (TSH) and free thyroxine (fT4) levels are normal. Pituitary protocol MRI is performed, which identifies a 1-cm intrasellar lesion concerning for a macroadenoma. The patient is not interested in fertility at this time.

What is the next best step in her management?

A. Initiate cabergoline 0.5 mg weekly
B. Initiate combined oral contraceptive pill (OCP)
C. Initiate levothyroxine 88 μg daily
D. Refer to neurosurgery for lesion removal

10. A 21-year-old woman presents to the ED for evaluation of fatigue and frequent urination. The patient reports experiencing constant fatigue and brain fog over the past year. She required an emergency room visit 6 months ago because of abdominal pain and was diagnosed with a kidney stone. She has also developed a worsening headache as well as a lack of menses over the past year. She is currently taking no medications. She denies alcohol or tobacco use. She is adopted and does not know her family history. On examination, the patient appears tired with dry mucous membranes. Her vital signs are as follows: BP 100/70 mmHg, HR 85 beats/min, T 36.8°C, and RR 18 breaths/min. Her abdomen is soft and nontender to palpation. She has trace nonpitting edema in her legs bilaterally.

Laboratory evaluations include:
- Calcium: 11.6 mg/dL (normal: 8.5-10.5 mg/dL)
- Creatinine: 0.9 mg/dL
- Parathyroid hormone (PTH): 75 pg/mL (normal: 10-65 pg/mL)
- 25-hydroxy (OH) vitamin D: 30 ng/dL (normal: 20-80 ng/dL)
- TSH: 0.4 mU/L (normal: 0.4-5.0 mU/L)
- fT4: 0.7 ng/dL (normal: 0.9-1.8 ng/dL)
- Prolactin: 10 ng/mL (normal: <22 ng/mL)

The patient receives aggressive hydration in the ED with reduction in her calcium. A brain MRI is performed because of headache, and a 1-cm pituitary lesion is noted that abuts the cavernous sinus but does not compress the optic chiasm. A thyroid ultrasound is performed, which shows a normal-sized thyroid with enlarged masses in each lobe concerning for parathyroid enlargement.

What is the most important screening test for this patient after management of her acute presentation?

A. Abdominal MRI
B. Colonoscopy
C. Echocardiogram
D. Pelvic ultrasound

11. A 36-year-old woman with no chronic medical conditions presents to her PCP with weight gain, fatigue, and dry skin.

What is the appropriate screening test(s) for hypothyroidism?

A. TSH
B. TSH and fT4
C. TSH, fT4, and free triiodothyronine (T3)
D. TSH, fT4, and total T3

12. A 39-year-old man with a medical history including obesity is diagnosed with primary hypothyroidism after presenting to his PCP with fatigue and constipation. His TSH is 29 mU/L (ref. 0.4-5 mU/L) and fT4 is 0.6 ng/dL (ref. 0.9-1.8 ng/dL). His weight is 80 kg.

How should his hypothyroidism be managed?

A. Levothyroxine 50 μg
B. Levothyroxine 88 μg
C. Levothyroxine 125 μg daily
D. Levothyroxine 150 μg daily

13. A 79-year-old man with a medical history including obesity, heart failure (HF), and coronary artery disease (CAD) is diagnosed with primary hypothyroidism after presenting to his PCP with fatigue and constipation. His TSH is 29 mU/L (ref. 0.4-5 mU/L) and fT4 is 0.6 ng/dL (ref. 0.9-1.8 ng/dL). His weight is 80 kg.

How should his hypothyroidism be managed?

A. Levothyroxine 25 μg
B. Levothyroxine 50 μg
C. Levothyroxine 88 μg daily
D. Levothyroxine 120 μg daily

14. A 35-year-old woman with a medical history of obesity and hypothyroidism is admitted to the medical intensive care unit with altered mental status, hypothermia, and bradycardia. Laboratory evaluation is notable for creatinine 0.8 mg/dL, TSH 30.4 mU/L (ref. 0.4-5 mU/L), fT4 0.2 ng/dL (ref. 0.9-1.8 ng/dL), and white blood cell (WBC) count 15 500/μL.

What is the most appropriate next best step in her management?

A. Restart home levothyroxine
B. Start broad-spectrum antibiotics
C. Start hydrocortisone 100 mg every 8 hours and 100 μg T4 IV daily
D. Start 200 μg T4 IV and T3 10 μg IV

15. A 55-year-old woman with a medical history of multiple sclerosis was admitted to the medical intensive care unit with *Staphylococcus aureus* pneumonia complicated by bacteremia and infective endocarditis. One week into her hospitalization, thyroid function studies are checked and she is found to have a TSH of 0.3 mU/L (ref. 0.4-5 mU/L) with fT4 of 0.7 ng/dL (ref. 0.9-1.8 ng/dL).

What is the appropriate management?

A. Repeat thyroid tests after recovery
B. Start levothyroxine 25 μg IV daily
C. Start levothyroxine 25 μg IV daily and T3 10 μg IV daily
D. Start levothyroxine 50 μg oral daily

16. A 45-year-old woman presents to the ED complaining of palpitations. She reports heat intolerance and unintended 5-lb weight loss in the past month. She has no chronic medical conditions and denies ingestions. Her laboratory evaluation is notable for undetectable TSH with fT4 of 4.1 ng/dL (ref. 0.9-1.8 ng/dL). On examination, the thyroid is not enlarged, is nontender, and no nodules are appreciated.

What is the next best diagnostic step?

A. Order radioiodine uptake and scan
B. Order thyroid ultrasound
C. Order thyrotropin receptor antibodies
D. Repeat TSH and fT4

17. A 55-year-old man presents for evaluation of hyperthyroidism discovered during evaluation for palpitations. Laboratory evaluation was notable for undetectable TSH with fT4 of 3.8 ng/dL (ref. 0.9-1.8 ng/dL). Radioiodine uptake and scan is performed, revealing absent radioiodine uptake.

Which of the following is the most likely diagnosis?

A. Graves disease
B. Painless thyroiditis
C. Toxic adenoma
D. TSH-producing pituitary adenoma

18. A 35-year-old woman presents for treatment of newly diagnosed Graves disease with eye irritation without vision changes, diplopia, or restriction of extraocular movements. She is the sole caregiver for a 12-month-old child and desires pregnancy in the next 6 to 12 months.

Which of the following would be the best treatment option?

A. Methimazole for 1 year
B. Propranolol alone
C. Radioiodine
D. Surgery

19. A 56-year-old man presents after CT scan with contrast with agitation, tachycardia, hypotension, and fever to 40.5°C. Laboratory evaluation is notable for TSH of 0.05 mU/L (ref. 0.4-5 mU/L), fT4 of 3.7 ng/dL (ref. 0.9-1.8 ng/dL), and total T3 of 360 ng/dL (ref. 60-181 ng/dL).

All EXCEPT which of the following are recommended as initial treatment?

A. β-Blocker
B. Glucocorticoids
C. Selenium
D. Thionamide

20. A 65-year-old woman presents to primary care clinic after a thyroid nodule is seen incidentally on a CT scan while she was hospitalized for pulmonary nodular amyloidosis. She has a history of well-controlled hypertension. She underwent a thyroid ultrasound that revealed a single 10-mm hypoechoic nodule with microcalcifications. Her TSH is within normal limits.

What is the most appropriate management?

A. No further evaluation indicated
B. Refer for fine needle aspiration (FNA)
C. Repeat TSH and ultrasound in 6 months
D. Repeat ultrasound in 6 months

21. A 42-year-old female with a minimal past medical history presents for evaluation of a nodule located in her neck. She has spent most of her life living near Chernobyl and has recently moved to the United States. Upon further examination, she is found to have a left thyroid nodule with no associated cervical lymphadenopathy. Thyroid function tests are normal.

    What sonographic findings would warrant FNA for a nodule that is ≥1 cm?

    A. Solid hypoechoic nodule with microcalcifications
    B. Purely cystic nodules
    C. Partially cystic nodules with normal margins
    D. All of the above

22. A 70-year-old man undergoes FNA of a 1.5 cm solid, hypoechoic nodule with irregular margins. Cytologic results show atypia of undetermined significance (Bethesda III).

    What is the next appropriate step?

    A. Perform surgery
    B. Repeat FNA with sample for molecular testing
    C. Repeat TSH and ultrasound in 6 months
    D. Repeat ultrasound in 6 months

23. A 79-year-old man with atrial fibrillation is started on amiodarone.

    Which of the following is NOT true regarding amiodarone and thyroid function?

    A. Amiodarone can result in destructive thyroiditis
    B. Amiodarone can result in hypo- and hyperthyroidism
    C. Amiodarone inhibits T4 to T3 conversion
    D. Each 100 mg amiodarone contains half of the iodine contained in the average diet daily

24. A 35-year-old man with newly diagnosed hypertension presents to clinic with ongoing elevated BPs at home despite maximum dose triple therapy. He is currently taking metoprolol, amlodipine, and hydrochlorothiazide with minimal effect. He has no family history of hypertension and denies symptoms. On examination, he is well appearing. BP is 165/95 mmHg, HR 80 beats/min, T 37°C, and RR 16 breaths/min. Laboratory evaluation is notable for creatinine 0.8 mg/dL, potassium 3.6 mmol/L, and sodium 141 mmol/L. He denies weight gain, bruising, muscle weakness, or skin changes.

    Evaluation for the most likely secondary cause would involve which of the following?

    A. Dexamethasone suppression test (DST)
    B. Morning plasma renin and aldosterone
    C. Renal ultrasound
    D. Twenty-four hours urinary fractionated metanephrines and catecholamines

25. An aldosterone/renin ratio is checked in the patient in Question 24 with appropriate technique and was found to be 25 (<10) with a plasma aldosterone concentration of 13 ng/dL (ref. <21 ng/dL).

    What is the next appropriate step in his management?

    A. Abdominal CT adrenal protocol
    B. Adrenal venous sampling
    C. Initiate spironolactone 100 mg daily
    D. Salt suppression test

26. The patient in Questions 24 and 25 receives a salt suppression test via saline infusion in clinic and has an aldosterone level of 12 ng/dL (ref. <5 ng/dL) after 4 hours. An abdominal CT is performed, which shows the right adrenal gland with a 6-mm nodule and the left adrenal gland with mild hypertrophy and a 1.1-cm nodule. Hounsfield units are consistent with adrenal adenomas.

    What is the next best step in his management?
    A. Adrenal venous sampling
    B. Initiate spironolactone 100 mg daily
    C. Left-sided adrenalectomy
    D. Right-sided adrenalectomy

27. A 67-year-old woman presents to the clinic because of 1 year of weight gain. The patient had mild weight gain after menopause but noted a sudden increase in weight of 20 lb over the past year. She has also noted increased fatigue and difficulty climbing the stairs. On examination, she exhibits mild facial plethora and rounding as well as prominent central adiposity. She has 1+ pitting edema in her legs with occasional bruises on her arms. Vital signs show a BP of 150/95 mmHg, HR 78 beats/min, RR 16 breaths/min, and body mass index (BMI) 32 kg/m^2. Laboratory values show a creatinine of 1.1 mg/dL, potassium of 3.5 mmol/L, and sodium of 138 mmol/L. Cushing syndrome is suspected and the patient receives a dexamethasone suppression test (DST). A morning cortisol level after a 1-mg dexamethasone dose the night before is 6.2 μg/mL (ref. <1.8 μg/mL).

    What is the next best step in her management?
    A. Refer for abdominal CT scan adrenal protocol
    B. Refer for high-dose (8 mg) DST
    C. Refer for inferior petrosal sinus sampling
    D. Repeat DST with dexamethasone level and obtain ACTH

28. The patient in Question 27 receives a repeat 1-mg dexamethasone suppression test (DST), which shows a morning cortisol of 7.3 μg/dL (<1.8 μg/dL) and an ACTH level of 1 pg/mL (<0.6 pg/mL), with an appropriate dexamethasone level. She undergoes an abdominal CT scan, which shows a nodular right adrenal gland containing an 8-mm and a 1.2-cm lesion and a nodular left adrenal gland containing a 1.4-cm lesion.

    What is the next best step in her management?
    A. Adrenal venous sampling
    B. Bilateral adrenalectomy
    C. Initiation of ketoconazole 200 mg twice daily
    D. Initiation of metyrapone 500 mg three times daily

29. A 40-year-old woman with a history of hypertension and hypothyroidism presents for management of her hypertension. She is well controlled on levothyroxine and maximum dose of amlodipine. Her last TSH was checked 4 weeks ago and was normal. She undergoes screening metabolic panel.

    Laboratory evaluation reveals:

    Sodium 138 mEq/L
    Potassium 3 mEq/L
    Creatinine 0.8 mg/dL

What is the next best step in her management?

A. Obtain TSH with reflex
B. Obtain morning cortisol
C. Obtain morning plasma renin and aldosterone
D. Obtain dexamethasone suppression test (DST)

30. A 53-year-old man with hypertension and obesity is admitted to the hospital for an episode of dizziness, nausea, and vomiting. On examination, he appears in mild distress, BP 170/100 mmHg, HR 100 beats/min, RR 20 breaths/min, and T 36.6°C. His abdomen is soft and mildly tender in the epigastric region. During his workup, he has a CT of his abdomen and pelvis that is notable for a 4.2 × 3.5 cm left adrenal mass with smooth borders.

    What is the next best step in the management of this finding?

    A. Abdominal MRI with adrenal protocol
    B. No further evaluation required given benign features of nodule
    C. Twenty-four-hour urine fractionated metanephrines now, with plans for aldosterone, renin, and overnight 1 mg dexamethasone suppression test (DST) in the outpatient setting
    D. Twenty-four-hour urine fractionated metanephrines, aldosterone, renin, and overnight 1 mg DST now

31. The patient in Question 30 is successfully discharged home and receives hormonal testing. The results are: urine fractionated metanephrines and catecholamines are within normal range, an aldosterone/renin ratio of 35 (ref. <10) with aldosterone level of 10 ng/dL and a cortisol level of 5.7 µg/dL (ref. <1.8 µg/dL) after dexamethasone suppression test (DST).

    What is the next best step in his management?

    A. Repeat abdominal CT adrenal protocol in 6 months
    B. Repeat abdominal CT adrenal protocol in 12 months
    C. Repeat imaging and biochemical testing in 6 months
    D. Surgical referral

32. A 25-year-old woman with no chronic medical conditions presents to primary care with intermittent headache, associated sweating, and palpitations over the past 3 months. She states that these episodes occur randomly and are not associated with hunger, anxiety symptoms, or panic. She does not experience any flushing, diarrhea, or abdominal pain with the episodes. She does not use alcohol or illicit drugs and is not on any medications. In the office, she is afebrile with HR of 90 beats/min and BP 135/90 mmHg. Her abdomen is soft with no masses palpated. Laboratory findings show a creatinine of 1.0 mg/dL and normal electrolytes.

    What is the next best step in her management?

    A. Insulin and glucose check during the next episode
    B. Renin/aldosterone ratio
    C. Twenty-four-hour urinary fractionated metanephrines and catecholamines
    D. Urinary 5-hydroxyindoleacetic acid, chromogranin, and gastrin levels

33. The urinary metanephrines of the patient in Question 32 were measured and were 3000 µg/24 h (normal: <1000 µg/24 h in hypertensive patients). The patient received an abdominal CT scan, which revealed normal adrenal glands and otherwise was unremarkable.

What is the next best step in her management?

A. Initiation of terazosin
B. Metaiodobenzylguanidine (MIBG) I-123 scan
C. Serial monitoring of urinary metanephrines
D. Whole-body CT scan

34. MIBG scan was performed in the patient in Questions 32 and 33 that identified a lesion in the left neck. The patient was referred to an endocrine surgeon and is pending surgery.

What is the next best step in her management?

A. Initiate metoprolol 50 mg twice daily
B. Initiate metyrapone 250 mg four times daily
C. Initiate nifedipine 30 mg every 8 hours
D. Initiate prazosin 1 mg every 4 hours

35. The patient in Questions 32-34 successfully receives surgery and a 2.3-cm paraganglioma is resected from the left neck, with negative lymph nodes and local margins. The patient is now pending discharge from the hospital.

What is the recommended follow-up?

A. Benign tumor, no follow-up indicated
B. Genetics referral, repeat imaging, and catecholamines in 1 year
C. Repeat imaging and catecholamine levels in 1 year
D. Repeat imaging in 1 year

36. A 23-year-old woman with a history of hypothyroidism presents to clinic with symptoms of extreme fatigue. The patient has noted markedly low energy levels and is barely able to get out of bed. She is experiencing dizziness when standing and walking. She also has been craving very salty foods like pretzels and chips. She denies illness, sick contacts, traveling abroad, or camping. She denies alcohol, tobacco, or illicit drug use. She has a history of hypothyroidism diagnosed at age 21 and has been on LT4 100 μg daily with stable TSH. On examination, the patient appears ill, BP 85/60 mmHg, HR 110 beats/min, T 37.6°C, and RR 15 breaths/min. Her abdomen is soft and nontender. She has dry, tan skin, which she reports is darker than usual. Her examination is otherwise unremarkable.

What is the next best step in her management?

A. Cosyntropin stimulation test and thyroid function studies
B. Dexamethasone 2 mg oral dose and cosyntropin stimulation test with baseline ACTH
C. Hydrocortisone 20 mg oral dose and encourage fluids
D. Referral to the emergency room

37. The patient in Question 36 is sent to the ED where she receives IV hydrocortisone and 3 L normal saline. She was noted to have a potassium of 5.6 mmol/L, which recovered to 4.0 mmol/L after the hydrocortisone. She is feeling much better.

What is the next appropriate step in her management?

A. Check aldosterone and renin levels
B. Check antiadrenal antibodies
C. Check baseline ACTH and perform cosyntropin stimulation test
D. Refer for abdominal CT scan adrenal protocol

38. The morning ACTH of the patient in Questions 36 and 37 returns at 300 pg/mL (ref. 10-60 pg/mL). A cosyntropin stimulation is performed, which shows maximal cortisol stimulation to 1.3 µg/dL (ref. >18 µg/dL).

What is the most appropriate treatment for her Addison disease?

A. Dexamethasone 1 mg daily
B. Fludrocortisone 0.1 mg daily
C. Hydrocortisone 20 mg daily
D. Prednisone 5 mg daily and fludrocortisone 0.1 mg daily

39. A 29-year-old carpenter broke his radius after a fall from a ladder. His calcium was found to be elevated at 11.3 mg/dL (normal: 8.5-10.5 mg/dL), PTH 75 pg/mL (normal: 10-65 pg/mL), and 25(OH)D 20 ng/mL (normal: 20-80 ng/mL).

What is the next best diagnostic step?

A. Check dual-energy x-ray absorptiometry (DXA)
B. Neck ultrasound and sestamibi scan
C. Check serum and 24-hour urine calcium and creatinine
D. Check serum phosphate and magnesium

40. A 70-year-old man with a history of hypertension, remote history of Graves disease and total thyroidectomy, and a 25-pack-year history of smoking presents with increasing fatigue, thirst, frequent urination, weight loss, and confusion. He drinks several liters of water every day. On examination, he has double vision and is not oriented to time.

Which of the following diagnoses is highest in the differential?

A. Hypercalcemic crisis
B. Hyperosmolar hyperglycemic state (HHS)
C. Hyperthyroid crisis
D. Stroke

41. TSH in the patient in Question 40 was found to be 0.9 mU/L (ref. 0.4-5 mU/L), calcium 15.0 mg/dL (ref. 8.5-10.5 mg/dL), albumin 3.0, albumin-corrected calcium 15.8 mg/dL (ref. 8.5-10.5 mg/dL), creatinine 2.0 mg/dL, head CT normal, and glucose 80 mg/dL. His calcium was normal a year ago at a routine blood check.

What is the most likely etiology of the hypercalcemia?

A. Graves disease
B. Lung cancer
C. Multiple endocrine neoplasia type 1 (MEN1)
D. Primary hyperparathyroidism

42. Chest x-ray and subsequent chest CT in the patient in Questions 40 and 41 show a central 4-cm spiculated tumor with cavitation.

How would you treat the hypercalcemia?

A. Calcitonin 200 mg IM every 12 hours
B. Infusion of PTH/PTH-related protein (PTHrP) receptor antibody
C. Normal saline IV
D. Treatment of the underlying lung tumor

43. A 40-year-old woman presents with dry cough for several months, fatigue, and mild dyspnea on exertion. Chest x-rays and subsequent CT show bilateral hilar lymphadenopathy and micronodules. Laboratory evaluation shows normal renal function, calcium 11.5 mg/dL (8.5-10.5 mg/dL), and albumin 3.9 g/dL. PTH is 5 pg/mL (10-60 pg/mL), PTHrP is undetectable, 25(OH)D is 30 ng/mL (20-80 ng/mL), and 1,25(OH)$_2$D is 110 pg/mL (19-70 pg/mL).

What is the most likely diagnosis?

A. Humoral hypercalcemia of malignancy
B. Primary hyperparathyroidism
C. Sarcoidosis
D. Secondary hyperparathyroidism

44. A 51-year-old woman presents with tingling in her hands and feet and numbness around her mouth several times a week. She has had these symptoms for about 2 months, and she has not identified any particular triggers. She is worried about multiple sclerosis and would like to be tested for it. She only takes a multivitamin and levothyroxine since a total thyroidectomy 3 months ago. There is no family history of any neurologic disease. Her recent TSH was normal.

What tests would you order?

A. Calcium and albumin
B. Complete blood count (CBC)
C. Lumbar puncture with cerebrospinal fluid (CSF) evaluation
D. Urinalysis

45. A 45-year-old healthy computer engineer has a serum calcium of 8.6 mg/dL (ref. 8.5-10.5 mg/dL), phosphorus of 1.7 mg/dL (2.5-4.5 mg/dL), and normal renal function. He is asymptomatic but worried about his low phosphorus.

What is the next best diagnostic test?

A. Check vitamin D and PTH
B. Genetic test for *PHEX* mutation
C. Measure fasting blood glucose and insulin
D. Measure fibroblast growth factor (FGF)23

46. A 35-year-old woman with chronic postsurgical hypoparathyroidism is in her second trimester of pregnancy. Her serum calcium is low at 6.8 mg/dL (8.5-10.5 mg/dL). She takes calcium 500 mg TID and calcitriol 0.25 μg QD.

What is the next best step?

A. Increase her calcitriol to 0.25 μg BID
B. Increase her calcium to 1000 mg TID
C. A and B and recheck calcium 2-3 days later
D. Check serum calcium and albumin
E. Check serum phosphate and magnesium

47. A 76-year-old female with a history of hypertension, hyperlipidemia, and atrial fibrillation presents to the ED after a fall from standing height in her home. She sustained a left femur fracture. It is determined that she would benefit from bisphosphonate therapy.

What factors should be considered before initiating bisphosphonate therapy?

A. History of esophageal stricture
B. Imminent invasive dental procedure
C. Vitamin D level
D. All of the above

48. A 52-year-old woman with a history of hypertension and alcohol use disorder presents to the ED with new-onset tetany. She is also noted to be newly bradycardic. Laboratory work reveals calcium 6.5 mg/dL (normal 8.5-10.5 mg/dL) and magnesium 0.5 mg/dL (normal 1.7-2.4 mg/dL).

What is the next best step in management?

A. Treat hypomagnesemia
B. Initiate oral vitamin D
C. Initiate oral calcium
D. Obtain TSH level

49. A 65-year-old asymptomatic woman with osteoporosis (T-score in the femoral neck -2.8) is found to have a calcium of 10.9 mg/dL (normal: 8.5-10.5 mg/dL), albumin of 3.7 g/dL, PTH of 70 pg/mL (normal: 10-65 pg/mL), estimated glomerular filtration rate (eGFR) of 70 mL/min/1.73 m², and 25(OH)D of 32 ng/mL (normal: 20-80 ng/mL). Calcium-to-creatinine clearance ratio (CCCR) is 0.04 (ref. >0.02).

What is the next best step?

A. Recommend genetic testing
B. Recommend parathyroid surgery
C. Recommend watchful waiting
D. Recommend vitamin D_3 50 000 IU weekly

50. A 65-year-old man comes into clinic for follow-up of his type 2 diabetes mellitus (T2DM). He has been on metformin 1000 mg twice daily for 1 year and his HbA_{1c} recently was 8.2%. He has modified his diet and has lost 10 lb. His past medical history is notable for CAD and hypertension. He underwent percutaneous coronary intervention with placement of drug-eluting stent (DES) to the right coronary artery 6 months ago.

What would be the next best drug to add?

A. Basal insulin
B. Glipizide 2.5 mg daily
C. Liraglutide daily
D. Rosiglitazone 4 mg daily

51. A 75-year-old man with a history of T2DM and hypertension is admitted to the hospital for a urinary tract infection and acute kidney injury, with creatinine increased to 3.5 mg/dL from baseline of 0.85 mg/dL. His home diabetes medications include metformin 1000 mg BID and empagliflozin 25 mg daily, with blood glucose levels ranging from 150 to 200 mg/dL. His most recent HbA_{1c} was 8.2% 1 month ago. On examination, he is in mild distress from abdominal pain. He weighs 100 kg, and BMI is 35 kg/m². His blood sugar level is persistently elevated to over 300 mg/dL in the hospital after holding home medications.

In order to improve glycemic control, you make which of the following changes to his current therapy?

A. Initiate 5 U regular insulin TID with regular sliding scale
B. Initiate sliding scale aspart insulin
C. Resume home medications and start sliding scale regular insulin
D. Start 15 U insulin glargine nightly with sliding scale aspart insulin

52. A 35-year-old woman with T2DM and obesity (BMI $=$ 44 kg/m²) presents to clinic for routine follow-up. Her laboratory evaluation reveals HbA_{1c} of 8.5%, creatinine 0.75 mg/dL, and is otherwise unremarkable. Her current medications include metformin 1000 mg twice daily and daily multivitamin. Since her last visit 3 months ago, she has modified her diet and increased her physical activity to 30 minutes of moderate exercise three times weekly. She has lost 2 lb.

What changes would you recommend?

A. Continue current medical therapy and encourage lifestyle modification
B. Start glargine 20 U nightly
C. Start glipizide 2.5 mg daily
D. Start liraglutide 0.6 mg subcutaneous (SC) once daily

53. A 27-year-old man with type 1 diabetes mellitus (T1DM) presented to ED with nausea, vomiting, and altered mental status after missing 2 days of insulin because of insurance issues. He received fluid resuscitation, potassium repletion to maintain serum potassium between 3.3 and 5.3 mEq/L, and was started on insulin IV infusion after receiving IV bolus of 0.1 U/kg. Initial labs with venous pH of 7.15, anion gap of 30, and bicarbonate of 12 improved after 12 hours to pH of 7.38, anion gap of 12, and bicarbonate of 21. The insulin IV infusion was discontinued and home regimen of insulin glargine daily in the morning with insulin Humalog at meals was restarted.

What parameters, in addition to blood glucose <200 mg/dL, do the American Diabetes Association (ADA) recommend be met when tapering IV insulin and overlapping with SC insulin?

A. Able to eat and hemodynamically stable
B. Hemodynamically stable, venous pH >7.30
C. Serum anion gap <12 mEq/L and serum bicarbonate ≥15 mEq/L
D. Venous pH >7.3, K >3.3 and <5.3 mEq/L

54. A 54-year-old man with a history of hypertension presents with an episode of confusion and slurred speech. In the ED, he is found to have fingerstick glucose of 33 mg/dL. His confusion improves after he drinks 8 ounces of orange juice. Additional history gathered from the patient's wife reveals the patient has had episodes of confusion often in the morning for about 1 month.

Which of the following labs drawn during hypoglycemia are most consistent with endogenous hyperinsulinemia (insulinoma)?

	Insulin (pmol/L)	Proinsulin (pmol/L)	C-peptide (ng/mL)	β-hydroxybutyrate (mmol/L)	Oral hypoglycemic agent screen
A.	3	4	0.4	6.5	Negative
B.	20	14	0.6	<2.7	Positive
C.	36	<2	<0.2	<2.7	Negative
D.	38	25	0.8	<2.7	Negative

55. A 75-year-old woman with unknown medical history presents to the emergency room with altered mental status. Her family states she has been visiting for Thanksgiving and has been feeling unwell for several days. On examination, her BP is 105/75 mmHg, HR is 115 beats/min, and RR is 18 breaths/min. She is stuporous with dry mucous membranes and tachycardia, but otherwise the examination is unremarkable. Her laboratory evaluation is most notable for venous blood gas (VBG) with pH of 7.35, basic metabolic panel (BMP) with glucose of 738 mg/dL, serum bicarbonate of 22 mEq/L, and anion gap of 12. Serum osmolality is 330 mOsm/kg and β-hydroxybutyrate is negative.

Initial management involves all BUT which of the following?

A. Electrocardiogram (ECG)
B. Infectious disease evaluation
C. IV fluid resuscitation
D. Transthoracic echocardiogram

56. A 56-year-old man with T2DM on metformin and stage 3 chronic kidney disease (CKD) presents to clinic for follow-up of diabetes care. His most recent HbA_{1c} is 8.0%. He is exercising 30 minutes, five times per week, and has made dietary changes to improve his glycemic control. He is interested in the medications he has heard about that protect the kidneys and treat diabetes.

All of the following are true regarding diabetic nephropathy and sodium-glucose cotransporter 2 (SGLT2) inhibitors EXCEPT:

A. Diabetic nephropathy is the most common cause of end-stage renal disease worldwide
B. SGLT2 inhibitors have been shown to reduce urinary albumin-to-creatinine ratio
C. SGLT2 inhibitors increase hyperfiltration
D. Studies evaluating SGLT2 inhibitors in patients with moderate renal impairment have shown an initial decrease in eGFR, but then a lesser decrease over time compared with placebo

57. A 65-year-old woman presents to clinic for follow-up of T2DM. She is currently taking metformin at maximum dose and dulaglutide 4.5 mg weekly. Her most recent HbA_{1c} is 9.5% while on this regimen regularly for 5 months. She wakes up several times during the night to urinate and is willing to start daily injections for improved glycemic control and to improve nocturia.

What are the appropriate instructions for starting insulin?

A. Start long-acting insulin at 0.1 to 0.2 IU/kg/day and prandial insulin at 4 U per meal
B. Start long-acting insulin at 0.1 to 0.2 IU/kg/day with instructions to increase 2 U every 3 days until reaching fasting glucose target
C. Start long-acting insulin at 20 U/day and continue this dose until follow-up while keeping glucose log
D. Start long-acting insulin at 20 U/day and reduce metformin dose to 500 mg twice daily

58. A 58-year-old man with T2DM and HF with ejection fraction of 35% presents for follow-up. He is physically active, and his diabetes is well controlled with HbA_{1c} of 7.0% on maximally tolerated metformin. He has no history of kidney disease or atherosclerotic heart disease.

What changes would be appropriate to make to antihyperglycemic agents today?

A. Continue metformin and add dapagliflozin
B. Continue metformin and add sitagliptin
C. Stop metformin and start dapagliflozin
D. Stop metformin and start basal insulin

59. A 19-year-old woman presents to clinic after recent hospitalization for diabetic ketoacidosis (DKA) during which she was diagnosed with T1DM.

What additional screening tests are recommended at the time of diagnosis?

A. Lipid profile
B. Lipid profile and TSH
C. Lipid profile, tissue transglutaminase, and TSH
D. TSH

60. A 58-year-old man with T2DM on basal-bolus insulin regimen presents for an urgent visit after 1 week of worsened hyperglycemia and variable response to prandial insulin injections (he uses vial and syringe). He otherwise feels well and has changed his injection sites. He had left his insulin vial overnight in the car on a cold night.

What should have been done with this insulin vial?

A. Allow insulin to thaw in refrigerator
B. Allow insulin to warm to room temperature before administration
C. Discard vial and open new vial
D. Shake insulin thoroughly before use

61. A 35-year-old man with a history of T1DM managed with insulin pump presents to the emergency room obtunded after an MVA. His temperature is 36°C, BP is 80/55 mmHg, HR is 120 beats/min, and RR is 22 breaths/min. The initial fingerstick glucose is 150 mg/dL and his labs are not consistent with DKA.

What is the appropriate management of this patient's diabetes?

A. Continue insulin pump at current settings
B. Continue insulin pump at current settings and provide correctional with SC insulin on sliding scale
C. Discontinue insulin pump and administer long-acting insulin based on weight
D. Discontinue insulin pump and transition to IV insulin infusion

62. A 64-year-old male with a history of T2DM and CKD (stage 2), presents for evaluation in outpatient clinic. He recently completed a test measuring the level of albumin in his urine. He was found to have albuminuria >300 mg/g creatinine. The patient is on an angiotensin-converting enzyme (ACE) inhibitor. His most recent HbA_{1c} was 7.5%.

What is the next best step in his management for renal protective benefits?

A. Initiate basal insulin
B. Initiate SGLT2 inhibitor
C. Initiate angiotensin II receptor blocker (ARB)
D. Initiate calcium channel blocker (CCB)

63. A 58-year-old male with a history of obesity (BMI 30), T2DM, hypertension, bilateral carotid stenosis, prior transient ischemic attack, and hyperlipidemia presents for an evaluation in outpatient clinic. His BP and low-density lipoprotein (LDL) are medically managed and at goal. His HbA_{1c} is 6.8% on metformin 1000 mg twice daily.

What is the next best step in his management for his diabetes mellitus?

A. Initiate glucagon-like peptide-1 receptor agonist (GLP-1 RA)
B. No change recommended
C. Initiate sulfonylurea
D. Referral to bariatric surgery

64. The patient in Question 63 is started on semaglutide once-weekly injection. It is confirmed that he has no history of pancreatitis.

This patient should be counseled regarding which side effects when initiating semaglutide?

A. Increased risk of amputation
B. Genital yeast infections
C. Nausea, vomiting
D. Increased risk of HF

65. A 76-year-old female with a history of T2DM presents as an outpatient to clinic for management of her diabetes. Her blood sugar is 250 mg/dL. She denies weight loss, dysphagia, polyuria, and polydipsia. Her HbA$_{1c}$ is 9.8%.

What is the next best step in her management?

A. Initiate basal insulin
B. Direct to the ED
C. Initiate insulin pump
D. Initiate GLP-1 RA

66. The same patient returns to clinic. Repeat laboratory work reveals HbA$_{1c}$ 13%. She is now reporting weight loss, polyuria, polydipsia, and malaise.

What is the next best step in her management?

A. Initiate basal insulin at 0.1-0.2 U/kg/day
B. Initiate sulfonylurea
C. Initiate trimethoprim/sulfamethoxazole empirically
D. Send a urine analysis

67. A 65-year-old woman presents to the emergency room with nausea, vomiting, and abdominal pain 24 hours after undergoing a routine colonoscopy for colorectal cancer screening. Her medical history is notable for hypertension and type 2 diabetes for which she takes lisinopril, metformin, and empagliflozin. Her labs on admission are notable for anion gap 22 mmol/L (normal 3-17 mmol/L), bicarbonate 15 mmol/L (ref. 23-32 mmol/L), glucose 209 mg/dL, lactic acid 2.4 mmol/L (normal 0.5-2.0 mmol/L), and β-hydroxybutyrate 2.8 mmol/L (normal <0.4 mmol/L).

What medication put her at risk for this condition?

A. Fentanyl used for sedation for colonoscopy
B. Lisinopril
C. Metformin
D. Empagliflozin

68. A 67-year-old man with a history of hypertension and CAD presents for evaluation regarding lipid management. He experienced a myocardial infarction (MI) 6 months ago requiring two DESs. He was placed on atorvastatin 80 mg at that time, which he has been taking consistently. His pretreatment LDL was 162 mg/dL, and a lipid panel checked 2 weeks ago showed an LDL of 85 mg/dL. He currently feels well with no chest pain, myalgias, or leg cramping.

What is the next best step in his management?

A. Continue atorvastatin 80 mg daily and add ezetimibe 10 mg daily
B. Continue atorvastatin 80 mg daily and add fenofibrate 145 mg daily
C. Discontinue atorvastatin and initiate evolocumab 140 mg every 2 weeks
D. Switch to pravastatin 40 mg

69. A 28-year-old man presents to lipid clinic because of concerns regarding family history. His father experienced an MI at age 40 and died at age 48 from cardiovascular causes. His 34-year-old brother also recently experienced an MI requiring stent placement. He feels well and has no chest pain. On examination, there is no evidence of tendon xanthomas. A lipid panel is performed, which shows a total cholesterol of 350 mg/dL, LDL of 250 mg/dL, high-density lipoprotein (HDL) of 35 mg/dL, and triglycerides of 200 mg/dL.

What would be the recommended treatment at this time?

A. Atorvastatin 80 mg daily
B. Evolocumab 140 mg every 2 weeks
C. No treatment indicated
D. Simvastatin 10 mg daily

70. A 45-year-old man with a history of T2DM, hypertension, and nonalcoholic fatty liver disease presents with acute-onset abdominal pain radiating to his back with nausea and vomiting. A CT scan is performed in the ED, which shows evidence of acute pancreatitis. On examination, the patient is in distress because of abdominal pain; T 37.7°C, HR 115 beats/min, RR 25 breaths/min, and BP 110/75 mmHg. Laboratory work shows a creatinine of 1.5 mg/dL, blood glucose of 230 mg/dL, and a WBC of 20 000/μL. A lipid panel is performed, which shows a triglyceride level of 2000 mg/dL.

Other than aggressive hydration and NPO status, what is the next best step in management for this patient's triglycerides?

A. Initiate apheresis
B. Initiate fenofibrate 145 mg daily
C. Initiate fenofibrate 145 mg daily and atorvastatin 80 mg daily
D. Initiate IV insulin and dextrose

ANSWERS

1. **The correct answer is: A. Administer IV hydrocortisone 50 mg.** The patient is experiencing pituitary apoplexy and requires glucocorticoid therapy; doses of hydrocortisone between 50 and 100 mg IV are typically given. The patient will require evaluation by neurosurgery to determine management of the pituitary lesion and the hemorrhage; however, the patient will require medical stabilization first. This patient has hypotension, tachycardia, and mild hyponatremia, thus exhibiting symptoms concerning for adrenal insufficiency. Acute adrenal insufficiency can be life-threatening and requires immediate attention to prevent hemodynamic collapse. Administration of IV fluids is often needed but was not offered as a choice here. Evaluations for adrenal insufficiency are important but should occur after medical stabilization to prevent delay in the administration of glucocorticoids.

2. **The correct answer is: B. Baseline: 0.5; 30 min: 15.3; 60 min: 20.5.** The patient is experiencing acute central adrenal insufficiency, whereby sudden loss of pituitary function prevents the release of ACTH. Under these conditions, the adrenal glands have not yet atrophied from lack of stimulation and thus remain sensitive to ACTH. Answer B is correct because the patient should exhibit no stimulation at baseline with a low-morning cortisol; however, her adrenal glands are responsive to cosyntropin (an ACTH analog). Answer A suggests primary adrenal pathology because of profound lack of cortisol production. Answer C suggests chronic secondary adrenal insufficiency with some evidence of adrenal atrophy. Answer D represents a normal stimulation test. It is important to remember that cosyntropin stimulation tests can be falsely reassuring in situations of acute central adrenal insufficiency, as the adrenal glands have not had time to atrophy.

3. **The correct answer is: A. Order a low-dose dexamethasone suppression test (DST).** This patient is exhibiting classic signs and symptoms of Cushing syndrome, including hypertension, hyperglycemia, abdominal adiposity, easy bruising, and edema. She warrants confirmation of these clinical findings and assessment of the etiology of her hypercortisolism. Screening examinations for Cushing syndrome include the DST, the late-night salivary cortisol test, or the 24-hour urinary cortisol collection. It is important to note that a random or morning cortisol is not a helpful tool in diagnosing Cushing syndrome. Imaging should be performed only after biochemical confirmation of disease and testing to suggest a pituitary source.

4. **The correct answer is: D. Refer to radiology for inferior petrosal sinus sampling.** This patient has clinical and biochemical evidence of Cushing syndrome. Once hypercortisolemia is confirmed, the diagnostic evaluation focuses on whether the disease is due to a central or peripheral cause. The ACTH level measured during the dexamethasone suppression test (DST) was detectable, suggesting an ACTH-dependent process. This could be either a pituitary source (adenoma) or Cushing syndrome from an ectopic ACTH-producing tumor. The method to determine if the ACTH production localizes to the pituitary gland is through inferior petrosal sinus sampling, which measures ACTH values in the venous beds of the pituitary. Moving forward with medical or surgical therapy might lead to misdiagnosis of the etiology of hypercortisolemia. Of note, the presence of a lesion on pituitary MRI does not guarantee that it is the source of hypercortisolism, as incidental lesions are not uncommon.

5. **The correct answer is: D. Measurement of serum IGF-1.** This patient is exhibiting classic signs of acromegaly, including enlargement of the hands and feet, soft tissue edema, changes in facial structure, and development of skin tags. The patient has strong clinical findings of acromegaly; however, they require laboratory confirmation. The first test is to

measure a serum IGF-1 level. If the IGF-1 level is elevated or equivocal, confirmatory testing with oral glucose tolerance test is recommended. Lack of suppression after a glucose load is diagnostic for acromegaly. Random growth hormone levels are not diagnostic in acromegaly because of their large physiologic variability. The glucagon stimulation test is used for the diagnosis of growth hormone deficiency.

6. **The correct answer is: C. Refer to neurosurgery for resection.** Acromegaly is almost always caused by excess growth hormone secretion from a pituitary adenoma. The first-line therapy is surgical resection, as it may lead to cure. If the tumor is inoperable because of size or involvement of central nervous system (CNS) structures, or incomplete resection is achieved, then medical therapy can be added for control of symptoms. Pegvisomant is a growth hormone receptor blocker and lanreotide is a somatostatin analog, both of which can successfully reduce IGF-1 levels in uncontrolled acromegaly.

7. **The correct answer is: B. Initiate desmopressin.** Central diabetes insipidus (DI) is the result of decreased release of ADH, resulting in water diuresis. It can be idiopathic, because of tumors or infiltrative diseases, neurosurgery, or trauma. Severe hypernatremia can occur if a patient has an impaired thirst mechanism, is unable to access free water, or has a cognitive impairment. Typically, a patient with an appropriate thirst mechanism can generally stay eunatremic with DI. In this case, normal saline would worsen this patient's hypernatremia, given increased solute. D5W would provide free water and stabilize sodium levels; however, it would not address the lack of ADH.

8. **The correct answer is: C. Pituitary mass.** The patient is exhibiting signs and symptoms of hyperprolactinemia, including amenorrhea, galactorrhea, and headaches. Hyperprolactinemia is frequently due to prolactin-secreting pituitary adenomas: prolactinomas. Other pituitary pathologies that can produce elevations in prolactin include empty sella syndrome and stalk compression/deviation. Ovarian tumors and adrenal hyperplasia are more commonly associated with hyperandrogenism, rather than hyperprolactinemia. Medication-induced prolactin elevations are common; however, there is no evidence this patient is taking such a medication. It is always important to evaluate for use of dopamine antagonists, as these frequently raise prolactin.

9. **The correct answer is: A. Initiate cabergoline 0.5 mg weekly.** This patient has evidence of a macroprolactinoma. Prolactin-secreting adenomas frequently respond excellently to dopamine agonist therapy and do not require surgical management as first-line therapy. The patient's symptoms of amenorrhea and galactorrhea are suggestive that she is experiencing symptomatic hyperprolactinemia and should receive treatment. Cabergoline is a once-weekly dopamine agonist that is a well-tolerated treatment for hyperprolactinemia. If the patient was experiencing only amenorrhea as a symptom and was not interested in conceiving, then an OCP would be a reasonable alternative.

10. **The correct answer is: A. Abdominal MRI.** This patient's presentation is consistent with hyperparathyroidism, with symptomatic hypercalcemia in the context of elevated PTH levels. She also is exhibiting headache and amenorrhea, which are concerning for a pituitary lesion. This is further supported by the evidence of hypothyroidism that is central in origin with low TSH and low fT4. The combination of hyperparathyroidism and pituitary mass is concerning for MEN1. Patients with MEN1 are at risk for developing neuroendocrine tumors of the pancreas as well, and should be screened for pancreatic neuroendocrine tumors at the time of diagnosis. This is best done with abdominal MRI. Pelvic ultrasound and colonoscopy are important for screening tumors in other oncogenic syndromes but are not indicated here, nor is an echocardiogram. Referral for genetic testing for MEN1 with a genetic counselor would be appropriate but was not offered as a choice.

11. **The correct answer is: A. TSH.** In most patients with signs or symptoms of hypothyroidism, TSH should be the initial test. At some hospitals, TSH can be ordered with reflexive testing, meaning that fT4 is checked only if the TSH is elevated or TSH can be ordered alone and can be repeated with fT4 if the initial TSH is elevated. T3, either total or free, is not helpful in the management of outpatient hypothyroidism.

12. **The correct answer is: C. Levothyroxine 125 μg daily.** The formula 1.6 μg/kg body weight per day is used to estimate the initial replacement dose in adults. The full estimated dose can be used in young and healthy patients without history of cardiac disease.

13. **The correct answer is: A. Levothyroxine 25 μg.** Initial levothyroxine dosing for older adults with a history of CAD or cardiopulmonary disease should be low (12.5-25 μg daily), with gradual increases based on symptoms and TSH levels. Full calculated daily levothyroxine dose based on weight is not recommended to minimize the risk of precipitating cardiac events by increasing myocardial demand.

14. **The correct answer is: C. Start hydrocortisone 100 mg every 8 hours and 100 μg T4 IV daily.** Myxedema coma is an endocrine emergency. Until coexisting adrenal insufficiency is ruled out, patients should be empirically treated for adrenal insufficiency while treating severe hypothyroidism. As myxedema coma is associated with high mortality (~40%), treatment should be initiated based on clinical suspicion, even prior to return of laboratory results. Supportive care and evaluation for triggers are fundamental for the management of myxedema coma, in addition to treatment of hypothyroidism and possible adrenal insufficiency.

15. **The correct answer is: A. Repeat thyroid tests after recovery.** In critically ill patients, assessment of thyroid function is difficult, as nonthyroidal illness can cause acquired central hypothyroidism that resolves with treatment of primary illness. Thyroid studies should be checked in critically ill patients only if there is high suspicion for thyroidal illness. This patient's thyroid studies likely reflect nonthyroidal illness (sick euthyroid) and will resolve with treatment of her infection.

16. **The correct answer is: A. Order radioiodine uptake and scan.** For the evaluation of hyperthyroidism, indicated in this patient by decreased TSH and elevated fT4, radioiodine and uptake scan is the appropriate first test. The most common etiology of hyperthyroidism is Graves disease. Radioactive iodine uptake in Graves disease shows diffuse homogeneous uptake.

17. **The correct answer is: B. Painless thyroiditis.** Painless thyroiditis is a transient hyperthyroidism resulting from release of stored thyroid hormone and is thought to be a form of Hashimoto thyroiditis. Radioiodine uptake indicates synthesis of thyroid hormone within the gland, so causes of hyperthyroidism resulting from excess stimulation or de novo synthesis of thyroid hormone have high radioiodine uptake. Low radioiodine uptake is seen in hyperthyroidism caused by destruction or inflammation of the thyroid and release of preformed hormone or exogenous thyroid hormone.

18. **The correct answer is: D. Surgery.** The American Thyroid Association (ATA) emphasizes discussing all treatment options for Graves disease with patients as there is no best treatment. In this patient, radioiodine would be contraindicated, as she is the sole caregiver of a child and would not be able to follow radiation precautions. Antithyroid drugs are teratogenic and should be avoided when possible in women desiring pregnancy. Surgery provides cure of hyperthyroidism and would be the best option for this patient.

19. **The correct answer is: C. Selenium.** Thyroid storm is an endocrine emergency that requires prompt treatment. The ATA recommends multimodal treatment with β-adrenergic blockade, thionamide, inorganic iodide, corticosteroids, cooling with acetaminophen and cooling blankets, volume resuscitation, nutritional support, and respiratory care. Selenium may improve symptoms in patients with mild thyroid eye disease, but it is not used for the treatment of thyroid storm.

20. **The correct answer is: B. Refer for fine needle aspiration (FNA).** FNA should be performed on nodules ≥1 cm if they are solid or hypoechoic and they have one or more suspicious sonographic characteristics: irregular margins, microcalcifications, taller than wide shape, and/or rim calcifications. In this patient, who has a 10-mm hypoechoic nodule with microcalcifications, FNA should be pursued.

21. **The correct answer is: A. Solid hypoechoic nodule with microcalcification.** The ATA has recommendations for diagnostic FNA of a thyroid nodule based on sonographic patterns. High-suspicion features include: solid hypoechoic nodule/component with irregular margins, microcalcifications, taller than wide shape, rim calcifications with small extrusive soft tissue component, or extra thyroid extension. These high-suspicion nodules require FNA if ≥1cm. Low-suspicion nodules are described as isoechoic or hyperechoic solid nodules without any of the high-risk features described earlier. For low-suspicion nodules, FNA is recommended at ≥1.5 cm.

22. **The correct answer is: B. Repeat FNA with sample for molecular testing.** When the results of FNA are indeterminate (atypia of unknown significance, follicular lesion of undetermined significance), additional evaluation is required. After a biopsy with indeterminate cytology, the ATA recommends either molecular testing, if an extra sample was collected during initial biopsy, or repeat FNA at a 6- to 12-week interval. If the repeat cytology is indeterminate, molecular testing is performed.

23. **The correct answer is: D. Each 100 mg amiodarone contains half of the iodine contained in the average diet daily.** Amiodarone is ~37% iodine by weight. Each 100 mg tablet contains 3 mg of inorganic iodine, which is 10 times the amount of iodine consumed daily by the average American. Amiodarone can cause hypo- or hyperthyroidism and inhibits T4 to T3 conversion. It is recommended that patients have thyroid function checked prior to starting amiodarone therapy and at least every 6 months while on treatment.

24. **The correct answer is: B. Morning plasma renin and aldosterone.** Hyperaldosteronism is present in 11% of patients with hypertension refractory to three drugs. In this patient, with resistant hypertension without a family history and without symptoms to suggest hypercortisolism or a pheochromocytoma, the most likely etiology of secondary hypertension is primary hyperaldosteronism. The first step in the evaluation of hyperaldosteronism is measurement of morning plasma renin and aldosterone as a screening test.

25. **The correct answer is: D. Salt suppression test.** This patient exhibits an aldosterone/renin ratio that is elevated; a ratio >20 is suspicious of primary hyperaldosteronism. In the rare cases where the diagnosis is unequivocal (frank hypokalemia on presentation, aldosterone >20 μg/mL, and renin suppressed), no further testing is required. In this case, however, confirmation of primary aldosteronism is recommended. This can be done with the salt suppression test. Salt suppression test can be performed in the ambulatory setting with salt tablets or via infusion of IV saline in clinic. The administration of saline over 4 hours should suppress aldosterone levels <5 ng/dL in normal individuals. Lack of suppression is diagnostic of primary hyperaldosteronism.

26. **The correct answer is: A. Adrenal venous sampling.** Imaging reveals multiple adrenal adenomas of unclear significance. Assuming that the larger lesion or more hypertrophied/nodular adrenal gland is the source of the aldosterone may lead to erroneous diagnosis. The correct approach would be to perform adrenal venous sampling to determine the source of the aldosterone. Once the source is localized, then the patient can be referred to surgery for subtotal or total adrenalectomy. Medical therapy is utilized in situations where surgical management is technically difficult or refused.

27. **The correct answer is: D. Repeat DST with dexamethasone level and obtain ACTH.** The patient's DST is concerning for lack of suppression, as dexamethasone would expect to bring morning cortisol levels to <1.8 µg/dL. It is important to evaluate whether the patient appropriately took, absorbed, and metabolized dexamethasone, however, as compliance or hypermetabolism may explain the failed test. If cortisol levels are confirmed to not suppress with adequate dexamethasone level, then it would be necessary to determine whether the hypercortisolism is ACTH dependent or independent. A nonsuppressed ACTH level would suggest an ACTH-dependent process such as a pituitary mass or ACTH-producing tumor. A suppressed ACTH would suggest an autonomous source of cortisol production such as an adrenal adenoma.

28. **The correct answer is: A. Adrenal venous sampling.** The patient has ACTH-independent Cushing syndrome and received abdominal imaging to look for adrenal sources. Bilateral nodularity and lesions in this patient make it difficult to localize the main source for the glucocorticoids. As with mineralocorticoid excess, adrenal venous sampling can be helpful to determine which adrenal gland is most involved in excess production of glucocorticoids. If the source is not lateralized, then the other three options (one surgical, two medical) are reasonable to manage the hypercortisolism.

29. **The correct answer is: C. Obtain morning plasma renin and aldosterone.** Primary aldosteronism should be suspected in patients with hypertension and unexplained hypokalemia. The hypokalemia can be spontaneous or low-dose diuretic induced. Initial evaluation includes obtaining a plasma renin and aldosterone level. This patient's TSH was recently checked and found to be normal. Given the patient's lack of thyroid-related symptoms, TSH does not warrant repeat check.

30. **The correct answer is: C. Twenty-four-hour urine fractionated metanephrines now, with plans for aldosterone, renin, and overnight 1 mg dexamethasone suppression test (DST) in the outpatient setting.** All patients with adrenal incidentalomas should be evaluated for hormonal hyperfunction. Hormonal evaluation includes workup for pheochromocytoma, subclinical Cushing syndrome, and, if hypertensive or with unexplained hypokalemia, hyperaldosteronism. In this scenario, given the high degree of clinical suspicion for pheochromocytoma and the seriousness of the condition, it would be recommended to perform evaluation for pheochromocytoma as soon as possible. The rest of the workup should be performed in the outpatient setting when the patient is at his baseline health, as acute illness may induce false positives. An abdominal MRI does not add further information at this time.

31. **The correct answer is: D. Surgical referral.** Imaging characteristics that suggest malignancy include irregular shape, heterogeneous density, diameter >4 cm, and calcifications. For nodules with benign appearance (<10 HU or relative washout $>40\%$), repeat imaging after 6 to 12 months should be performed. In this case, the tumor is >4 cm, making the risk for adrenocortical carcinoma much higher and warranting prophylactic adrenalectomy to prevent progression to adrenocortical carcinoma. Of note, the patient failed the dexamethasone suppression test (DST) and had elevated aldosterone/renin ratio, suggesting

overproduction of glucocorticoids and mineralocorticoids. Adrenocortical carcinomas can produce multiple hormones, unlike adenomas which, when active, usually secrete only one.

32. **The correct answer is: C. Twenty-four-hour urinary fractionated metanephrines and catecholamines.** The patient's presentation is most concerning for catecholamine excess. Although sweating and palpitations may be associated with hypoglycemia, the patient is not describing Whipple triad. The symptoms are also less likely due to a gut neuroendocrine tumor or carcinoid syndrome, as there is no flushing or gastrointestinal (GI) symptoms. The patient warrants evaluation for pheochromocytoma and paraganglioma by measuring urinary fractionated metanephrines and catecholamines. An elevated value warrants further evaluation with imaging.

33. **The correct answer is: B. Metaiodobenzylguanidine (MIBG) I-123 scan.** Elevated catecholamines can also be produced by tumors of the sympathetic chain known as paragangliomas. They are extra-adrenal and require broader imaging to identify. Frequently multiple modalities are required until they are identified, with MIBG, fluorodeoxyglucose-positron emission tomography (FDG-PET), and octreotide scans having different sensitivities for identifying paragangliomas. As catecholamine excess has been confirmed, serial monitoring or prophylactic treatment is inappropriate at this time.

34. **The correct answer is: D. Initiate prazosin 1 mg every 4 hours.** The current preoperative practice for catecholamine-secreting tumors is to provide α-blockade, preventing catastrophic α-adrenergic stimulation during manipulation of the tumor. This can be performed with nonselective α-blockers, such as phenoxybenzamine, or with selective agents, such as prazosin. Patients need dose titration until they develop orthostatic hypotension as a marker for sufficient blockage. Exclusive β-blockade should not be performed in patients with catecholamine-secreting tumors to prevent cardiovascular collapse from unopposed α-stimulation. Metyrosine prevents the production of catecholamines and is used in the management of metastatic pheochromocytoma.

35. **The correct answer is: B. Genetics referral, repeat imaging, and catecholamines in 1 year.** As the field of genetics has advanced, more gene mutations have been identified that increase the risk for paraganglioma/pheochromocytoma. It is estimated that >20% of pheos are genetic/familial in origin; therefore, genetic counseling and testing are of high value in this patient population. Patients with catecholamine-secreting tumors should be regularly screened with imaging and catecholamine levels to ensure no evidence of recurrence, particularly in those with known genetic mutations such as MEN2A, Von Hippel-Lindau syndrome, and succinate dehydrogenase mutations.

36. **The correct answer is: D. Referral to the emergency room.** The patient is presenting with signs of adrenal insufficiency, including fatigue, hypotension, and orthostasis. The presence of hyperpigmentation and salt cravings suggests both a glucocorticoid and mineralocorticoid deficit. In the context of a young woman with hypothyroidism, the most likely cause would be Addison disease. The patient is exhibiting significant hemodynamic symptoms and may also have underlying severe electrolyte abnormalities such as hyperkalemia and hyponatremia. Her presentation is concerning for adrenal crisis and requires prompt management with IV hydrocortisone, fluid resuscitation, and correction of electrolyte abnormalities.

37. **The correct answer is: C. Check baseline ACTH and perform cosyntropin stimulation test.** The clinical picture is strongly suggestive of Addison disease; however, the patient requires biochemical confirmation of adrenal insufficiency. An elevated ACTH (frequently in the hundreds) is consistent with adrenal failure. A cosyntropin stimulation test

would be expected to show a minimal response to cosyntropin. Once the diagnosis is confirmed, the patient will require discussions regarding appropriate glucocorticoid and mineralocorticoid replacement. 21-Hydroxylase antibodies can also be checked, as their presence is associated with Addison disease but is not necessary for diagnosis. An abdominal CT scan can be used to identify other etiologies of adrenal failure but is of low utility for known autoimmune adrenalitis.

38. **The correct answer is: D. Prednisone 5 mg daily and fludrocortisone 0.1 mg daily.** With her new diagnosis, the patient will require replacement of both glucocorticoids and mineralocorticoids for life. Prednisone and fludrocortisone cover this requirement. Although hydrocortisone has both glucocorticoid and mineralocorticoid effects, the replacement dose of hydrocortisone is unlikely to provide sufficient mineralocorticoid coverage and is typically supplemented with fludrocortisone. Hydrocortisone is often used (together with fludrocortisone), but it needs to be administered in two (or three) divided doses, which was not an available choice. The lowest possible dose of both is recommended to prevent the complications of excess glucocorticoid use and aldosteronism.

39. **The correct answer is: C. Check serum and 24-hour urine calcium and creatinine.** Primary hyperparathyroidism is unusual in young men and raises the possibility of a familial form of hypercalcemia. Familial hypocalciuric hypercalcemia (FHH) needs to be ruled out, as parathyroidectomy should be avoided in FHH. In FHH, all parathyroid cells have a defect in the calcium-sensing receptor and removing a parathyroid gland will not change the disease. Currently, calculating the calcium-to creatinine clearance ratio (CCCR) CCCR is the standard test, and a 24-hour urine calcium, creatinine, and concomitant serum calcium and creatinine measurements are needed. Magnesium and phosphate, although typically checked, will not contribute much to the diagnostic question. Imaging tests for parathyroid gland localization may be performed after FHH is ruled out. He suffered a traumatic, but not a fragility, fracture (defined as a fall from standing height). DXA is not indicated at this stage of diagnostic workup.

40. **The correct answer is: A. Hypercalcemic crisis.** This patient's presentation with acute neurologic symptoms and signs requires emergent evaluation. Although his presentation could be associated with hyperthyroidism, the history of thyroidectomy without mentioning medication changes makes this diagnosis unlikely. The fact that he is able to drink a lot of water makes HHS less likely. Thirst, frequent urination, and weight loss are not characteristics of a stroke. Hyponatremia should be ruled out, but this was not a choice given. Hypercalcemia can cause all of the symptoms and is high on the differential diagnosis. Lethargy and confusion can be seen in severe hypercalcemia, and weakness of extraocular muscles can lead to diplopia.

41. **The correct answer is: B. Lung cancer.** Severe hypercalcemia, or hypercalcemic crisis, can have several causes, but hypercalcemia of malignancy is most likely in this patient with a strong history of tobacco use. A normal calcium a year ago practically excludes primary hyperparathyroidism, including MEN1-associated hyperparathyroidism. His TSH is normal, presumably through appropriate therapy with levothyroxine, excluding hyperthyroidism (from Graves disease or other etiologies).

42. **The correct answer is: C. Normal saline IV.** Severe hypercalcemia needs to be treated immediately. Aggressive hydration with IV saline is the most effective intervention. Large doses are often needed. Calcitonin is sometimes used in the acute treatment of hypercalcemia, but its effect is relatively weak and does not last more than a few days because of tachyphylaxis. Bisphosphonates (if renal function allows) and denosumab are effective in the treatment of hypercalcemia of malignancy but do not work immediately. PTH/PTHrP

receptor antibodies are not clinically available. The management of the underlying lung tumor needs to be addressed but should not delay the acute treatment of the hypercalcemia.

43. **The correct answer is: C. Sarcoidosis.** Sarcoidosis, an inflammatory disease characterized by the presence of noncaseating granulomas, can affect almost all organs, can be asymptomatic, or is associated with a wide range of symptoms and presents a diagnostic challenge. Black women have a higher incidence of sarcoidosis. This patient's presentation is classic for pulmonary sarcoidosis, but a diagnostic evaluation that typically includes a tissue biopsy is needed. Hypercalcemia in sarcoidosis is due to the PTH-independent conversion of 25(OH)D to the active 1,25(OH)$_2$D. Primary or secondary hyperparathyroidism presents with elevated PTH (and serum calcium is not elevated in secondary hyperparathyroidism). Humoral hypercalcemia of malignancy is caused by elevated PTHrP.

44. **The correct answer is: A. Calcium and albumin.** This is a typical presentation of hypocalcemia with neuromuscular irritability. If her (albumin-adjusted) serum calcium turns out to be low and her PTH is low or inadequate, she has postsurgical hypoparathyroidism and not multiple sclerosis.

45. **The correct answer is: A. Check vitamin D and PTH.** This patient was found to have an undetectable vitamin D level with secondary hyperparathyroidism, a common condition that is characterized by low-to-normal serum calcium (because of low calcium absorption) and low serum phosphorus (because of the elevation of PTH). Treatment with vitamin D supplementation normalizes these findings. PHEX is mutated in X-linked hypophosphatemia, a hereditary form of rickets. FGF23 is elevated in several rare types of hypophosphatemia. Vitamin D deficiency is much more common and should be ruled out first. Insulin can lead to an intracellular shift of phosphate, but this is not relevant in this otherwise healthy patient.

46. **The correct answer is: D. Check serum calcium and albumin.** During pregnancy, serum albumin is typically decreased because of an increase in plasma volume. Total serum calcium must be corrected for albumin. Her albumin is 2.0 g/dL and her adjusted calcium is 8.4 mg/dL and, therefore, within range for hypoparathyroid patients who target low-normal calcium levels. In the absence of symptoms, no change in treatment is needed.

47. **The correct answer is: D. All of the above.** This patient, who has experienced an osteoporotic fracture, warrants therapy for osteoporosis. Bisphosphonates are often the initial therapy. Oral bisphosphonates should not be used in patients with esophageal disorders that put them at risk for the tablet to be stuck in the esophagus. Additionally, the risk of jaw osteonecrosis must be considered if patients will have imminent invasive dental procedures. A vitamin D level is checked prior to initiation of bisphosphonate therapy, as repletion is recommended prior to administration to avoid hypocalcemia.

48. **The correct answer is: A. Treat hypomagnesemia.** This patient is having severe symptomatic hypocalcemia, which includes tetany. Other symptoms include seizures and prolonged QT interval. This will require IV formulation of calcium with eventual addition of oral medication once the patient is able to safely take PO. In patients with concurrent hypocalcemia and hypomagnesemia, the serum magnesium levels should be corrected aggressively because hypocalcemia will otherwise be difficult to correct. Hypomagnesemia induces resistances to PTH and diminishes its secretion.

49. **The correct answer is: B. Recommend parathyroid surgery.** She has primary hyperparathyroidism, a disease with an incidence of >100 000 new cases annually in the United States. That primarily affects postmenopausal women. In FHH, a very rare disease,

CCCR typically is <0.01; genetic testing is, therefore, not indicated. Criteria for the surgical treatment of asymptomatic primary hyperparathyroidism include any of the following: age <50 years, serum calcium >11.5 g/dL, CrCl <60 or DXA T-score <−2.5, or history of fragility fracture. She has osteoporosis and parathyroidectomy is recommended.

50. **The correct answer is: C. Liraglutide daily.** In this patient with known cardiovascular disease, according to the 2022 ADA guidelines when adding a second medication to metformin and lifestyle management to improve glycemic control, it is recommended to add therapy validated to improve heart health. Of the listed options, GLP-1 RA liraglutide is the only agent approved by the Food and Drug Administration (FDA) to reduce the risk of cardiovascular death in adult patients with T2DM.

51. **The correct answer is: D. Start 15 U insulin glargine nightly with sliding scale aspart insulin.** This patient appropriately had his home antihyperglycemic medications held on admission, given his acute illness and kidney injury. The extent of his underlying insulin resistance, both because of metabolic factors and from his acute illness, suggests that he will require insulin during the hospitalization. In patients for whom a significant insulin requirement is anticipated, initiating standing insulin will provide better glycemic control than correctional doses alone. Starting basal insulin with insulin glargine or neutral protamine Hagedorn (NPH) would be a reasonable approach in someone with the glycemic pattern mentioned.

52. **The correct answer is: D. Start liraglutide 0.6 mg subcutaneous (SC) once daily.** This patient is not currently meeting her HbA$_{1c}$ goal of 7.0%, so it is appropriate to add an additional therapy for improved glycemic control. Given her comorbid obesity, liraglutide is the most appropriate option, as liraglutide is FDA approved for the treatment of obesity. Sulfonylureas and insulin are associated with weight gain.

53. **The correct answer is: C. Serum anion gap <12 mEq/L and serum bicarbonate ≥15 mEq/L.** The ADA guidelines for DKA recommend IV insulin be tapered and a multiple-dose SC insulin schedule be started when blood glucose is <200 mg/dL and at least two of the following parameters are met: (1) serum anion gap <12 mEq/L (or at the upper limit of normal for the local laboratory), (2) serum bicarbonate ≥15 mEq/L, and (3) venous pH >7.30. In addition, it is preferred for a patient to remain on IV infusion if unable to eat. The IV infusion should be continued for 1 to 2 hours after initiation of SC insulin.

54. **The correct answer is: D. Insulin = 38 pmol/L, proinsulin = 25 pmol/L, C-peptide = 0.8 ng/mL, β-hydroxybutyrate <2.7 mmol/L, oral hypoglycemic agent screen = negative.** In the evaluation of hypoglycemia in an adult without diabetes, it is necessary to document Whipple triad and collect the following labs at the time of symptoms: insulin, proinsulin, C-peptide, β-hydroxybutyrate, and oral hypoglycemic agent screen. In cases of endogenous hyperinsulinemia (insulinoma), there will be a low glucose with elevated insulin, proinsulin, and C-peptide, with suppressed β-hydroxybutyrate and negative oral hypoglycemic agent screen. The laboratory findings in hypoglycemia because of sulfonylureas will be identical, except the oral hypoglycemia agent screen will be positive.

55. **The correct answer is: D. Transthoracic echocardiogram.** The initial management of HHS, like the management of DKA, involves replacing volume and electrolyte deficits, insulin, and identification of any underlying illness that may have precipitated HHS. Common precipitants include infection, medication noncompliance, MI, and stroke. Although MI can be a precipitant of HHS, this would be evaluated initially with an ECG rather than an echocardiogram.

56. **The correct answer is: C. SGLT2 inhibitors increase hyperfiltration.** Animal models have suggested that SGLT2 inhibition reduces hyperfiltration and reduces albuminuria. In clinical trials, SGLT2 inhibitors cause a slight initial decrease in eGFR, but then lessen the decrease in eGFR over time compared with placebo. Canagliflozin, empagliflozin, and dapagliflozin have been approved to reduce the risk for kidney disease progression and cardiovascular death among adults with T2DM and diabetic kidney disease.

57. **The correct answer is: B. Start long-acting insulin at 0.1 to 0.2 IU/kg/day with instructions to increase 2 U every 3 days until reaching fasting glucose target.** The ADA recommends early introduction of insulin if there is evidence of ongoing catabolism (weight loss), if symptoms of hyperglycemia are present, or when A_{1c} level is >10%. In this patient, her nocturia likely reflects symptomatic hyperglycemia. Once initiated, metformin should be continued as long as tolerated with additional agents added as necessary. The ADA recommends initial basal insulin dosing of 0.1 to 0.2 IU/kg/day or 10 U/day with instructions for patient self-titration. Prior to initiation of prandial insulin, it would be reasonable to monitor response to basal insulin to simplify regimen and promote adherence.

58. **The correct answer is: A. Continue metformin and add dapagliflozin.** In individuals with T2DM with HF as the predominant comorbid condition, SGLT2 inhibitors are recommended as the second agent (in addition to metformin). SGLT2 inhibitors have been shown to significantly lower the risk of hospitalization because of HF. The ADA recommends the addition of SGLT2 inhibitors with proven benefit independent of HbA_{1c} in patients with HF.

59. **The correct answer is: C. Lipid profile, tissue transglutaminase, and TSH.** At the time of diagnosis of T1DM, screening for celiac disease, hypothyroidism, and dyslipidemia is recommended.

60. **The correct answer is: C. Discard vial and open new vial.** Unopened insulin should be stored in the refrigerator. Most insulin vials expire ~30 days after first use and do not require refrigeration after opening. Insulin should not be exposed to extremes of temperature as it can lead to significant changes in insulin action. It is recommended that insulin be stored at room temperature in a place away from direct heat and light, as long as the temperature is not >30°C. If a vial of insulin freezes or is exposed to extreme heat, it should be discarded.

61. **The correct answer is: D. Discontinue insulin pump and transition to IV insulin infusion.** The ADA advocates allowing patients who are physically and mentally able to continue to use their pumps when hospitalized. In this setting in which the patient is critically ill and unable to manage his insulin pump because of altered mental status, it would be appropriate to transition to IV insulin infusion. The ADA recommends transitioning to basal-bolus regimen in noncritically ill patients admitted to hospital but unable to safely operate the pump.

62. **The correct answer is: B. Initiate SGLT2 inhibitor.** Per the ADA, patients with type 2 diabetes who have established atherosclerotic cardiovascular disease (ASCVD) or indicators of high ASCVD risk (such as patients ≥55 years of age with coronary, carotid, or lower-extremity artery stenosis >50% or left ventricular hypertrophy), HF, or CKD, an SGLT2 inhibitor or GLP-1 RA with demonstrated CVD benefit is recommended as part of the glucose-lowering regimen independent of A_{1c}, independent of metformin use, and in consideration of patient-specific factors. For patients with T2DM and diabetic kidney disease, SGLT2 inhibitors are recommended to reduce CKD progression and cardiovascular events. Insulin is not indicated given this patient does not have evidence of ongoing catabolism. An ARB is not indicated, as the patient is already taking an ACE inhibitor.

63. **The correct answer is: A. Initiate glucagon-like peptide-1 receptor agonist (GLP-1 RA).** Per the ADA, patients with T2DM who have established ASCVD or indicators of high ASCVD risk (such as patients ≥55 years of age with coronary, carotid, or lower-extremity artery stenosis >50% or left ventricular hypertrophy), HF, or CKD, an SGLT2 inhibitor or GLP-1 RA with demonstrated CVD benefit is recommended as part of the glucose-lowering regimen independent of A_{1c}, independent of metformin use, and in consideration of patient-specific factors. In addition to this patient's established ASCVD, he also would benefit from a GLP-1 RA for its efficacy for weight loss regardless of his current HbA_{1c} level.

64. **The correct answer is: C. Nausea, vomiting.** When initiating GLP-1 RA, patients can experience nausea, vomiting, and diarrhea. Nausea may wane with duration and can be minimized with dose reduction. Pancreatitis has been reported to be associated with GLP-1 RA treatment; however, there are insufficient data to know if it is a causal relationship. If pancreatitis is suspected, the GLP-1 RA should be discontinued. Some studies regarding SGLT2 inhibitors have shown an increased risk of amputation, although this mechanism is not completely understood. SGLT2 inhibitors also increase the rate of genital yeast infections. Thiazolidinediones increase the risk of HF.

65. **The correct answer is: D. Initiate GLP-1 RA.** A GLP-1 RA should be considered prior to insulin in patients that require an injectable therapy to reduce HbA_{1c}. When compared to insulin, GLP-1 RAs have lower risk of hypoglycemia and beneficial effects on weight. Insulin should be considered if there is evidence of weight loss, symptoms of hyperglycemia, A_{1c} >10%, or blood glucose level >300 mg/dL.

66. **The correct answer is: A. Initiate basal insulin at 0.1-0.2 U/kg/day.** Insulin should be considered if there is evidence of weight loss, symptoms of hyperglycemia, HbA_{1c} >10%, or blood glucose level >300 mg/dL. Basal insulin should be initiated in this patient with symptoms of catabolism and an HbA_{1c} not at target despite treatment with GLP-1 RA.

67. **The correct answer is: D. Empagliflozin.** The patient is presenting with euglycemic DKA, which is characterized by euglycemia (<250 mg/dL) with metabolic acidosis and ketonemia. The FDA has issued a warning about an increased risk of euglycemic DKA in patients taking SGLT2 inhibitors. Patients taking SGLT2 inhibitors should be instructed to stop the medication 3 days prior to surgery or procedure, if unable to eat or drink, or feeling unwell with an infection. The patient's mild increase in lactic acid is likely due to dehydration and unlikely represents metformin-associated lactic acidosis, which is often a result of renal impairment and a concurrent illness. Lisinopril and fentanyl have not been shown to increase the risk of euglycemic DKA.

68. **The correct answer is: A. Continue atorvastatin 80 mg daily and add ezetimibe 10 mg daily.** The IMPROVE-IT trial showed the addition of ezetimibe to statin therapy decreased LDL and improved cardiovascular outcomes in patients with known CAD. As this patient has a more stringent LDL goal (<70 mg/dL), further therapy would be beneficial. He is currently on a high-potency statin and so switching to a moderate potency would not improve his LDL. It is unclear if the addition of the fibrate would add concomitant cardiovascular benefit and can increase the risk of myalgias and rhabdomyolysis with statins. It is reasonable to start by adding ezetimibe and see the resultant LDL cholesterol (LDL-C). U.S. guidelines recommend adding a PCSK9 inhibitor if the LDL-C remains 70 mg/dL or above; European guidelines recommend targeting an LDL-C <55 mg/dL.

69. **The correct answer is: A. Atorvastatin 80 mg daily.** The current recommendations are to initiate high-intensity statins as first-line therapy in patients thought to be

heterozygote carriers of familial hypercholesterolemia. High-intensity statin with or without the addition of ezetimibe would be a good first option to reduce LDL levels by >50%. If the patient shows evidence of cardiovascular disease or does not respond sufficiently to a statin, the addition of a PCSK9 inhibitor such as evolocumab would be reasonable.

70. **The correct answer is: D. Initiate IV insulin and dextrose**. This patient is experiencing severe hypertriglyceridemia and shows concerning symptoms such as tachycardia and leukocytosis in association with his pancreatitis. Rapid management of the metabolic insults associated with hypertriglyceridemia is needed. Insulin promotes expression of lipoprotein lipase, encouraging clearance of triglycerides from circulation. As this patient is hyperglycemic and can tolerate insulin therapy, initiation of IV insulin with sufficient glucose to preserve euglycemia would assist in decreasing triglycerides. If this patient does not respond to more conservative measures, then apheresis would be a reasonable next step.

QUESTIONS

1. A 42-year-old woman with an unremarkable medical history presents to her primary care doctor with discomfort along the radial side of her right wrist that started 1 week ago. She reports no injury or trauma to the hand or wrist and is otherwise healthy. She has a 6-month-old healthy boy. Physical examination reveals tenderness over the dorsal radial side of the wrist with fullness over the first dorsal compartment of the right wrist. Pain is reproduced with ulnar deviation of the wrist with the thumb grasped in her palm. Palpation of the first carpometacarpal (CMC) joint is not painful. A radiograph of the wrist is normal.

   Which of the following is the most likely diagnosis?

   A. De Quervain tenosynovitis
   B. Hand osteoarthritis
   C. Carpal tunnel syndrome
   D. Early presentation of inflammatory arthritis

2. A 64-year-old male with a history of hypertension, obesity, nonalcoholic fatty liver disease, and dyslipidemia presents to rheumatology clinic in November with a 2-month history of bilateral hand pain. He denies any rashes, oral or nasal ulcers, Raynaud phenomenon, proximal weakness, dyspnea, or pleuritic chest pain. Medications include amlodipine 10 mg daily, simvastatin 20 mg daily, and aspirin 81 mg daily. Examination is notable for swelling and tenderness of the bilateral hand proximal interphalangeal (PIP) joints and second through fourth metacarpophalangeal (MCP) joints. Labs show normal complete blood count (CBC). Aspartate aminotransferase (AST) is 130 and alanine aminotransferase (ALT) is 150, which are at baseline. Renal function is normal. Hepatitis serologies are negative, and a tuberculosis (TB) QuantiFERON test is negative. X-ray of hands do not show any erosive disease.

   Which of the following is the most likely diagnosis?

   A. Polyarticular gout
   B. Rheumatoid arthritis (RA)
   C. Parvovirus-associated arthritis
   D. Ankylosing spondylitis

3. Positive tests for which of the following will help to establish the diagnosis in the patient in Question 2?

   A. Rheumatoid factor (RF) and anti–cyclic citrullinated peptide (CCP) antibodies
   B. Human leukocyte antigen (HLA)-B27
   C. Acute parvovirus serologies
   D. Magnetic resonance imaging (MRI) of the hand
   E. Dual-energy computed tomography (CT) scan

4. The patient in Questions 2 and 3 is started on sulfasalazine 500 mg twice daily and hydroxychloroquine 400 mg daily. Three weeks later, during travel to Florida, the patient presents to the local emergency department (ED) with fever, cough, rash, myalgias, and diffuse arthralgias. On examination, there is a confluent maculopapular rash over the trunk and arms. He is noted to have bilateral MCP and PIP joint swelling and tenderness. Labs are

notable for AST of 400, ALT of 350, and alkaline phosphatase of 800. He has mild leukopenia. A chest x-ray is negative for any consolidation. A rapid flu test is negative.

Which of the following is the most appropriate next step in the management of this patient?

A. Stop sulfasalazine and start prednisone 0.5 mg/kg
B. Start oseltamivir for flu given high index of suspicion
C. Conservative management for viral syndrome with hydration, acetaminophen, and rest
D. Stop hydroxychloroquine
E. Start prednisone 0.5 mg/kg for flare of RA

5. A 32-year-old female was recently diagnosed with non-erosive seropositive RA. She is unable to tolerate methotrexate because of gastrointestinal intolerance even when switched to subcutaneous formulation and folinic acid is added. Her past medical history is notable for Stevens-Johnson syndrome that developed after a course of sulfamethoxazole/trimethoprim for the treatment of urinary tract infection 3 years ago. She is married and wants to have children. She is started on hydroxychloroquine but does not tolerate the medication because of gastrointestinal symptoms, and on follow-up 3 months later she continues to have joint pain and swelling.

Which of the following is an appropriate next agent?

A. Sulfasalazine
B. Leflunomide
C. Biologic disease-modifying antirheumatic drug (DMARD)
D. Penicillamine

6. You decide to start the patient in Question 5 on a biologic DMARD.

Which of the following agents is LEAST likely to achieve good disease control?

A. Anakinra (interleukin [IL]-1 receptor antagonist)
B. Infliximab (anti–tumor necrosis factor [TNF]-α)
C. Tocilizumab (anti-IL-6)
D. Abatacept (cytotoxic T lymphocyte–associated antigen-4 immunoglobulin [CTLA-4 Ig])

7. A 28-year-old otherwise healthy male presents to urgent care with a 6-week history of polyarticular pain involving his wrists, elbows, knees, and feet. He experiences daily febrile episodes up to 38.9°C occurring toward the end of the day. His mother, who accompanies him, notes a rash over his trunk during these episodes. A thorough review of systems is notable for a weight loss of 6 lb that is unintentional over the last 4 weeks and night sweats. He denies any sore throat, oral/nasal ulcers, cough, abdominal pain, diarrhea, or dysuria. He denies any recent travel or exposure to known sick contacts. On examination, he is afebrile and vital signs are normal. No rash is noted. There is tenderness to palpation of both wrists, without evidence of effusion, redness, or warmth. Firm, nontender matted cervical lymph nodes are palpable, the largest of which measures 2 cm in greatest diameter. The remainder of the examination is unremarkable. A CBC shows white blood cell (WBC) count of 14 000 cells/µL with neutrophil predominance. His AST and ALT are mildly elevated at 78 and 98, respectively. RF, CCP, and antinuclear antibody (ANA) are negative. X-rays of the wrists are normal. Blood cultures show no growth after 5 days.

Which of the following is NOT an appropriate step in evaluation and management?

A. Start prednisone 0.5 mg/kg
B. Start naproxen 500 mg twice daily with omeprazole 20 mg daily
C. Open biopsy of cervical lymph node
D. CT chest, abdomen, and pelvis

8. A 55-year-old woman presents to clinic with several weeks of right ear swelling. Over the past year, she has experienced several such episodes for which topical and oral antibiotics had not proven helpful. She experiences moderate relief of symptoms with naproxen 440 mg taken twice daily, though not complete resolution of symptoms. Other than a bout of vertigo earlier this year, she otherwise has been well. On examination, the upper portion of her right ear is swollen and erythematous, but the earlobe appears normal. A saddle nose deformity is also appreciated.

Suspicion is highest for which of the following?
  A. Relapsing polychondritis
  B. Scleroderma
  C. Cryoglobulinemia
  D. Infectious perichondritis
  E. Tophaceous gout

9. The most appropriate treatment for the patient in Question 8 is which of the following?
  A. Methotrexate
  B. Broader antibiotics
  C. Corticosteroids
  D. Allopurinol
  E. Cyclophosphamide

10. Workup for the patient in Questions 8 and 9 should additionally involve which of the following?
  A. Arthrocentesis and crystal analysis
  B. Blood cultures
  C. Anti-Scl-70 serology
  D. Evaluation of the larynx and large airways with CT
  E. Serum cryoglobulins, serum protein electrophoresis (SPEP), and serum free light chain (SFLC) assay

11. A 28-year-old male with a history of hypertension, obesity, and dyslipidemia presents to the ED with a 1-day history of severe right knee and left ankle pain. He is afebrile with normal vitals. Examination is notable for swelling and tenderness of the right knee and left ankle. Left knee examination is also notable for tenderness along the infrapatellar tendon, as well as small firm nodules in the left olecranon bursa. The remainder of the examination is normal. Labs in the ED show a normal CBC, normal comprehensive metabolic panel (CMP), and elevated erythrocyte sedimentation rate (ESR, 56 mm/h) and C-reactive protein (CRP, 80 mg/L). He reports two previous similar episodes of acute-onset knee pain and swelling that were treated with nonsteroidal anti-inflammatory drugs (NSAIDs) with complete resolution within 1 week. He denies any history of rash, inflammatory eye disease, low back pain, conjunctivitis, dysuria, heel pain, abdominal pain, or diarrhea. He does not recall any antecedent gastrointestinal, genitourinary, or sinopulmonary infections.

Which of the following is the most likely diagnosis?
  A. Acute gouty arthritis
  B. Septic arthritis
  C. Seronegative spondyloarthritis
  D. Systemic lupus erythematosus (SLE)
  E. RA

12. Which of the following is the next best step to establish the diagnosis in the patient in Question 11?

A. Arthrocentesis with cell count, differential, Gram stain, culture, and crystal examination
B. Dual-energy CT scan
C. Musculoskeletal ultrasound examination
D. Sacroiliac (SI) joint X-ray
E. HLA-B27 testing

13. A 50-year-old male with a history of hypertension, hyperlipidemia, type 1 diabetes mellitus (T1DM) on insulin pump, peptic ulcer disease, chronic kidney disease (CKD) stage 3, ischemic cardiomyopathy, and gout is admitted to the hospital with a 2-day history of worsening dyspnea on exertion. He is found to be in acute decompensated heart failure and is treated with intravenous (IV) furosemide. On the third day of hospitalization, the patient develops severe joint pain and swelling of multiple joints including the wrists, elbows, knees, ankles, and metatarsophalangeals (MTPs). On examination, he is afebrile. You note multiple subcutaneous painless hard masses within both olecranon bursae. His second and third MCPs, bilateral knees, and bilateral first through third MTP joints are swollen, tender, and warm. Arthrocentesis of the right knee is performed, with preliminary studies showing 36 000 cells/μL with 85% neutrophils. Crystal examination and Gram stain are pending. A CBC shows normal WBC and red blood cell (RBC) count. His glomerular filtration rate (GFR) is 18 mL/min. One month ago his GFR was 39 mL/min. His uric acid level is 5.7 mg/dL. A recent hemoglobin A_{1c} (HbA$_{1c}$) was 9.

Which of the following is the best treatment for his arthritis?

A. Indomethacin 50 mg three times daily
B. Start colchicine 1.2 mg followed by 0.6 mg 1 hour later
C. Administer intra-articular steroid injections
D. Administer subcutaneous adrenocorticotropic hormone (ACTH)
E. Start anakinra 100 mg subcutaneous daily

14. A 65-year-old male with a history of hypertension, hyperlipidemia, and tophaceous gout is being seen in follow-up for hypertension. His gout is stable, and he has not had any acute gouty arthritis in 2 years. His most recent uric acid level is 5.8 mg/dL. His blood pressure (BP) on multiple visits is elevated and you plan to make adjustments to the current regimen of amlodipine 10 mg daily.

Which antihypertensive medication adjustment would be LEAST likely to raise his uric acid level?

A. Stop amlodipine and start hydrochlorothiazide
B. Stop amlodipine and start lisinopril
C. Continue amlodipine and start lisinopril
D. Continue amlodipine and start losartan
E. None of the above, would recommend against changing his antihypertensive regimen as this is likely to worsen renal function and precipitate a gout attack

15. An 80-year-old male with a history of hypertension, stage 4 CKD, diabetes mellitus, and atrial fibrillation on coumadin presents to the ED with a 2-day history of right knee pain and swelling. He denies any prior episodes of joint pain. He reports a recent fall 1 week earlier but does not recall injuring the knee. He denies any fevers, chills, rashes, abdominal pain, diarrhea, dysuria, or eye pain. He has not received any antibiotics in the preceding 3 months. On examination, he is afebrile. BP is 130/85 mmHg. There is a moderate-sized knee effusion, redness, and warmth. Range of motion is limited by pain, but you are able to passively flex the knee to 45°. X-ray demonstrates moderate effusion and medial compartment joint space narrowing with calcification of the articular cartilage. His CBC is normal. Basic metabolic panel (BMP) is notable for GFR of 25 mL/min, and serum uric acid level is 6.7.

What of the following is NOT a likely cause of his presentation?

A. Septic arthritis
B. Acute gouty arthritis
C. Pseudogout
D. Hemarthrosis
E. An acute presentation of RA

16. What is the next best step in the management of the patient in Question 15?

A. Arthrocentesis with cell counts, crystal examination, Gram stain, and culture
B. MRI of the right knee
C. Dual-energy CT scan
D. Serum uric acid level
E. Start prednisone 40 mg daily.

17. Arthrocentesis is performed in the patient in Questions 15 and 16, and 20 mL of cloudy, yellow fluid is aspirated. Cell count shows 35 000 cells/μL, 75% neutrophils. Gram stain is negative for organisms and crystal analysis shows weakly positively birefringent rhomboid-shaped crystals. Joint fluid culture shows no growth after 3 days.

What is the diagnosis?

A. Gout
B. Pseudogout
C. Calcium hydroxyapatite arthritis
D. Cholesterol arthritis

18. What is the next best step in the management of the patient in Questions 15-17?

A. Start ceftriaxone and vancomycin
B. Intra-articular steroid injection with 80 mg methylprednisolone
C. Start naproxen 500 mg twice daily
D. Start colchicine
E. Repeat arthrocentesis

19. A 28-year-old male is referred to rheumatology for the evaluation of a 3-month history of low back pain. The patient notes the insidious onset of low back pain, associated with 60 minutes of morning stiffness. Pain improves with activity and is worsened with rest. He has tried naproxen 440 mg twice daily with good effect but with recurrence of pain upon discontinuation of therapy. The patient denies any rashes, visual blurring, red eyes, sensation of eye grittiness, dysuria, frequency, abdominal pain, or diarrhea. There is no history of antecedent genitourinary or gastrointestinal infections. His examination is notable for tenderness over the lower spine and paraspinal region, particularly over the SI joints. Flexion, abduction, and external rotation (FABER) of his hips reproduces low back pain.

What is the most likely diagnosis?

A. RA
B. Ankylosing spondylitis
C. Reactive arthritis
D. Inflammatory bowel disease (IBD)-associated axial spondyloarthritis

20. What is the next best diagnostic test to evaluate the low back pain of the patient in Question 19?

   A. SI joint radiographs
   B. Sacral MRI
   C. Colonoscopy
   D. RF and anti-CCP antibodies

21. SI joint x-rays with Ferguson views of the patient in Questions 19 and 20 show evidence of bilateral grade 2 SI joint disease (joint sclerosis and erosions). Lumbar spine radiographs reveal small erosions and sclerosis at the corners of vertebral bodies and a few symmetric marginal syndesmophytes. Laboratory evaluation shows a normocytic and normochromic anemia, normal renal and liver functions, and elevated inflammatory markers. He is HLA-B27 positive. You decide to start the patient on adalimumab 40 mg subcutaneous every 2 weeks.

Which of the following testing is necessary prior to starting adalimumab in this patient?

   A. Interferon-γ release assay
   B. Human immunodeficiency virus (HIV) antigen/antibody testing
   C. Treponema-specific antibodies
   D. Hepatitis C antibody

22. A 28-year-old male presents to the ED with a 3-day history of right knee pain and swelling. His medical history is notable for cocaine abuse complicated by levamisole-induced vasculitis and an episode of gonococcal urethritis 5 weeks ago treated with intramuscular ceftriaxone and azithromycin. Three weeks ago, he developed bilateral eye redness that has since resolved, a rash on the glans penis, as well as ongoing low back pain worse in the morning and improved with activity. He denies any other rashes, dactylitis, ongoing symptoms of dysuria, frequency, or urgency. He denies any heel pain. There is no personal history of psoriasis or IBD. Family history is unremarkable. On examination, he is afebrile. There are right knee and left ankle swelling and tenderness. He has an erythematous serpiginous rash over the glans penis without penile discharge. There are no other rashes. SI joint palpation is not painful. A left FABER test is negative; right-sided FABER is limited by knee pain and reduced range of motion. Labs are notable for WBC of 12.7 and Hb 9.9. His CRP is 127 mg/L and ESR 98 mm/h. A urinalysis (UA) is negative for WBC, RBC, and nitrites. Urine tox screen is negative. Synovial fluid analysis is performed in the ED, which shows 27 000 cells/μL with 71% neutrophils. Gram stain and crystal examination are both negative. Culture is pending.

What is the most likely diagnosis?

   A. Disseminated gonococcal arthritis
   B. Reactive arthritis
   C. Septic arthritis
   D. RA
   E. Gout

23. Which of the following is the most appropriate next step in the management of the patient in Question 22?

   A. Start ceftriaxone and vancomycin
   B. Start ceftriaxone and azithromycin
   C. Start IV ketorolac and transition to oral NSAIDs
   D. Start oral prednisone 40 mg daily
   E. Do nothing and wait for results of culture

24. A 24-year-old man with low back pain of insidious onset associated with morning stiffness and improvement with exercise, sacroiliitis on imaging, and positive HLA-B27 testing has been treated with weekly etanercept for 8 months. His father was diagnosed with ankylosing spondylitis at age 20 but requires no medication for management of his spine symptoms. The patient has been experiencing nonbloody diarrhea for 2 months, which he is concerned is a side effect of etanercept. He has not been taking NSAIDs, and he takes no other medications. He has no fever or abdominal pain, but he has lost a few pounds since the diarrhea started. His back pain remains well controlled on etanercept therapy. On laboratory testing, his CRP is newly elevated to 27.3 mg/L from 2.2 mg/L 6 months prior. Microbiologic analyses of a stool sample included negative *Clostridiodes difficile* toxin, negative bacterial culture, and negative stool ova and parasites. There were many fecal leukocytes present on microscopy and stool calprotectin was elevated to 2687 μg/g (normal range <50.0 μg/g).

What is the next best step in the management of his diarrhea?

A. Reduce the dose of etanercept
B. Send TB testing
C. Offer supportive treatment for an anticipated self-limited viral gastroenteritis
D. Refer to gastroenterology for suspected IBD
E. Recommend elimination of lactose from his diet

25. Which of the following would be the best next therapeutic step in the management of the patient in Question 24?

A. Restart an NSAID
B. Stop etanercept and start ustekinumab (IL-12/23 inhibitor)
C. Stop etanercept and start infliximab (TNF-α inhibitor)
D. Stop etanercept and start sulfasalazine
E. Stop etanercept and start secukinumab (IL-17A inhibitor)

26. A 23-year-old female presents to the ED with a 2-day history of left ankle and right hand pain. She reports feeling warm a few days earlier but has not checked her temperature. She denies any rashes, oral or nasal ulcers, chest pain, abdominal pain, dysuria, frequency, or eye redness, grittiness, or pain. She denies any history of trauma. She is sexually active with a single male partner. On examination, she is afebrile. Her left ankle is swollen, tender, and warm with severely limited range of motion. There is no other joint swelling or tenderness on the remainder of her examination, but passive extension of her right second finger reproduces pain along the second flexor tendon. A few pustular papules are noticed along the palms of her hands, bilaterally. A CBC is notable for mild leukocytosis, and her CMP is normal. Synovial fluid analysis shows a white cell count of 35 000 cells/μL, 84% neutrophil predominant. UA shows 20-50 WBCs.

Which of the following is the most likely diagnosis?

A. Reactive arthritis
B. Disseminated gonococcal infection
C. Syphilis
D. RA
E. Gout

27. Which of the following tests would have highest yield for diagnostic confirmation in the patient in Question 26?

A. Blood cultures
B. Serologic testing
C. Nucleic acid amplification testing
D. MRI

28. A 69-year-old male with type 2 diabetes mellitus (T2DM), RA, and crystal-proven gouty arthritis presents to the ED with a 2-day history of right knee pain. He denies any fever, chills, rashes, or other joint pain. He is historically seropositive for RF and anti-CCP antibodies. He is on methotrexate and infliximab therapy for his RA. He notes good control of his RA symptoms, which in the past have consisted of MCP and PIP joint and wrist pain. He discontinued his allopurinol some months ago, as his last gout flare (in his left first MTP joint) was 2 years ago. On examination, he is afebrile. His right knee is swollen, tender, and erythematous with significantly reduced range of motion. A CBC is notable for leukocytosis at 13 500 cells/μL. His renal function is reduced with a GFR of 35 mL/min. X-ray of his knee shows evidence of chondrocalcinosis.

Which of the following is the LEAST likely cause of his symptoms?

A. Gout
B. Pseudogout
C. Septic arthritis
D. RA

29. What is the next best step in diagnosis for the patient in Question 28?

A. Arthrocentesis with cell count, differential, crystal analysis, and Gram stain and culture
B. Blood cultures
C. X-ray of right knee
D. MRI of right knee

30. Arthrocentesis is performed in the patient in Questions 28 and 29 with complete evacuation of 40 mL of cloudy synovial fluid. Results of synovial fluid analysis show a WBC count of 49 000 cells/μL with 98% neutrophils. Crystal examination is positive for extracellular negatively birefringent, needle-shaped crystals. Gram stain is negative, and cultures are pending.

What is the next best step in the management of the patient?

A. Start oral prednisone
B. Administer intra-articular steroid injection
C. Resume allopurinol
D. Start indomethacin
E. Obtain blood cultures and start IV vancomycin/ceftriaxone

31. A 36-year-old female presents to urgent care in Massachusetts in the fall with a 3-week history of bilateral hand and wrist pain. She notes pain is worse in the morning, associated with 45 minutes of stiffness. Pain improves with activity and is associated with worsening and stiffness after rest. She has not noted any new rashes, oral or nasal ulcers, chest pain, abdominal pain, back pain, diarrhea, or dysuria. She denies any recent genitourinary or gastrointestinal infections. She is a mother of two healthy boys. The youngest, 2 years old, has been recovering from a febrile illness with upper respiratory symptoms and a malar rash after a family vacation to Florida. She denies any other known sick contacts. On examination, there is swelling and tenderness of the bilateral second through fifth MCP and PIP joints and both wrists. CBC and CMP are normal.

Which of the following tests is most likely to establish the diagnosis?

A. Lyme antibody testing with reflex western blot
B. Parvovirus B19 IgM/IgG
C. ANA and double stranded DNA (dsDNA)
D. Hepatitis B surface antibody IgG
E. Chikungunya virus polymerase chain reaction (PCR)
F. RF and anti-CCP

32. A 46-year-old female with a history of hypertension, hyperlipidemia, T2DM, and Raynaud disease presents to the ED with headache and blurred vision for the past 8 hours. On examination, she is noted to be afebrile with heart rate (HR) 100 beats/min, BP 170/95 mmHg, respiratory rate (RR) 18 breaths/min, and oxygen saturation 97% on room air. Skin examination is notable for small blanching dilated blood vessels on her hands and face, and examination of her hands reveals sclerodactyly and nailfold capillaries with dilated loops and dropout. Labs are notable for the following:

CBC: WBC 7, Hb 8.6, Plt 54
BMP: Na 144, K 4.0, Cl 108, bicarb 32, Cr 3.9, BUN 78
LFTs: total bilirubin (TBili) 4.5 (direct bilirubin [DBili] 0.4), AST 35, ALT 42, Alk Phos 86
UA: negative protein, negative blood, negative leukocyte esterase, negative nitrites

What is the next best step in management?

  A. Observation and supportive care
  B. Start IV steroids
  C. Start captopril
  D. Plasmapheresis
  E. Emergent hemodialysis

33. Which of the following autoantibodies puts the patient in Question 32 most at risk for developing this complication of her disease?

  A. ANA
  B. Anti-dsDNA
  C. Anti-histone antibody
  D. Anti-U1 ribonucleoprotein (RNP)
  E. Anti-RNA polymerase III

34. A 53-year-old male with a history of coronary artery disease, hypertension, hyperlipidemia, and gastroesophageal reflux disease presents to clinic with a chief complaint of progressive weakness over the past 5 weeks. He first noted increased fatigue when climbing the stairs to his second-floor apartment and recently developed difficulty combing his hair. On examination, the patient is noted to be afebrile with HR 63 beats/min and BP 130/72 mmHg. His examination is notable for 4/5 strength in his proximal muscles, poikiloderma of the upper chest and back, and fissured scaly plaques of the radial index fingers. The patient is given a diagnosis of new heart failure and is started on goal-directed medical therapy but unfortunately develops progressive shortness of breath over the next few months.

Which of the following antibodies is most closely associated with an increased risk of developing interstitial lung disease for patients with this condition?

  A. ANA
  B. Anti-dsDNA
  C. Anti-histone antibody
  D. Anti-topoisomerase I
  E. Anti-Jo-1
  F. Anti-RNA polymerase III

35. Given the new underlying diagnosis for the patient in Question 34, which of the following screening tests is indicated?

  A. Retinal examination
  B. Barium swallow
  C. Cardiac ultrasound
  D. Colonoscopy
  E. Bone marrow biopsy

36. A 34-year-old female with a history of obesity, hyperlipidemia, T2DM, and Raynaud disease presents to clinic with an 8-week history of arthralgias of the bilateral wrists, hands, and knees. She denies any recent fevers, chills, cough, nasal congestion, nausea, vomiting, diarrhea, or rash. The patient drinks two to three glasses of wine per night and denies smoking. Her grandmother has an unspecified history of arthritis. On examination, the patient is noted to be afebrile with a HR of 75 beats/min and BP of 107/53 mmHg. Her oxygen saturation is 98% on room air. Joint examination reveals no evidence of joint swelling or tenderness, but she is noted to have puffy fingers on examination. On further review of symptoms, the patient notes hair thinning and some difficulty putting on her shirts and jackets in the morning. Initial laboratory workup reveals the patient is ANA positive at 1:1280, SSA positive, SSB negative, Scl-70 negative, Jo-1 negative, U1 RNP positive, CCP negative, and RF positive.

What is the most likely diagnosis?

A. SLE
B. Mixed connective tissue disease (MCTD)
C. RA
D. Dermatomyositis
E. Scleroderma
F. Sjögren syndrome

37. The patient in Question 36 is most likely to develop which of the following complications of her condition?

A. Vision loss
B. Pulmonary hypertension
C. Acute renal failure
D. Lymphoma
E. Erosive arthritis

38. A 39-year-old G1P0010 woman with a history of ectopic pregnancy loss presents with complaint of vaginal dryness. Her menstrual periods remain regular, she and her partner continue to use condoms for contraception, and she has no family history of premature ovarian failure. On review of symptoms, she endorses recently having to stop wearing contacts because of dry eyes. She has had three dental fillings for caries in the past year despite never having had caries previously. She denies arthralgias, photosensitivity, rash, oral ulcers, chest pain, Raynaud disease, or muscle pain or weakness. She has no history of venous or arterial thrombus. On examination, she has reduced saliva pooling and bilateral parotid fullness.

Long term, which of the following does her underlying condition put her at highest risk of?

A. Malignancy
B. Joint destruction
C. Life-threatening infection
D. Pulmonary hypertension
E. Infertility

39. On further discussion, the patient in Question 38 reports that she and her partner are contemplating trying to conceive within the next 1 or 2 years. She asks about prenatal vitamins and pregnancy complications that increase with age.

It would additionally be important to know her antibody serologies because of risk of which of the following?

A. Bleeding
B. Fetal complete heart block
C. Neural tube defects on first-line therapy
D. Recurrent miscarriage
E. Recurrent ectopic pregnancy

40. A 65-year-old male with a history of RA, coronary artery disease, hyperlipidemia, atrial fibrillation, hepatic steatosis, CKD, and benign prostatic hypertrophy presents to clinic with 3 weeks of low-grade fever, arthralgias, rash, and right-sided chest pain on inspiration. Prior to this episode, he was in his usual state of health and had been taking all his home medications as prescribed. Review of symptoms is negative for recent sick contacts, chills, upper respiratory symptoms, nausea/vomiting, or diarrhea. Vitals show temperature 100.3°F, HR 93 beats/min, and BP 143/89 mmHg. On examination, the patient is noted to have faint erythematous macular rash overlying the sun-exposed areas of his arms with no evidence of synovitis. Notable labs include WBC 4.3, Hb 11.2, Plt 95, Cr 0.65, ANA positive at 1:640, anti-dsDNA positive, anti-Smith negative, anti-histone positive, and normal complement levels.

Which of the following medications from the patient's home medication list may be responsible for his clinical presentation?

A. Methotrexate
B. Adalimumab
C. Aspirin
D. Atorvastatin
E. Rivaroxaban

41. Which of the following is most likely to differentiate the presentation of the patient in Question 40 from a diagnosis of new-onset SLE?

A. Clinical history
B. Skin biopsy
C. ANA pattern
D. Anti-histone antibody status

42. A 32-year-old female with a history of SLE manifesting in the past with pericarditis and deep vein thrombosis for which she is now on warfarin presents with increasing fatigue, low-grade fevers, rash, and bilateral wrist pain and swelling for the past 2 weeks. The patient has been adherent to her home hydroxychloroquine regimen but continues to smoke on a regular basis. On examination, the patient is noted to be febrile to 100.8°F with HR 98 beats/min and BP 128/68 mmHg. Joint examination reveals symmetric bilateral swelling and tenderness of the wrists with associated edema, and she has been taking ibuprofen 600 mg three times daily with little effect on her symptoms. The patient is also noted to have a bright red rash overlying her nose and bilateral cheeks. Labs are notable for creatinine 0.84, UA with no proteinuria or hematuria, weakly positive dsDNA, normal C3 and C4, and elevated ESR and CRP.

What is the next best step in her management?

A. Provide reassurance
B. Renal biopsy
C. Start steroids
D. Stop hydroxychloroquine
E. Start methotrexate

43. The patient in Question 42 unfortunately goes on to develop renal involvement and is noted to have a Cr 2.8, UA with 3+ protein and 2+ blood, and a spot urine total protein to creatinine ratio of 2.7.

    Which of the following would be the most appropriate treatment for a patient newly diagnosed with lupus nephritis?
    A. IV cyclophosphamide
    B. Azathioprine
    C. Methotrexate
    D. Rituximab
    E. Belimumab
    F. Plasmapheresis

44. A 56-year-old female with a history of SLE diagnosed 20 years ago and complicated by lupus nephritis requiring hemodialysis, antiphospholipid syndrome (APLS) with recurrent deep venous thrombosis and pulmonary embolism for which she is on anticoagulation, pericarditis, lupus arthritis, and anemia presents with a chief complaint of vision changes. The patient has noted increasing difficulty reading over the past 3 to 4 weeks and worsening night vision for the past 6 months that have led her to stop driving at night. Fundus examination is notable for bilateral parafoveal retinal pigment atrophy, and further ophthalmologic testing confirms these findings consistent with "bull's eye maculopathy." The patient is on appropriate medical therapy for her conditions.

    Which of the following medications is most likely responsible for her retinopathy?
    A. Prednisone
    B. Hydroxychloroquine
    C. Azathioprine
    D. Methotrexate
    E. Warfarin

45. How could the medication-related adverse event in Question 44 have been prevented?
    A. Regular monitoring of medication levels
    B. Tight blood glucose control
    C. Combination antioxidant and zinc vitamins
    D. Yearly ophthalmologic examinations
    E. Intraocular pressure monitoring

46. A 65-year-old man with a history of hypertension, hyperlipidemia, chronic obstructive pulmonary disease, current smoking, abdominal aortic aneurysm, nephrolithiasis, and benign prostatic hypertrophy presents to clinic with 1 week of painless jaundice. The patient denies fever, chills, weight loss, or night sweats and is otherwise in his usual state of health. Vitals: temperature 97.6°F, HR 75 beats/min, BP 150/93 mmHg, RR 16 breaths/min, and SpO_2 93% on room air. Examination reveals axillary lymphadenopathy and jaundice. Labs show WBC 8, Hb 12, Plt 274, lipase 130, AST 110, ALT 85, Alk Phos 218, TBili 4.3, DBili 3.8, Cr 0.78. CT scan of the chest, abdomen, and pelvis reveals a 3-cm mass in the pancreatic head with mediastinal, hilar, axillary, and retroperitoneal lymphadenopathy. Endoscopic retrograde cholangiopancreatography (ERCP) shows dilation of the bile duct but no gallstones. Serum IgG4 is elevated.

What is the next best step in management?

A. Observation
B. Magnetic resonance cholangiopancreatography
C. Endoscopic ultrasound with biopsy
D. Referral for Whipple procedure
E. Referral for radiation therapy
F. Smoking cessation counseling

47. Further workup for the patient in Question 46 reveals findings consistent with IgG4-related disease.

What is the first step in treatment?

A. Steroids
B. Methotrexate
C. Adalimumab
D. Rituximab
E. Surgical resection
F. Radiation therapy

48. A 75-year-old male with a history of hypertension, hyperlipidemia, T2DM, coronary artery disease, congestive heart failure (CHF), obstructive sleep apnea, asthma, CKD stage 3, osteoarthritis, gastroesophageal reflux disease, and allergic rhinitis presents to the ED with a chief complaint of hemoptysis for the past 6 hours. He describes three episodes where he coughed up approximately one tablespoon of bright red blood. He also notes 2 to 3 weeks of recurrent low-grade fevers at home, 15 lb of unintentional weight loss, and difficulty writing because of new-onset weakness of his right hand and wrist. Vitals show temperature 100.7°F, HR 105 beats/min, BP 160/83 mmHg, RR 20 breaths/min, and SpO$_2$ 91%. Examination is notable for a petechial rash of both lower extremities and wrist drop on the right. Laboratory workup is shown below:

CBC: Hb 10.9, Plt 165, WBC 16.9 (Diff %: 61% neutrophils, 22% lymphocytes, 12% eosinophils, 0.2% basophils)
BMP: Na 142, K 3.8, Cr 0.9
LFT: AST 32, ALT 25, TBili 1.0, DBili 0.3, Alk Phos 91
UA: negative blood, 1+ glucose, negative leukocyte esterase, negative protein, specific gravity 1.010

Which of the following is the most likely cause of his current symptoms?

A. Polyarteritis nodosa
B. Granulomatosis with polyangiitis
C. Eosinophilic granulomatosis with polyangiitis
D. Microscopic polyangiitis
E. Cryoglobulinemic vasculitis

49. What study is most likely to yield a diagnosis for the patient in Question 48?

A. Blood smear
B. Bronchoscopy
C. Allergy testing
D. Nerve biopsy
E. Electromyography (EMG)

50. A 54-year-old homeless male who is not well known to the medical system presents to the ED with 1 week of diffuse abdominal pain and difficulty ambulating. His abdominal pain generally worsens with meals, and, although he denies nausea/vomiting, he has experienced three episodes of hematochezia in the past 24 hours. The patient also reports left ankle tingling and weakness for 2 weeks and has fallen twice after losing his balance. Review of systems is positive for subjective fever, malaise, myalgias, weight loss, and rash. Social history is notable for recent incarceration and IV drug use. Vitals: temperature 99.7°F, HR 112 beats/min, BP 170/95 mmHg, RR 16 breaths/min, SpO_2 98% on room air. Examination reveals mild-moderate diffuse abdominal pain, 3/5 strength on foot dorsiflexion, and palpable purpura over both lower extremities. Initial laboratories show WBC 15.8, Hb 7.5, Plt 115, ESR 61, CRP 15.8, Cr 2.3 (baseline 0.8), UA 1+ protein and 1+ blood without RBC casts. The patient is admitted to the hospital and undergoes renal artery angiography, which reveals multiple renal artery aneurysms with constrictions in the large vessels and occlusion of several smaller arteries.

What is the most likely diagnosis?

A. Polyarteritis nodosa
B. Granulomatosis with polyangiitis
C. Eosinophilic granulomatosis with polyangiitis
D. Microscopic polyangiitis
E. Cryoglobulinemic vasculitis

51. Which of the following infections is most closely associated with the condition that the patient in Question 50 has?

A. HIV
B. Hepatitis B
C. Hepatitis C
D. Epstein-Barr virus (EBV)
E. TB

52. A 69-year-old man with a history of chronic obstructive pulmonary disease, former tobacco use, alcohol use disorder, recurrent falls and traumatic subdural hematoma in the setting of intoxication, dementia, and leaking abdominal aortic aneurysm requiring endovascular repair presents with rash, joint pain, and abdominal pain. The patient was in his usual state of health until approximately 3 weeks prior to his presentation when he reports a sore throat, fevers, and mild neck tenderness. His symptoms resolved over the course of 3 to 4 days. Two days ago, the patient noted rash on his lower extremities and went on to develop colicky abdominal pain and joint pain affecting both ankles, knees, and hips. Vitals: Temperature 98.3°F, HR 94 beats/min, BP 115/65 mmHg, RR 14 breaths/min, SpO_2 90% on room air. Examination reveals violaceous purpura overlying the lower legs and distal thighs, swelling of the ankles and knees, and mild diffuse abdominal tenderness. Labs reveal WBC 12, Hb 13, Plt 170, and Cr 0.52, and UA is negative for both protein and blood. Skin biopsy demonstrates leukocytoclastic vasculitis with IgA deposition.

What is the most likely diagnosis?

A. Cryoglobulinemic vasculitis
B. Microscopic polyangiitis
C. IgA vasculitis
D. Granulomatosis with polyangiitis
E. Anti–glomerular basement membrane disease

53. What is the next best step in the management of the patient in Question 52?

A. Observation
B. Abdominal CT angiogram
C. Renal artery ultrasound
D. Colchicine
E. Steroids

54. A 65-year-old man with a history of T2DM, hypertension, stable thoracic aortic aneurysm, and chronic obstructive pulmonary disease presents to clinic endorsing worsening shoulder stiffness over the past 4 days. He reports that he awakens with pain and stiffness in his bilateral shoulders and hips that lasts for over an hour each morning but gets better as the day goes on. However, if he sits down for more than a few minutes, the stiffness returns. He denies fevers, headache, vision changes, scalp tenderness, or difficulty chewing. On examination, he exhibits restricted active abduction of his bilateral shoulders but full strength in his upper and lower extremities. ESR and CRP are elevated and creatine phosphokinase (CPK) is normal.

Treatment should begin with which of the following?

A. Rituximab (anti-CD20)
B. TNF-α inhibitor
C. Methotrexate
D. Physical therapy
E. Steroids

55. The symptoms of the patient in Question 54 markedly improved on therapy. Shortly after beginning to taper the regimen several weeks later, he develops a fever, headache, and transient vision changes.

This development is most concerning for which of the following?

A. Immunosuppression-related infection
B. Thrombosis secondary to hypercoagulability
C. Development of a large-vessel vasculitis
D. Recurrence of his original pathology
E. An occult malignancy

56. The next step for the patient in Questions 54 and 55 should be which of the following?

A. Increase his immunosuppression dose
B. Decrease his immunosuppression dose
C. Obtain blood cultures
D. Obtain a biopsy
E. Obtain imaging

57. A 45-year-old man with a history of alcoholic cirrhosis, alcohol withdrawal complicated by seizures, IV drug use, untreated hepatitis C, methicillin-resistant *Staphylococcus aureus* (MRSA), tricuspid valve endocarditis, and lumbar osteomyelitis presents to the ED with a chief complaint of new-onset rash involving both lower extremities for the past 2 days. The patient first began feeling unwell approximately 1 week ago when he developed generalized malaise, fatigue, arthralgias, and paresthesia with mild weakness in both lower legs. The patient was recently released from prison and has not been followed by a regular medical provider for several years. Vitals: temperature 99.3°F, HR 97 beats/min, BP 93/64 mmHg, RR 16 breaths/min, SpO$_2$ 95% on room air. Examination is notable for violaceous palpable purpura involving lower extremities, 2/6 systolic murmur best heard at the lower sternal border, nodular liver, splenomegaly, 4/5 strength to dorsiflexion and plantarflexion of both feet, and decreased sensation to light touch over the lower legs to mid-shin. Labs reveal WBC 11, Hb 8.5, Plt 69, AST 60, ALT 45, Alk Phos 115, TBili 1.5, DBili 0.8, Cr 0.75, UA 2+ protein, negative ANA, and positive RF.

All of the following would be reasonable next steps EXCEPT which?

A. Blood cultures
B. Echocardiogram
C. Complement levels
D. Cryoglobulin testing
E. Kidney biopsy

58. The patient in Question 57 is started on empiric broad-spectrum antibiotics without improvement. Three days later, multiple sets of blood cultures remain without growth. Transthoracic and transesophageal echocardiograms have revealed moderate tricuspid regurgitation but no other remarkable findings. Additional workup sent on admission has resulted showing normal C3, low C4, and positive cryoglobulins.

What is the patient's main risk factor for developing this condition?

A. Cirrhosis
B. Hepatitis C
C. Alcohol use disorder
D. IV drug use
E. History of endocarditis

59. A 21-year-old woman presents to clinic for a new patient visit. On review of her past medical history, she reports that, as a young child, beginning shortly after her family immigrated from Armenia, she experienced multiple episodes of fever with severe abdominal pain prompting multiple exploratory laparotomies without identification of the cause of her symptoms. However, she reports it has been over 2 years since the last such episode, and her main current concern today is pain in her calf muscles when she attempts to exercise. She is currently on no medications other than an oral contraceptive pill.

Without additional medical therapy, she is at risk of all of the following EXCEPT which?

A. Systemic infection
B. Recurrent episodes of fever
C. Infertility
D. Recurrent episodes of abdominal pain
E. Renal failure

60. With which medication should the patient in Question 59 be treated?

A. Aspirin
B. Colchicine
C. Prednisone
D. Antibiotics
E. Anti-TNF-α inhibitor

61. A 65-year-old woman with a history of carpal tunnel syndrome, stress urinary incontinence, and anxiety presents to clinic as a triage visit with a chief complaint of bilateral lower extremity pain for the past 6 weeks. She describes the pain as a "tingling, electricity-like sensation" affecting both feet and both ankles. The pain is always present, but she reports she notices it most frequently at night. The patient is followed regularly by her primary care doctor, and she had not had any recent medical issues until she developed right-sided carpal tunnel syndrome approximately 6 months ago. Since that time, the patient describes various complaints, including worsening bilateral shoulder pain for the past 3 months, easy bruising, and 10 lb weight gain. Vitals: temperature 98.5°F, HR 65 beats/min, BP 120/70 mmHg, RR 14 breaths/min, SpO_2 98% on room air. Examination is notable for hepatosplenomegaly, fullness of the anterior shoulder bilaterally, positive Phalen and Tinel sign of the right wrist, decreased sensation to light touch of the feet and ankles, 2+ pitting lower extremity edema to the knees, and periorbital bruising with additional scattered bruising over both upper and both lower extremities. Labs reveal WBC 8, Hb 12, Plt 95, Cr 1.6, and UA 3+ protein.

What is the next best step in her management?

A. EMG
B. SPEP and urine protein electrophoresis (UPEP) with immunofixation
C. Hepatitis B testing
D. Liver biopsy
E. Venous ultrasound of the lower extremities
F. Coronary angiogram

62. After pursuing the testing indicated for the patient in Question 61, the decision is made to perform a fat pad biopsy.

Pathologic evaluation of the tissue is most likely to show what?

A. Interface dermatitis
B. Focal lymphocytic sialadenitis
C. Dense lymphoplasmacytic infiltrate with "storiform fibrosis"
D. Positive Congo red staining with "apple green" birefringence
E. Excessive organized collagen deposition with expansion of the dermis

ANSWERS

1. **The correct answer is: A. De Quervain tenosynovitis.** The clinical history of atraumatic radial wrist pain and examination findings of fullness and tenderness over the dorsal radial wrist and a positive Finkelstein maneuver are suggestive of De Quervain tendinopathy. The etiology is not completely understood, but observational data suggest repetitive activities maintaining the thumb in extension and abduction predispose to this condition. The tendinopathy affects the abductor pollicis longus and the extensor pollicis brevis as they pass through the first dorsal compartment from the forearm into the hand. Treatment is conservative with application of ice to area, immobilization with a forearm-based thumb spica splint, and NSAIDs. Glucocorticoid injection may be considered in patients who do not respond to these measures, whereas surgery may be offered in resistant cases.

2. **The correct answer is: B. Rheumatoid arthritis (RA).** The patient's presentation is notable for a chronic, symmetric, small-joint predominant inflammatory arthritis consistent with RA. Parvovirus arthritis may have a similar presentation, but the duration of symptoms is longer than would be expected for parvovirus infection. Gout typically presents with an acute inflammatory arthritis, which may be polyarticular, but a chronic small-joint polyarthritis is a much less likely presentation for gout. Ankylosing spondylitis can be associated with an inflammatory arthritis that is typically oligoarticular, asymmetric, and large-joint predominant. A polyarticular small-joint arthritis without inflammatory-type low back pain does not suggest ankylosing spondylitis.

3. **The correct answer is: A. Rheumatoid factor (RF) and anti–cyclic citrullinated peptide (CCP) antibodies.** The next best step in the evaluation of suspected RA is to check serologic tests for RF and anti-CCP antibodies.

4. **The correct answer is: A. Stop sulfasalazine and start prednisone 0.5 mg/kg.** The constellation of fever, maculopapular rash, arthralgias, myalgias, and transaminitis occurring 2 to 3 weeks after initiation of sulfasalazine should raise concern for an allergic hypersensitivity syndrome related to sulfasalazine, and the medication should be discontinued immediately. Systemic steroids may be used to control the acute inflammatory state and to allow for resolution of hypersensitivity symptoms. Although symptoms and findings are nonspecific and may suggest a viral exanthem, empirically treating for a viral etiology without discontinuing sulfasalazine is not the correct answer, particularly given the severe and potentially fatal consequences of sulfasalazine allergy. The patient's symptoms are unlikely to be caused by hydroxychloroquine, nor can they be explained by a flare of his underlying RA, which would not be expected to cause fever, rash, myalgias, and transaminitis.

5. **The correct answer is: C. Biologic disease-modifying antirheumatic drug (DMARD).** DMARD options in RA include conventional DMARDs (including sulfasalazine, hydroxychloroquine, methotrexate, leflunomide), targeted synthetic DMARDs (JAK/STAT inhibitors), and biologic DMARDs (such as anti-TNF-α, anti-IL-6). Given her intolerance of methotrexate and persistent disease activity, she requires adjustment of therapy. Her history of a severe reaction to a sulfa-containing medication precludes the use of sulfasalazine, and her desire to have children would make the use of leflunomide undesirable given its teratogenicity. Of the choices provided, the next best step would be to initiate a biologic therapy.

6. **The correct answer is: A. Anakinra (interleukin [IL]-1 receptor antagonist).** Anakinra is least likely to achieve symptom control in this patient with RA. Anakinra is a recombinant human IL-1 receptor antagonist that is effective in the treatment of autoinflammatory conditions that involve, in part, the overproduction of IL-1 through dysregulated or aberrant activation of the inflammasome, a multimeric platform that converts pro-IL-1 to IL-1. Although anakinra is available for the treatment of RA, it is significantly less effective for RA as compared to other biologic agents including anti-TNF-α therapies.

7. **The correct answer is: A. Start prednisone 0.5 mg/kg.** The constellation of daily fevers, night sweats, unintentional weight loss, and lymphadenopathy in an otherwise healthy adult should prompt a broad evaluation for infectious, malignant, and inflammatory noninfectious etiologies. Adult-onset Still disease (AOSD), an inflammatory disease of unknown etiology, may account for many of the features, including the rash concurrent with fevers, polyarthralgias, and transaminitis. However, this diagnosis requires exclusion of malignant, infectious, and other inflammatory conditions. Appropriate next steps in the evaluation include additional imaging of chest, abdomen, and pelvis to evaluate for localizing pathology. An excisional biopsy of a cervical or other accessible lymph node to evaluate for lymphoma, other malignancy, and atypical infectious etiologies would be appropriate. Judicious use of NSAIDs may be pursued for symptomatic control while additional evaluation is pursued. Empiric treatment for AOSD with steroids would not be appropriate at this stage given the potential for steroids to obscure underlying pathology.

8. **The correct answer is: A. Relapsing polychondritis.** Relapsing polychondritis arises from autoimmune destruction of cartilage. It most commonly presents with painful ear inflammation (frequently bilateral) that spares the cartilage-free lobe. Involvement of other cartilaginous structures can result in saddle nose deformity, chondromalacia or stricture of large airways, joint pain, costochondritis, and cardiac valvulopathies. Eye inflammation, in particular episcleritis, is also common. Some develop vertigo symptoms thought possibly to be caused by either inner ear/eustachian tube inflammation or vasculitis affecting cranial nerve VIII. Ear involvement, especially unilateral involvement, often is mistaken for infection of the ear (infectious perichondritis), but biopsies with cultures fail to reveal an organism and the symptoms remain unresponsive to antibiotics.

9. **The correct answer is: C. Corticosteroids.** Steroids are first-line treatment for relapsing polychondritis, and some patients experience partial relief with NSAIDs. Methotrexate could be considered later for steroid-sparing effect if unable to adequately taper steroids. Cyclophosphamide (CYC) would be the treatment of choice for severe life-threatening organ involvement, such as severe laryngotracheal involvement.

10. **The correct answer is: D. Evaluation of the larynx and large airways with CT.** All new diagnoses should be accompanied by evaluation of the larynx and major airways via ear, nose, and throat (ENT) referral, CT, or bronchoscopy. Up to 40% of relapsing polychondritis cases are associated with another systemic disease (vasculitis, connective tissue disease, myelodysplastic syndrome, or VEXAS), so further workup should be pursued if the history, review of symptoms, or examination is suggestive; however, in this case, Scl-70 antibody testing in the absence of symptoms suggestive of scleroderma would be premature. Type 1 cryoglobulinemia can cause acrocyanosis or purpura of acral sites, including ears, but there would be an association of symptoms with cold exposure, and involvement of portions of distal extremities (such as the toes) would be expected. Tophi can be deposited in the ears in gout but are typically not painful and would be unexpected in an individual without a history of gouty arthritis.

11. **The correct answer is: A. Acute gouty arthritis.** The recurrent acute intermittent inflammatory asymmetric oligoarthritis that resolves completely with anti-inflammatory therapy, as well as evidence of firm nodules in the olecranon bursa, is suggestive of crystal-induced arthritis, specifically tophaceous gout. The intermittent resolving nature of these episodes and the absence of extra-articular or axial features argue against peripheral arthritis associated with seronegative spondyloarthropathies.

12. **The correct answer is: A. Arthrocentesis with cell count, differential, Gram stain, culture, and crystal examination.** Confirmation of the diagnosis with crystal examination of a synovial fluid sample would be the most appropriate next step. Septic arthritis is less likely given normothermia, polyarticular involvement, relapsing course, and resolution of past episodes without antimicrobial treatment, but it is prudent to send Gram stain and culture from synovial fluid to further exonerate infection. If arthrocentesis is not possible, or crystal examination is negative, evaluation for the presence of monosodium urate crystal deposition with imaging may be pursued, but this would not be the first step in evaluation. As the symptoms are not consistent with a seronegative spondyloarthropathy, SI joint films or HLA-B27 testing is not necessary.

13. **The correct answer is: E. Start anakinra 100 mg subcutaneous daily.** The patient has developed an acute inflammatory polyarthritis in the setting of multiple comorbidities including CKD, T1DM, and ischemic cardiomyopathy. The differential diagnosis for an acute polyarthritis includes crystalline arthritis, viral arthritis, immune complex arthritis, or acute presentation of a chronic inflammatory arthritis. The patient has multiple risk factors for hyperuricemia, and the clinical finding of bilateral tophi suggests a considerable burden of chronic hyperuricemia. Diuresis with loop diuretics is a risk factor for fluctuation in serum uric acid levels that can precipitate an acute gouty arthritis. A uric acid level within normal range does not exclude an acute gouty arthritis because of the uricosuric effect of inflammatory cytokines. Septic arthritis is less likely given the polyarticular involvement and absence of fever. For these reasons, the most likely diagnosis is acute polyarticular gouty arthritis.

    Treatment of gout involves (1) the acute management of gouty arthritis and (2) determination of whether the patient will benefit from urate-lowering therapy. Options for the acute management of gout include NSAIDs, intra-articular steroids, colchicine, systemic steroids, or anti-IL-1 therapy, and the choice is often determined by severity of symptoms, number of involved joints, and presence of comorbidities that may preclude the safe use of certain therapies. NSAIDs are contraindicated because of CKD and peptic ulcer disease, intra-articular or systemic steroids will cause acute blood sugar elevations with his T1DM, and colchicine is relatively contraindicated because of severe renal insufficiency. Anakinra, an IL-1 receptor antagonist, has been demonstrated to be efficacious for the treatment of severe gouty arthritis flares, and its use is not precluded by the patient's comorbidities. The number of involved joints—particularly the number of small joints involved—makes intra-articular steroid injections not practical. If anakinra's cost is prohibitive or it is otherwise unavailable, oral steroids can be given with close attention to subsequently increased insulin needs. ACTH could be considered as an alternative to exogenous steroids to minimize the impact on glucose homeostasis, with the downsides of increased cost and more limited clinical familiarity compared to steroids.

14. **The correct answer is: D. Continue amlodipine and start losartan.** Multiple risk factors including hypertension, hyperlipidemia, T2DM, obesity, and CHF have been identified for hyperuricemia and gout. The presence of hyperuricemia has also been linked to adverse cardiovascular outcomes. Thus modification of risk factors for hyperuricemia and

gout, including appropriate control of hypertension, is necessary to reduce cardiovascular risk. Losartan is the only angiotensin II receptor blocker (ARB) that has been shown to have uricosuric effects and reduce uric acid levels. This effect is hypothesized to be related to the inhibition of URAT1 transporters in the kidney that are involved in reabsorption of filtered uric acid. Hydrochlorothiazide would increase serum uric acid levels through promoting net uric acid reabsorption. Angiotensin-converting enzyme (ACE) inhibitors, including lisinopril, have not been shown to reduce uric acid levels.

15. **The correct answer is: E. An acute presentation of RA.** The differential diagnosis for an acute monoarthritis is limited and includes crystal-induced inflammatory arthritis, including gout and pseudogout, bacterial septic arthritis, and an acute monoarticular presentation of a chronic inflammatory arthritis. However, an acute presentation of RA is the least likely diagnosis.

16. **The correct answer is: A. Arthrocentesis with cell counts, crystal examination, Gram stain, and culture.** Arthrocentesis MUST be performed to exclude an infectious etiology; clinical features alone, including absence of fever, examination findings (degree of pain, swelling, loss of range of motion), and absence of leukocytosis are not sensitive enough to exclude an infectious process, particularly in elderly patients with immunosuppressive comorbidities.

17. **The correct answer is: B. Pseudogout.** The presence of crystals on arthrocentesis does not exclude the possibility of infection. The synovial fluid cell count of 35 000 cell/μL is reassuring but neither does it rule out a septic process. Likewise, Gram stain is only 30% to 50% sensitive for the detection of septic arthritis. However, synovial fluid cultures have sensitivity greater than 75% to 90% in nongonococcal septic arthritis. Taken together, calcium pyrophosphate deposition (CPPD) crystal-induced arthritis (pseudogout) is the most likely diagnosis given the absent evidence of infection from synovial fluid analysis and culture and the multiple findings and risk factors associated with CPPD: chondrocalcinosis on x-ray; knee osteoarthritis (as evidenced by x-ray with joint space narrowing; CPPD is frequently superimposed on osteoarthritis); age (CPPD increases with age); and a first presentation with knee involvement (which is common in CPPD but relatively uncommon in gout). Crystal examination showing weakly positively birefringent rhomboid-shaped crystals establishes the diagnosis.

18. **The correct answer is: B. Intra-articular steroid injection with 80 mg methylprednisolone.** The patient's advanced CKD would preclude the safe use of NSAIDs. Colchicine may be used if adjusted for renal function but is less likely to be effective given the duration of the patient's symptoms. Colchicine may be started while waiting for results of synovial fluid analysis to rule out a septic etiology. In this case, based on results of cell counts, Gram stain, and culture, an infectious etiology is unlikely, and an intra-articular steroid injection is likely to provide the most rapid and complete resolution of joint inflammation.

19. **The correct answer is: B. Ankylosing spondylitis.** This 28-year-old patient is presenting with low back pain with insidious progression, prolonged morning stiffness improved with activity, and a good response to NSAID therapy, which are suggestive of inflammatory-type low back pain. The differential for this includes the axial spondyloarthritides including ankylosing spondylitis, reactive arthritis, IBD-associated spondyloarthritis, psoriatic arthritis, non-radiographic axial spondyloarthritis, and undifferentiated spondyloarthritis. In this patient, there are no historical or examination findings to suggest the presence of underlying IBD or psoriasis, or preceding infectious etiologies to suggest another type of spondyloarthritis. Inflammatory involvement of the lower axial skeleton is not typically associated with RA.

20. **The correct answer is: A. SI joint radiographs.** The next best step in the evaluation is a plain radiograph of the SI joints to evaluate for radiographic involvement of the SI joints. SI joint abnormalities are typically graded from 0 to 4 based on severity, with grade 4 defined as total ankylosis, and the grade indicating the degree of confidence that the changes seen reflect sacroiliitis. MRI of the SI joints may be considered if radiographs do not suggest sacroiliitis or when findings are uncertain. Lumbar spine radiographs are also helpful, as they may reveal erosions and reactive sclerosis of the corners of vertebral bodies ("shiny corners"), squaring of vertebral bodies, and syndesmophytes (ossification of the annulus fibrosus or spinal ligaments of the spine). Syndesmophytes in ankylosing spondylitis are classically at the margins of vertebral bodies and symmetric. In more advanced cases, syndesmophytes can bridge vertebral bodies (ankylosis) and give the appearance of a rigid fused "bamboo" spine.

21. **The correct answer is: A. Interferon-γ release assay.** Anti-TNF-α therapy is associated with a high risk of *Mycobacterium tuberculosis* reactivation in patients with a history of latent TB. Therefore, excluding latent TB infection PRIOR to anti-TNF-α initiation is critical, especially if the patient is from an area TB is endemic and would therefore be at high risk for TB infection. Several tests are available to assess for immunologic response to TB that indicates exposure to TB in the past. These tests include the tuberculin skin test, which involves the intradermal injection of purified protein derivative which stimulates a delayed-type hypersensitivity response mediated by T-lymphocytes at the injection site within 48 to 72 hours. Other tests include the interferon-γ release assays, which measure T-cell release of interferon-γ following stimulation by antigens from TB. Both assays can produce false-positive and false-negative results. The other tests are not required prior to initiation of anti-TNF-α therapy but may be checked depending on additional risk factors or age-appropriate screening.

22. **The correct answer is: B. Reactive arthritis.** The clinical picture of an acute oligoarticular inflammatory arthritis with asymmetric large-joint involvement and inflammatory-type low back pain in the setting of recent suspected genitourinary infection and symptoms compatible with conjunctivitis and circinate balanitis is consistent with a diagnosis of reactive arthritis. Although septic arthritis is a possibility given the acuity of the presentation and because a synovial fluid cell count of 27 000 cells/μL does not exclude a septic process, the clinical picture of oligoarticular involvement, extra-articular features (conjunctivitis, balanitis), and a negative Gram stain reduces the pretest probability that this is a bacterial septic process. Disseminated gonococcal infection must always be considered in any sexually active individual. Disseminated gonococcal infection can present as either a triad of tenosynovitis, dermatitis (painless pustular rash), and non-purulent polyarthralgias (typically migratory and asymmetric) ("arthritis-dermatitis syndrome") or as a purulent arthritis. The absence of evidence of tenosynovitis or pustular rash; the clinical picture of balanitis, conjunctivitis, and inflammatory low back pain; and recent history of appropriate treatment for suspected gonococcal urethritis with intramuscular ceftriaxone make a diagnosis of disseminated gonococcal infection unlikely.

23. **The correct answer is: C. Start IV ketorolac and transition to oral NSAIDs.** NSAIDs are considered first-line treatment for reactive arthritis. Most cases tend to resolve within 1 year of diagnosis. Conventional DMARDs or biologic DMARDs may be added depending on clinical response. Prednisone may be considered in patients who have an inadequate response to NSAIDs, though clinical response to steroids is usual suboptimal.

24. **The correct answer is: D. Refer to gastroenterology for suspected IBD.** This patient with inflammatory back pain, sacroiliitis on imaging, HLA-B27 positivity, a family history of ankylosing spondylitis, and a good response to a TNF-α inhibitor was previously

diagnosed with ankylosing spondylitis. However, the development of inflammatory diarrhea, as evidenced by chronic diarrhea, fecal leukocytes but negative infectious workup, and positive stool calprotectin, is worrisome for the development of IBD, and therefore suggests this patient has a different type of spondyloarthritis, namely, IBD-associated arthritis (also called enteropathic arthritis). Patients with spondyloarthritis who develop signs of IBD, such as diarrhea, abdominal pain, unexplained anemia, and/or weight loss, should be referred to a gastroenterologist for workup of possible IBD.

25. **The correct answer is: C. Stop etanercept and start infliximab (TNF-α inhibitor).** Although effective for ankylosing spondylitis, etanercept is not effective for the gastrointestinal manifestations of IBD. Other TNF-α inhibitors are effective for both axial spondyloarthritis and IBD. Therefore, this patient should be switched to another TNF-α inhibitor such as infliximab, adalimumab, or certolizumab. Although sulfasalazine is an appropriate choice for the treatment of IBD and NSAID-resistant IBD-associated peripheral arthritis, sulfasalazine is ineffective for axial inflammation. IL-12/23 inhibitors (eg, ustekinumab), although effective for IBD, have been shown to be ineffective for axial spondyloarthritis, so likewise would not be the best choice for monotherapy for this patient with sacroiliitis. Despite efficacy of secukinumab, an anti-IL-17A antibody, in spondyloarthritis, it has been shown to be ineffective for IBD. TNF-α inhibitors increase the risk of reactivation of TB, and patients should be screened for latent TB prior to initiation; but, in the absence of risk factors for TB acquisition, his current symptoms are more likely attributable to development of IBD because of underlying IBD-associated spondyloarthritis than to intestinal reactivation of TB or to primary extrapulmonary TB infection.

26. **The correct answer is: B. Disseminated gonococcal infection.** The clinical picture is suggestive of an acute inflammatory monoarthritis of the left ankle and tenosynovitis of the second flexor tendon. Other notable findings include a pustular eruption on the palms, leukocytosis, and pyuria. In a sexually active person, this constellation is highly concerning for disseminated gonococcal infection. Reactive arthritis can present with an acute monoarthritis but would not account for her pustular rash.

27. **The correct answer is: C. Nucleic acid amplification testing.** Nucleic acid amplification testing on bodily fluid from multiple sources including oropharynx, rectum, urethra, and synovial fluid has the highest diagnostic yield. Serologic testing does not have a role in the diagnosis, and MRI does not show specific findings for disseminated gonococcal infection. Blood cultures should be obtained, but culture has a lower diagnostic yield than nucleic acid amplification testing.

28. **The correct answer is: D. RA.** The differential diagnosis of an acute monoarthritis is rather limited and includes crystal-associated inflammatory arthritis (gout and pseudogout), bacterial infectious arthritis, and an acute presentation of a chronic inflammatory arthritis (eg, RA pseudosepsis). Risk factors for septic arthritis in this patient include immunosuppressed status (diabetes, immunosuppressive medications, age). Risk factors for gouty arthritis include prior history of crystal-proven gout, cessation of urate-lowering therapy, and renal dysfunction. The presence of chondrocalcinosis on x-ray suggests CPPD. Although a flare of his RA is possible, he notes good symptom control on his current regimen of methotrexate and infliximab, and an acute monoarthritis should therefore raise suspicion for an alternative process.

29. **The correct answer is: A. Arthrocentesis with cell count, differential, crystal analysis, and Gram stain and culture.** The next best step would be an arthrocentesis with cell counts/differential, crystal analysis, Gram stain, and culture.

30. **The correct answer is: E. Obtain blood cultures and start IV vancomycin/ceftriaxone.** Septic arthritis caused by most bacterial organisms is typically associated with high synovial fluid WBC counts, often >50 000 cells/μL. Lower cell counts may be observed, particularly in immunosuppressed patients, and thus the results of the fluid analyses must be interpreted in the clinical context. In this patient, the pretest probability for septic arthritis is high, so a cell count of 49 000 cells/μL does NOT rule out a septic process. Furthermore, a neutrophil percentage >90% is concerning for a septic process. Gram stain has a sensitivity of only 30% to 50%. The presence of crystals in the fluid DOES NOT rule out the presence of a concomitant septic process. Additionally, extracellular urate crystals are less specific for a flare than intracellular crystals. Given the overall high pretest probability of a septic bacterial arthritis, and the results of the synovial fluid analysis, the most appropriate next step would be to start empiric antibiotics after obtaining blood cultures. If a septic process is excluded based on cultures, then antibiotics can be discontinued, and the patient can be treated for a flare of gouty arthritis.

31. **The correct answer is: B. Parvovirus B19 immunoglobulin (Ig)M/IgG.** The patient is presenting with an acute symmetric small-joint predominant polyarthritis occurring in the absence of extra-articular features, known comorbidities, or antecedent infections. The differential diagnosis for such a presentation includes acute viral arthritides, such as those caused by parvovirus, acute hepatitis B or C, cytomegalovirus, EBV, or chikungunya. An acute presentation of a chronic process such as RA, a peripheral spondyloarthritis, or an immunologic connective tissue disease with arthritis is possible. Of these, a viral arthritis is favored given acuity, absence of extra-articular features, and history of likely viral infection in her son.

The son's exanthema presenting as a febrile illness with malar rash is consistent with acute parvovirus B19 infection, also known as fifth disease. In adults, acute parvovirus infection is often associated with an acute polyarthritis that may mimic RA in the pattern of joint involvement. Serologic testing with IgM and IgG is likely to lead to correct diagnosis; presence of positive IgM antibodies is suggestive of an acute infection. The pattern of joint symptoms in this patient is not consistent with a presentation of Lyme arthritis, which more typically involves a large-joint monoarthritis (most commonly of the knee) or large-joint asymmetric oligoarthritis. Hepatitis B surface antibody IgG would document presence of protective immunity and not acute infection. Although chikungunya virus arthritis can present with this clinical picture, pain is often more severe and virtually all chikungunya infections are acquired outside of the United States.

32. **The correct answer is: C. Start captopril.** This patient with a history of Raynaud disease presents with hypertension and is found to have an acute kidney injury with evidence of thrombotic microangiopathy (TMA) on laboratory testing with anemia, thrombocytopenia, and an elevated indirect bilirubin. Her presentation is most consistent with scleroderma renal crisis (SRC). SRC occurs in 10% to 15% of patients with systemic sclerosis and is more frequent in diffuse cutaneous systemic sclerosis compared to limited cutaneous systemic sclerosis. It often occurs early in the disease and generally occurs within a median duration of 7.5 months from the first non-Raynaud clinical manifestation of the disease. In this case, the patient's sclerodactyly, telangiectasias, and dilated capillary loops with dropout on examination suggest the diagnosis of scleroderma. UA is usually normal in SRC but may show proteinuria if severe hypertension is present. SRC is a TMA, and it is important to consider other causes of TMA such as thrombotic thrombocytopenic purpura (TTP, because of hereditary or acquired deficiency of ADAMTS13, which manifests as fever and mild acute kidney injury with or without neurologic symptoms), hemolytic uremic

syndrome (which is most commonly associated with hereditary complement or coagulation abnormalities or exposure to certain infectious agents, chiefly Shiga toxin–producing *Escherichia coli* in the form of a severe gastrointestinal infection with abdominal pain, nausea, vomiting, and diarrhea a few days prior to onset of the TMA), and drug-induced TMA (associated with exposure to quinine, or less likely gemcitabine or oxaliplatin).

SRC is a rheumatologic emergency and should be treated without delay, most commonly in an intensive care unit. An ACE inhibitor, such as captopril, is the mainstay of therapy for SRC. Steroids (>20 mg prednisone per day equivalents) are thought to provoke SRC and should be avoided in patients with scleroderma. Patients with SRC often require hemodialysis, but our patient has no current indication for emergent hemodialysis. Plasmapheresis is used to treat immune-mediated TTP, which could present similarly.

33. **The correct answer is: E. Anti-RNA polymerase III.** Scleroderma patients with antibodies against RNA polymerase III are at increased risk of developing SRC by comparison to patients with either anti-Scl-70 or anti-centromere antibodies. ANA is often positive in scleroderma, but a positive ANA does not increase the risk of SRC. Anti-dsDNA antibodies are associated with lupus, anti-histone antibodies are found in patients with drug-induced lupus and systemic lupus erythematosus (SLE), anti-Jo-1 antibodies can be seen in dermatomyositis, and anti-U1 RNP antibodies are seen in MCTD and some patients with lupus.

34. **The correct answer is: E. Anti-Jo-1.** The patient presents with progressive weakness and is found to have a history and physical examination that are consistent with proximal muscle weakness. This, combined with the patient's skin findings, is highly characteristic of dermatomyositis. Proximal muscle weakness is the most common presentation of dermatomyositis or polymyositis (PM). Patients often have difficulty performing tasks with their arms above their heads (eg, combing their hair, putting on shirts or jackets, etc), and proximal leg weakness may manifest as difficulty standing from a chair or climbing up stairs. Skin findings commonly seen in dermatomyositis include small purple or red papules on the extensor surfaces of the joints of the hand and elbows (Gottron papules), a violaceous rash affecting the upper eyelids (heliotrope sign), and poikiloderma of the neck (V-sign), back (shawl sign), and hips (holster sign).

A subset of patients may also have fissured scaly plaques on the radial surfaces of the fingers and palms with hyperpigmentation of the palmar creases known as mechanic's hands. Mechanic's hands are commonly seen in an aggressive form of dermatomyositis or polymyositis known as anti-synthetase syndrome (which is characterized by myositis, interstitial lung disease, arthritis, Raynaud disease, and/or fever). Patients with anti-synthetase syndrome may develop rapid onset interstitial lung disease and present with shortness of breath as their initial symptom in the absence of prominent muscle weakness or rash. Anti-Jo-1 is the most common antibody associated with anti-synthetase syndrome, and it is often ordered after a diagnosis of dermatomyositis or polymyositis is made to assess the risk of developing rapidly progressive lung disease.

ANAs are nonspecific and can be seen in a variety of different connective tissue diseases. Anti-dsDNA is associated with lupus, and anti-histone antibodies are seen in drug-induced as well as idiopathic lupus. Anti-topoisomerase I antibodies are also known as anti-Scl-70 antibodies and are seen in certain types of scleroderma. Anti-RNA polymerase III antibodies are also associated with scleroderma and their presence is associated with an increased risk of developing SRC.

35. **The correct answer is: D. Colonoscopy.** Because of its strong association with malignancy, all patients with a new diagnosis of dermatomyositis should undergo thorough cancer screening. This includes low-dose chest CT (as indicated for lung cancer screening),

mammogram, Papanicolaou smear, and colonoscopy. Many rheumatology providers will also obtain a transvaginal ultrasound to screen for ovarian cancer.

36. **The correct answer is: B. Mixed connective tissue disease (MCTD).** MCTD is a unique condition that represents an overlap of lupus, systemic sclerosis, and polymyositis. Patients often present with vague symptoms, including fatigue, arthralgias, myalgias, Raynaud disease, hand edema, puffy fingers, synovitis, and low-grade myositis with muscle weakness. Patients rarely present with clear overlap from multiple diseases initially but often develop these features over several years. A diagnosis of MCTD requires positive anti-U1 RNP antibodies by definition. MCTD falls into the connective tissue disease family and patients generally have a positive ANA and may have SSA or SSB positivity as well. RF is a nonspecific marker and may be seen in up to 50% of patients with MCTD.

37. **The correct answer is: B. Pulmonary hypertension.** Pulmonary hypertension is the major cause of death in these patients.

38. **The correct answer is: A. Malignancy.** The patient presents with sicca symptoms including xerophthalmia (dry eyes), xerostomia (dry mouth), and vaginal dryness. Her increased number of dental caries is due to salivary gland inflammation (parotid fullness) and destruction. Her review of symptoms suggests she has primary Sjögren syndrome rather than Sjögren syndrome associated with a second rheumatologic condition. ANA is positive in the majority but can be negative. Anti-Ro and anti-La antibodies have greater specificity for Sjögren syndrome but will be negative in about a third of patients. Workup would be anticipated to show reduced tear production on Schirmer test and lymphocytic infiltration on salivary gland biopsy. Primary Sjögren syndrome carries a greatly elevated risk of B-cell lymphoma (~5-44 times that of the general population). Sjögren's can predispose to suppurative parotitis and oral candidiasis but these are typically readily manageable with appropriate antimicrobials.

39. **The correct answer is: B. Fetal complete heart block.** Knowing her serologies would be important when planning a pregnancy, as passive transfer of anti-Ro (and less so anti-La) antibodies is associated with fetal heart block, requiring fetal monitoring for development of bradycardia. APLS is an important consideration in pregnancy planning given its association with recurrent miscarriage as well as premature birth, low weight for gestational age, thrombosis, and pre-eclampsia. Additionally, those with APLS on warfarin need to switch to heparin and aspirin during pregnancy. However, this patient does not have a history of clotting or recurrent miscarriage suggestive of APLS. Many rheumatologic medications are teratogenic, including methotrexate, mycophenolate mofetil, and cyclophosphamide. However, first-line treatment for this patient's primary Sjögren syndrome without extraglandular manifestations would not involve these agents. Initial treatment would generally involve artificial tears or eye drops that are not absorbed systemically (eg, cyclosporine) and topical saliva stimulants and substitutes, which do not pose a risk of harm to a fetus. Muscarinic agonists, sometimes prescribed to relieve dry mouth when these regimens fail, have unclear safety in pregnancy but do not cause neural tube defects.

40. **The correct answer is: B. Adalimumab.** The patient presents with fevers, arthralgia, rash, and chest pain upon inspiration, consistent with pleuritis. Laboratory testing is notable for a positive ANA with negative anti-dsDNA and anti-Smith testing. His symptoms and labs are most consistent with a diagnosis of drug-induced lupus caused by anti-TNF-α therapy. Drug-induced lupus is a relatively uncommon disorder caused by an autoimmune response triggered by certain medications. Common medications known to be associated with classic drug-induced lupus include isoniazid, chlorpromazine, hydralazine, methyldopa, procainamide, minocycline, and penicillamine, in addition to TNF-α inhibitors. Formation

of autoantibodies is characteristic, with anti-histone antibodies frequently seen in drug-induced lupus triggered by many medications, and anti-dsDNA antibodies particularly common in TNF inhibitor-induced lupus. From this patient's potential medication list described in the question above, adalimumab (TNF-α inhibitor) is the only medication known to be associated with drug-induced lupus.

41. **The correct answer is: A. Clinical history.** Although it shares many features in common with lupus (SLE), drug-induced lupus occurs with equal frequency in males and females, often occurs in older adults because of increased exposure to causative medications, and generally has a more abrupt onset. The most common symptoms of drug-induced lupus include fever, malaise, arthritis, rash, and serositis. The classic malar and discoid rashes seen in SLE are uncommon in drug-induced lupus and renal disease is rare. The skin biopsy for both SLE and drug-induced lupus would show interface dermatitis. Laboratory testing is generally positive for anti-histone antibodies in patients with classic drug-induced lupus (>90%), but anti-histone antibody positivity rates can be as high as 80% in patients with SLE, so a positive anti-histone antibody result does not help differentiate between drug-induced lupus and spontaneous SLE. Anti-dsDNA positivity rates are much lower in drug-induced lupus than in SLE and may serve to differentiate the two diseases, though anti-TNF-α-induced lupus and drug-induced lupus because of minocycline may also be characterized by the presence of anti-dsDNA antibodies. The diagnosis of drug-induced lupus relies on a plausible clinical syndrome, consistent laboratory testing, and a clear medication exposure.

42. **The correct answer is: C. Start steroids.** This patient with a known history of lupus (SLE) presents with fatigue, low-grade fevers, rash, and synovitis. Her symptom constellation is most consistent with a mild-to-moderate lupus flare. In addition to symptoms observed in our patient, lupus flares can also present with malaise, headache, oral or nasal ulcers, photosensitivity, shortness of breath, chest pain, decreased urine output, hematuria, confusion, and memory loss. Some lupus flares are asymptomatic and may only be suggested by abnormal results of laboratory testing, such as acute kidney injury or worsening anemia. Her symptoms certainly warrant treatment, and a short course of prednisone is most appropriate. Hydroxychloroquine is the foundation of lupus treatment and should not be stopped in the setting of an acute flare. If her symptoms were to persist despite prednisone therapy, or if the patient were to develop organ involvement, IV steroid therapy and/or the addition of other immunosuppressive agents may be warranted.

43. **The correct answer is: A. IV cyclophosphamide.** Lupus nephritis is a serious complication of SLE. The diagnosis is made by kidney biopsy, and aggressive treatment is generally warranted. Pending the patient's age and medication adherence history, new-onset lupus nephritis is generally treated with either oral mycophenolate mofetil or IV cyclophosphamide therapy. Newer agents, such as voclosporin or belimumab, have been shown to increase renal response when added to these standard induction regimens.

44. **The correct answer is: B. Hydroxychloroquine.** Hydroxychloroquine is the foundation of lupus treatment, and it is the only medication that provides a significant survival and morbidity benefit across the lupus spectrum. Hydroxychloroquine therapy is known to cause retinopathy, and fundoscopic examination often reveals parafoveal retinal pigment atrophy and "bull's eye maculopathy." The risk of retinopathy is dependent on both the cumulative dose of hydroxychloroquine and duration of exposure.

45. **The correct answer is: D. Yearly ophthalmologic examinations.** Patients should have a baseline screening fundoscopic examination with an ophthalmologist to rule out preexisting retinal disease within a few months of starting hydroxychloroquine. They should

then undergo annual screening with automated visual field testing and spectral domain optical coherence tomography beginning 5 years after initiation of hydroxychloroquine. Yearly examinations should commence earlier if there are any high-risk features (abnormalities on baseline retinal examination, high hydroxychloroquine dose, kidney disease, concurrent tamoxifen use, etc). Regular ophthalmologic examinations help identify hydroxychloroquine-induced retinopathy before vision changes occur so that risk of further damage can be reduced by stopping hydroxychloroquine, though retinopathy may in some cases continue to progress.

46. **The correct answer is: C. Endoscopic ultrasound with biopsy.** This patient presents with painless obstructive jaundice and is found to have a 3-cm mass in the pancreatic head with widespread lymphadenopathy and elevated serum IgG4 levels. Although a similar presentation could be seen in pancreatic cancer, the elevated IgG4 levels and widespread lymphadenopathy without additional evidence of metastatic disease suggest IgG4-related disease. Biopsy remains the gold standard for diagnosis, and endoscopic ultrasound is the preferred method for accessing lesions within the pancreas. Histopathologic examination in IgG4-related disease typically shows a dense lymphoplasmacytic infiltrate, storiform fibrosis, increased abundance of IgG4-positive plasma cells, and obliterative fibrosis. IgG4-related disease was only recently recognized as a distinct rheumatic condition. Patients may present with painless obstructive jaundice from a mass in the pancreas, but recurrent episodes of autoimmune pancreatitis are the most common presentation. Patients also typically have lymphadenopathy and may develop disease in several other organ systems including, but not limited to, sclerosing cholangitis, retroperitoneal fibrosis, sclerosing sialadenitis of the salivary glands, and orbital disease.

47. **The correct answer is: A. Steroids.** Steroids are the first line of treatment for IgG4 disease, and a lack of response to steroids suggests the presence of another disease process.

48. **The correct answer is: C. Eosinophilic granulomatosis with polyangiitis.** The patient presents with fevers, unintentional weight loss, hemoptysis, petechial rash, and mononeuritis multiplex, concerning for development of a new small vessel vasculitis. Given his history of allergic rhinitis, asthma, and the peripheral eosinophilia seen on his WBC differential, his clinical presentation is most consistent with eosinophilic granulomatosis with polyangiitis (formerly Churg-Strauss syndrome). Eosinophilic granulomatosis with polyangiitis is a rare form of antineutrophilic cytoplasmic antibody (ANCA) vasculitis that causes granulomatous inflammation of small- and medium-sized vessels in the body. The disease most commonly affects the lungs and the skin but can cause damage to any organ in the body.

49. **The correct answer is: D. Nerve biopsy.** Laboratory testing for p-ANCA is only positive in 30% to 60% of patients, and the majority with positive p-ANCA testing have a myeloperoxidase antigen–specific perinuclear staining pattern. Biopsy of affected tissue remains the gold standard for diagnosis and shows necrotizing vasculitis and/or perivascular necrotizing eosinophilic granulomas or eosinophilic infiltration. A significant history of asthma or rhinosinusitis with peripheral eosinophilia on laboratory testing can help differentiate eosinophilic granulomatosis with polyangiitis from other forms of ANCA vasculitis, such as granulomatosis with polyangiitis and microscopic polyangiitis.

50. **The correct answer is: A. Polyarteritis nodosa.** The patient presents with fever, malaise, weight loss, abdominal pain, hematochezia, and myalgias and is found to have purpura and mononeuritis multiplex on examination. The patient is also noted to be hypertensive with elevated inflammatory markers and an acute kidney injury on laboratory testing.

His clinical presentation is concerning for a medium vessel vasculitis, and the presence of renal artery aneurysms with large-vessel constrictions and occlusion of the small arteries confirms a diagnosis of polyarteritis nodosa (PAN). PAN is a medium vessel vasculitis that often presents with nonspecific systemic symptoms, hypertension because of renin-angiotensin-aldosterone system (RAAS) activation by renal artery disease, acute kidney injury, abdominal pain especially after meals (mesenteric arteritis), gastrointestinal bleeding, mononeuritis multiplex, and myalgias. When attempting to differentiate PAN from the other causes of vasculitis, PAN importantly tends to spare the lungs.

51. **The correct answer is: B. Hepatitis B.** The majority of cases of PAN are idiopathic, but hepatitis B is also known to cause PAN in up to one-third of cases. Hepatitis C and hairy cell leukemia are less common causes of secondary PAN.

52. **The correct answer is: C. IgA vasculitis.** The patient presents with petechial rash, lower extremity arthritis, and abdominal pain 3 weeks after having streptococcal pharyngitis. Skin biopsy shows leukocytoclastic vasculitis with positive IgA staining, confirming the diagnosis of IgA vasculitis (formerly Henoch-Schönlein purpura). IgA vasculitis is typically a self-limited disease and often resolves spontaneously without intervention within approximately 1 month. More severe disease can sometimes lead to an acute kidney injury requiring temporary dialysis and gastrointestinal complications including intussusception (generally in children), gastrointestinal bleeding, bowel ischemia and necrosis, and bowel perforation. Thankfully, serious complications are relatively rare, and this patient appears to have a milder case of the disease.

53. **The correct answer is: A. Observation.** Patients without renal involvement are generally managed symptomatically, and NSAIDs can be used to treat arthritis in the absence of renal disease. The use of steroids to treat IgA vasculitis is controversial. In adults, a prolonged steroid taper is generally only considered in patients with severe renal disease or if the patient has a contraindication to receiving NSAIDs.

54. **The correct answer is: E. Steroids.** The patient presents with classic symptoms of polymyalgia rheumatica (PMR), including pain and stiffness of his bilateral shoulders and hips. This stiffness improves with activity and returns with rest ("gelling" phenomenon). Inflammatory markers are typically elevated in PMR, but CPK is normal because, unlike myositis, inflammatory muscle damage is not a feature. Upon first presentation, the patient's symptoms were consistent with PMR, and first-line treatment is with steroids. PMR typically responds rapidly and dramatically to low-dose corticosteroids ($\leq$20 mg prednisone daily), which are then gradually tapered.

55. **The correct answer is: C. Development of a large-vessel vasculitis.** Given its close association with giant cell arteritis (GCA), a large-vessel vasculitis that can precede, accompany, or follow diagnosis of PMR, it is necessary to ask about GCA symptoms whenever PMR is suspected. Development of fever, jaw claudication, headache, temple or scalp tenderness, or vision symptoms (including diplopia and transient or permanent monocular vision loss) is worrisome for development of GCA.

56. **The correct answer is: A. Increase his immunosuppression dose.** Given the risk of vision loss because of GCA, it must be treated immediately with high-dose steroids. When suspected, treatment should be started empirically and not await results of diagnostics. For this reason, temporal artery biopsy does not impact immediate decision-making, but it can still be helpful for diagnostic support. The yield of temporal artery biopsy is minimally affected by the first 1 to 2 weeks of treatment.

57. **The correct answer is: E. Kidney biopsy.** The patient presents with general malaise, arthralgias, palpable purpura, and new-onset peripheral neuropathy. His symptom constellation is concerning for a small vessel vasculitis, and his history raises suspicion for mixed cryoglobulinemia syndrome. Other supporting lab testing for mixed cryoglobulinemia includes a positive RF and low C4 levels. Mixed cryoglobulinemia refers to a small vessel vasculitis caused by immune complex deposition. The disease can present in a number of ways but is most commonly associated with palpable purpura, joint pain (arthralgia or arthritis), and weakness (Meltzer triad). It may also be associated with peripheral neuropathy, renal disease, or a variety of other systemic manifestations. Cryoglobulin testing and biopsy can confirm the diagnosis of mixed cryoglobulinemia. Cryoglobulins can precipitate at room temperature, so blood samples must be collected in warmed tubes that remain warm until processed by the lab to prevent false-negative cryoglobulin testing. Leukocytoclastic vasculitis is generally seen on skin biopsy, and most patients with renal disease present with membranoproliferative glomerulonephritis. Because the patient is not exhibiting signs of renal disease, kidney biopsy would not be appropriate at this time.

58. **The correct answer is: B. Hepatitis C.** A patient with a history of untreated hepatitis C presenting with a symptom constellation concerning for a small vessel vasculitis suggests mixed cryoglobulinemia syndrome. When the patient initially presents, given his multiple risk factors for endocarditis, including history of IV drug use and history of endocarditis, it is imperative to rule out infectious endocarditis as a cause of his acute malaise, murmur, and petechiae. Moreover, a mixed cryoglobulinemia can also be secondary to chronic infections such as endocarditis. However, the absence of fever, multiple negative blood cultures, echocardiograms without vegetations, and progression of symptoms through broad antibiotics make endocarditis a less likely cause.

59. **The correct answer is: A. Systemic infection.** Familial Mediterranean fever (FMF) is a hereditary autoinflammatory syndrome caused by autosomal recessive mutations in the *MEFV* gene. The syndrome manifests as recurrent episodes of fever and serositis, most commonly causing abdominal pain that can mimic an acute (surgical) abdomen. Symptoms typically last for 1 to 3 days and can variably include chest pain because of pleuritis and/or pericarditis, arthritis (often monoarticular), and an erythematous rash (typically of the lower extremities). The interval between episodes can be variable, from weeks to years. The chronic inflammation of the disorder is strongly associated with secondary amyloid (AA), putting the individual at risk for end-stage renal disease from renal amyloidosis. Other complications include abdominal adhesions from repeated episodes of peritonitis (and abdominal surgeries) and infertility from scarring of fallopian tubes from chronic abdominopelvic inflammation.

60. **The correct answer is: B. Colchicine.** Colchicine is very effective in reducing inflammation, flares, and the risk of end-organ damage from AA amyloidosis, and therefore typically is recommended as a lifelong treatment for all FMF patients. Anti-IL-1 therapy is an alternative if colchicine is not tolerated. Exertional myalgia is also a common manifestation of FMF but is not episodic and generally does not respond to colchicine, though it may respond to NSAIDs.

61. **The correct answer is: B. SPEP and urine protein electrophoresis (UPEP) with immunofixation.** The patient presents with peripheral neuropathy, recent carpal tunnel syndrome, volume overload, and easy bruising. Examination is notable for enlargement of the anterior shoulder ("shoulder pad sign"), hepatosplenomegaly, and periorbital bruising. Laboratory testing reveals an elevated creatinine with significant proteinuria. The patient's

presentation is most concerning for immunoglobulin light chain (AL) amyloidosis. AL am-yloidosis is a primary amyloidosis caused by an overproduction of monoclonal light chains that cause complications when deposited in various tissues of the body. The presenting symptoms of AL amyloidosis differ depending on which organs are most affected. If the kidneys or heart are primarily involved, AL amyloidosis can present with volume overload because of nephrotic syndrome or restrictive cardiomyopathy. The majority of patients with AL amyloidosis have hepatic involvement, which can present with hepatomegaly or elevated liver enzymes in a cholestatic pattern. Patients may also have musculoskel-etal involvement leading to findings such as macroglossia, tongue scalloping, muscular pseudohypertrophy, shoulder arthropathy ("shoulder pad sign"), carpal tunnel syndrome, or involvement of other joints or connective tissues. Other potential findings include sple-nomegaly, anemia, thrombocytopenia, easy bruising or bleeding, peripheral neuropathy, and periorbital purpura ("raccoon eyes"). In this patient with renal involvement, mono-clonal light chains are likely to be identified in both serum and urine using electrophoresis (SPEP and UPEP, respectively) and immunofixation. SFLC ratio is also expected to be abnormal.

62. **The correct answer is: D. Positive Congo red staining with "apple green" birefringence.** Histopathologic examination is vital in the diagnosis of AL amyloidosis. The most common and least invasive procedure used to obtain a tissue diagnosis is an ab-dominal fat pad biopsy. A bone marrow biopsy is also commonly performed. Pathology of the affected tissue will show infiltration of an amorphous, waxy substance that will demon-strate positive staining with Congo red with apple green birefringence under polarized light. Though liver biopsy may be considered if the initial testing is equivocal, it would likely be considered only after SPEP, UPEP, and the less invasive abdominal fat pad biopsy were obtained. Interface dermatitis is associated with cutaneous lupus, focal lymphocytic sialad-enitis is seen on salivary gland biopsy in Sjögren syndrome, a dense lymphoplasmacytic infiltrate with "storiform fibrosis" is seen in IgG4-related disease, and excessive organized collagen deposition with expansion of the dermis is associated with scleroderma.

1. A 78-year-old woman with a history of Alzheimer disease, hypertension, atrial fibrillation on apixaban, and type 2 diabetes on insulin presents with a sudden change in mental status. At baseline, she has short-term memory difficulties with trouble remembering names. Her family helps her with medications and preparing meals, but she feeds and dresses herself, and has been able to remain in her home. Her daughter came to bring dinner and found her sitting at the kitchen table in her nightgown, disheveled-appearing, withdrawn, and unable to answer questions appropriately. She was brought to the emergency room. On examination, she was found to have a low-grade fever with otherwise normal vital signs, dry mucous membranes, clear lungs, and a soft, nontender, and nondistended abdomen. She was drowsy, often falling asleep unless constantly stimulated. She was able to give her name, but she stated that she was at home and was not oriented to month or year. She was able to name the days of the week forward, but not backward. The remainder of the neurologic examination was normal.

   What is the next best step in her management?
   A. Basic metabolic panel and complete blood count
   B. Blood glucose fingerstick
   C. Noncontrast head computed tomography (CT)
   D. Routine electroencephalogram (EEG)
   E. Urinalysis and urine culture

2. The labs of the patient in Question 1 return and are notable for a normal blood glucose, serum white blood cell (WBC) count of 12 000/μL and urinalysis showing 50 to 100 WBC/high-power field (hpf), positive leukocyte esterase, and positive nitrites. She has a head CT that shows stable, moderate atrophy most predominant in the temporal and parietal lobes, without any hemorrhage or other acute findings.

   Which of the following is NOT true about the cause of her mental status change?
   A. Advanced patient age and underlying neurologic disease are risk factors
   B. Inattention is a hallmark feature
   C. It is associated with increased mortality
   D. Symptoms are slowly progressive
   E. There is often an identifiable trigger

3. A 56-year-old man presents for evaluation of behavioral changes. His wife reports that the patient has become a "different person" over the past 2 years. He used to be a very calm and pleasant person, but over that period of time he has become "nasty." He curses in public, spits on the bus, and makes unwanted sexual advances toward women. He has also been less able to complete tasks at work and was recently given a formal warning by his employer that he is at risk of losing his job if he does not change his behavior and meet deadlines. During the neurologic examination, he calls the neurologist "honey"

and "gorgeous" and asks if he can use the reflex hammer to "hit the doctor back." He undergoes brain imaging, which is depicted below:

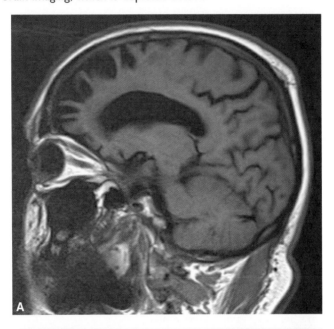

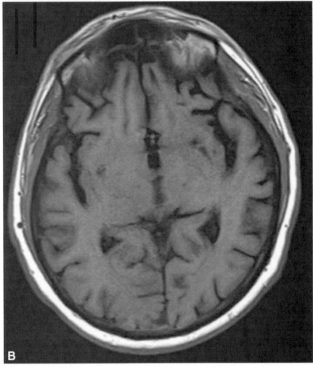

A: Sagittal view. **B:** Axial view. Courtesy of Dr. Omar Al-Louzi, Harvard Neurology Residency Program, Brigham and Women's & Massachusetts General Hospitals.

What is the most likely diagnosis?

A. Alzheimer disease
B. Behavioral variant of frontotemporal dementia
C. Corticobasal degeneration
D. Lewy body disease
E. Primary progressive aphasia

4. A 25-year-old woman presents to the hospital after a first-time seizure.

Which of the following could have contributed to her seizure risk?

A. Alcohol withdrawal
B. Bupropion
C. Hypoglycemia
D. Hyponatremia
E. All of the above

5. Which of the following is NOT consistently associated with an increased risk of seizure recurrence after an unprovoked first-time seizure in an adult?

A. Family history of seizure
B. Nocturnal seizure
C. Abnormal brain imaging
D. Prior brain insult
E. EEG with epileptiform abnormalities

6. Which of the following is the first step if you believe someone is in status epilepticus?

A. Administer intravenous (IV) lorazepam
B. Administer IV phenytoin
C. Administer stat naloxone
D. Ensure proper oxygenation
E. Refer for head CT

7. A 23-year-old man with no past medical history presents after losing consciousness at the supermarket. He recalls feeling flushed and slightly anxious in the moments before the event, and his next memory is of being on the ground attended to by a bystander. This bystander reported that the patient had lost consciousness for roughly 30 seconds, during which time he had occasional symmetric convulsions. He was drowsy and slightly confused for 10 to 15 minutes following this event, after which he returned to baseline. He notes that his tongue is sore. He is brought to the hospital and testing is ordered to investigate for possible seizure versus syncope.

Which of the following statements is FALSE?

A. A normal routine EEG excludes the possibility of an underlying seizure disorder
B. Echocardiogram should be performed to assess for structural cardiac disease
C. Syncope is frequently accompanied by convulsions
D. The patient should be counseled to refrain from driving for as long as is required by the driving regulations of his state
E. Tongue laceration increases the probability of seizure

8. A 39-year-old woman with a history of migraine, alcohol use disorder, and major depressive disorder with a prior suicide attempt presents to the emergency department (ED) with a first-time seizure, characterized by sudden loss of consciousness, rightward head turn, and rhythmic convulsions of the right arm lasting 2 minutes with a prolonged period of somnolence and confusion following the event. Laboratory studies reveal Na 132 mEq/L, aspartate transaminase (AST) 178 U/L, alanine aminotransferase (ALT) 98 U/L,

and platelets 118×10^9/L. Electrocardiogram (ECG) reveals first-degree heart block and is otherwise normal. Brain magnetic resonance imaging (MRI) is unremarkable. EEG shows infrequent epileptiform discharges originating from the left temporal lobe.

Which of the following is a relative contraindication to starting levetiracetam in this patient?

A. First-degree heart block
B. Hepatic disease
C. History of major depression
D. Hyponatremia
E. Thrombocytopenia

9. Deficiency in which of the following vitamins results in a syndrome characterized by ophthalmoparesis, ataxia, and altered mental status?

A. Cyanocobalamin
B. Pantothenic acid
C. Pyridoxine
D. Riboflavin
E. Thiamine

10. A 55-year-old man with a history of depression and alcohol abuse presents to the hospital for a planned surgery. About 72 hours after the surgery, the patient tells his nurse that he is hearing his friends tell him that he has been abducted by aliens. There is no one else in his room. He is shaky, hypertensive, and tachycardic on examination. His blood work is normal.

What is the most likely diagnosis?

A. Delirium tremens
B. Depression
C. Posttraumatic stress disorder
D. Schizoaffective disorder

11. A 48-year-old man with a history of chronic alcohol use disorder presents 36 hours after his last drink. He is tremulous, diaphoretic, and anxious. Heart rate (HR) is 110 to 120 beats/min and blood pressure (BP) is 177/93 mmHg.

All of the following medications would be appropriate for treating this patient's alcohol withdrawal EXCEPT:

A. Alprazolam
B. Chlordiazepoxide
C. Diazepam
D. Lorazepam
E. Phenobarbital

12. A 25-year-old woman presents to the ED with dizziness and vomiting since the morning. She reports that she was sick with a cold about a week ago, but otherwise had been healthy. On examination, you notice she has horizontal gaze-evoked nystagmus beating to the right that is worse when looking to the right and goes away when looking to the left. A catch-up saccade was seen with left head thrust. No skew was noted on the cover-uncover test. Her hearing and the rest of her neurologic examination are normal.

What is the most likely diagnosis?

A. Benign paroxysmal positional vertigo
B. Labyrinthitis
C. New posterior circulation stroke
D. Vestibular neuritis

13. A 78-year-old woman comes to clinic with repeated episodes of falls. On history she tells you that every morning when she wakes up and attempts to get out of bed, she has an episode of feeling very dizzy and is unable to walk for 30 seconds. She has a normal neurologic examination.

What is the most likely diagnosis?

A. Benign paroxysmal positional vertigo
B. Concussion
C. Migraine
D. Vertebrobasilar insufficiency
E. Vestibular neuritis

14. A 53-year-old woman with type 2 diabetes presents with sudden onset of dizziness and nausea, which began when she was eating breakfast. She has a constant feeling of spinning toward the right. The symptoms did not resolve after a period of lying down and she presented to the ED for evaluation.

All of the following findings would be concerning for a posterior circulation stroke EXCEPT:

A. Diminished hearing
B. Direction-changing nystagmus
C. Double vision
D. Dysarthria
E. Limb ataxia

15. Each of the following is a component of the HINTS test for sudden-onset dizziness EXCEPT:

A. Finger-to-nose coordination test
B. Head impulse test
C. Nystagmus
D. Test of skew

16. A 65-year-old man with a history of hypertension and dyslipidemia was brought to the hospital when his family found him unable to speak, eyes deviated to his left side, with right facial drooping, and inability to move his right arm.

The most likely location of his stroke is in the distribution of which of the following?

A. Left middle cerebral artery (MCA)
B. Left posterior cerebral artery
C. Right anterior cerebral artery
D. Right MCA
E. Right posterior inferior cerebellar artery

17. Which of the following patients is best qualified to receive tissue plasminogen activator?

A. A 40-year-old woman with no past medical history who presents with left-sided whole-body weakness, which she noticed when she woke up. She last felt normal at 8 PM the night before
B. A 55-year-old man with orthopedic surgery 1 week ago who presents with whole-body weakness on the right side that started 3 hours earlier
C. A 60-year-old man with an intracerebral hematoma 4 weeks ago who presents with acute onset of incoordination and dizziness that started 30 minutes prior to arrival
D. A 68-year-old woman with a history of hypertension and diabetes who presents to the hospital with sudden onset of left face and arm weakness that started 4 hours ago
E. A 92-year-old man with a history of hypertension who presents with 5 hours of difficulty seeing things off to his left side

18. A 68-year-old woman with a history of hypertension, hyperlipidemia, type 2 diabetes, and coronary artery disease presents with sudden onset of expressive aphasia and right face and arm weakness. She is brought to the ED 60 minutes after symptom onset. Her National Institutes of Health Stroke Scale (NIHSS) score is 17. CT with angiography of the head and neck is ordered.

    This test does all of the following EXCEPT:

    A. Assess for a proximal large-vessel occlusion that could warrant endovascular thrombectomy

    B. Assess the cervical and intracranial vasculature for atherosclerotic disease as a possible stroke etiology

    C. Determine the extent of an acute infarct

    D. Be contraindicated in patients with end-stage renal disease (ESRD) or allergy to iodine

    E. Rule out intracranial hemorrhage

19. A 74-year-old man with hypertension and hyperlipidemia presents with sudden onset of left face, arm, and leg weakness, which began suddenly while the patient was on the toilet. He is found by his wife to be dysarthric, weak throughout the left side, and unable to stand. The patient is brought to the ED, where noncontrast head CT reveals a 2 × 3 × 2 cm hemorrhage in the right basal ganglia.

    Which of the following is the most likely etiology?

    A. Aneurysm rupture

    B. Arteriovenous malformation

    C. Cerebral amyloid angiopathy

    D. Hemorrhage of a neoplastic lesion

    E. Hypertension

20. All of the following are similarities in tenecteplase (TNK) and alteplase EXCEPT:

    A. They are both thrombolytic agents

    B. They are both one single bolus

    C. They must be given within 4.5 hours of onset of stroke symptoms

    D. They both have a small bleeding risk

21. A 55-year-old woman with no significant past medical history had fever, malaise, and sore throat that was treated with antibiotics and analgesics. Ten days later, her legs "buckled" underneath her, she had difficulty climbing stairs, and she noticed tingling in both hands. She awoke the next morning and could not stand. She was brought to the hospital, where vital signs were normal. Neurologic examination was notable for weakness of eye closure bilaterally with otherwise intact cranial nerves, symmetric proximal more than distal weakness (neck flexion 4+/5, shoulder abduction 4/5, 5−/5 more distally in the upper extremities, hip flexion 3/5, 4+/5 more distally in the lower extremities), diffuse areflexia, decreased sensation to light touch and pinprick in both hands, and inability to sit or stand independently. Lumbar puncture was performed and showed 0 WBCs × 10^6/L, 4 red blood cells × 10^6/L, protein of 86 mg/dL, and glucose of 65 mg/dL.

    What is the next best step in her management?

    A. Electromyography (EMG)/nerve conduction studies

    B. IV corticosteroids

    C. Intravenous immunoglobulin (IVIG)

    D. MRI of the lumbar spine

    E. Vancomycin, ceftriaxone, and acyclovir

22. A 63-year-old, black female with a history of hypertension and tension-type headaches presents to your clinic complaining of numbness and pain in her feet for the past 2 years. This initially began as an abnormal sensation as though her socks were bunched up over the balls of her feet, but has progressed slowly over time to numbness and a burning sensation in the toes and soles of both feet. She denies back pain, leg weakness, or gait difficulties. There are no similar symptoms in her hands. You make a diagnosis of a distal, painful, sensory-predominant polyneuropathy.

Which of the following blood tests is NOT appropriate as part of an initial screening for this form of neuropathy?

A. Hemoglobin A1c
B. Serum protein electrophoresis and immunofixation
C. Heavy metals screening including mercury, arsenic, and lead
D. Vitamin B12

23. A 57-year-old man with a history of poorly controlled type 2 diabetes presents to clinic complaining of a burning pain in his feet, which is worse at night and sometimes prevents him from falling asleep. He endorses some numbness in the bilateral toes but denies any weakness or sensory symptoms in the hands. On examination, he has mildly decreased sensation to vibration at the bilateral great toes, with normal joint position sense. Vibration is normal at the ankles. Strength and reflexes are normal. Labs show hemoglobin A1c 8.2%, vitamin B12 723 ng/mL, thyroid-stimulating hormone (TSH) 1.16 mU/L, and serum protein electrophoresis (SPEP) with immunofixation normal without M-spike. You diagnose him with diabetic peripheral neuropathy and plan to optimize his glucose control. You would also like to address his pain.

Which of the following is NOT an effective option for treating neuropathic pain?

A. Nonsteroidal anti-inflammatory drugs (NSAIDs)
B. Nortriptyline
C. Pregabalin
D. Topical capsaicin
E. Venlafaxine

24. A 60-year-old day laborer had difficulty climbing stairs and getting up from the toilet seat for the last 5 months, particularly in the morning on waking up, which improves slightly throughout the day. He also complained of dry mouth and fatigue. There was no dysphagia or dysarthria. He had borderline diet-controlled diabetes and angina. He had smoked two packs of cigarettes per day for 30 years. He consumed several alcoholic drinks a day. The neurologic examination showed that the cranial nerves were intact, except for questionable sluggish pupils. Neck flexion was weak, deltoids were 4/5, and hip flexion was 3/5. He could hardly walk on his heels and toes. Deep tendon reflexes (DTRs) were trace, with an absent ankle jerk bilaterally. His gait was cautious and slightly wide-based. Nerve conduction studies showed diffusely reduced motor amplitudes (compound muscle action potentials). After rapid repetitive nerve stimulation (30-50 Hz) or brief (10 sec), intense contractions, a marked increase of the compound muscle action potential amplitude was seen.

What treatment would be most effective in reducing symptoms in this condition?

A. 3,4-Diaminopyridine (3,4-DAP)
B. IVIG
C. Pyridostigmine
D. Rituximab
E. Steroids

25. A 71-year-old woman notices difficulty reading her book at the end of the day. She goes to the optometrist who thinks that her prescription is correct. One evening, she goes out to a celebratory dinner with her family and feels that chewing her steak is more difficult than before. At the end of the long dinner, she sees double while reading the dessert menu and her husband asks if she had too much wine because her speech sounds slurred. Examination by a neurologist shows intact extraocular movements, but fatigable ptosis and a Cogan lid twitch as well as fatigability of the deltoid muscle. You discuss a possible diagnosis and treatment options.

What additional testing might you want to obtain to help aid management?

A. Brain MRI
B. CT scan of the chest
C. Anti–acetylcholine receptor (AChR) and anti–muscle-specific kinase (MuSK) antibodies
D. Erythrocyte sedimentation rate (ESR) and C-reactive protein (CRP)
E. Both B and C

26. A 63-year-old right-handed retired masonry worker presented to the clinic for evaluation regarding gait dysfunction with neck, shoulder, and leg weakness over the past 2 years. He reported experiencing a gradual deterioration in his gait as well as difficulty going up and down stairs. On examination, his vital signs were normal, and he was breathing on room air without excessive work of breathing or usage of accessory muscles. There was evidence of moderate erythema and papules over the extensor surfaces of his fingers and an erythematous rash on his upper chest and back. Motor examination was notable for mild atrophy of the periscapular muscles without apparent fasciculations. Neck flexion and extension were mildly weak (4+/5). There was evidence of proximal greater than distal weakness of the upper and lower extremities (4/5 in shoulder abduction, 4/5 in shoulder external rotation, and 4+/5 in hip flexion and abduction). DTRs were 2+ throughout with downgoing toes. He had a stooped posture with standing. His creatine kinase (CK) level was mildly elevated. Nerve conduction studies were normal, and EMG showed prominent spontaneous activity (fibrillation potentials and positive sharp waves).

Which of the following findings on muscle biopsy would be most consistent with his diagnosis?

A. Nodular collections of immune cells and degeneration with rimmed vacuoles
B. Perifascicular atrophy and perivascular inflammation
C. Prominent myofiber necrosis
D. Ragged red muscle fibers
E. Type 2 muscle fiber atrophy

27. A 28-year-old man with a history of smoking and heavy alcohol use comes to clinic complaining of daily headaches. Every evening at about 10 PM, he develops a left-sided stabbing pain in the front of his head that intensifies over 5 minutes to an excruciating level. The pain lasts about 30 minutes and then resolves. He also reports tearing and redness in the left eye and rhinorrhea. He has had these symptoms nightly for the last 2 weeks, although he recalls a similar period of headaches 1 year ago that resolved.

This patient's symptoms are most consistent with which of the following?

A. Cluster headache
B. Secondary headache
C. Short-lasting unilateral neuralgiform pain with conjunctival injection and tearing
D. Tension headache
E. Trigeminal neuralgia

28. A 28-year-old woman with no past medical history on oral contraceptive pills comes to clinic complaining of daily headaches. For the past 3 months, she has had a continuous daily left-sided headache. The headache intensity is typically moderate, although she does have exacerbations with severe pain that she likens to an ice pick stabbing pain behind the left eye. During these exacerbations, she has rhinorrhea and left-sided tearing and redness in the eye. Her neurologic examination is normal and she has had an MRI of the brain with a venogram that did not show a structural lesion or venous sinus thrombosis.

What is the best initial treatment?

A. Indomethacin
B. Sumatriptan
C. Topiramate
D. Tricyclic antidepressant
E. Verapamil

29. A 32-year-old woman with a past medical history of depression and migraine with aura presents to your office. She was recently in a car accident resulting in mild traumatic brain injury, and worsening of her baseline migraines. She is now having migraines three to four times a week, and has had to miss work once a week because of the severity of her head-aches. She is currently taking fluoxetine for her depression and has experienced significant weight gain, which she is also upset about.

What is the best course of action?

A. Monitor conservatively
B. Start an NSAID for breakthrough migraines
C. Start duloxetine
D. Start topiramate
E. Start propranolol

30. A 47-year-old woman is seen in clinic for evaluation of multiple subcortical ischemic strokes and abnormal brain imaging. She has experienced three separate subcortical strokes over the past 5 years, despite no known stroke risk factors and good adherence to healthy lifestyle habits. Her personal medical history is notable for migraine with aura dating back to adolescence; family history is remarkable for severe migraines in her sister and early strokes and cognitive impairment in her mother. Brain MRI is shown below:

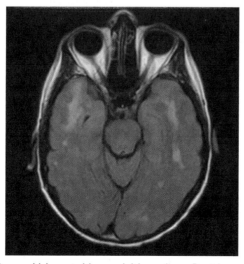

Courtesy of Dr. Omar Al-Louzi, Harvard Neurology Residency Program, Brigham and Women's & Massachusetts General Hospitals.

Genetic testing is most likely to show abnormalities in which of the following genes?

A. α-galactosidase A (GAL) gene
B. COL4A1 mutation
C. HtrA serine peptidase 1 (HTRA1) gene
D. NOTCH3
E. TREX1 gene

31. A 24-year-old woman with a history of polycystic ovarian syndrome on oral contraceptive pills presents with headache of 3 weeks' duration. She reported experiencing pressure-like, right occipital headaches for the prior 2 to 3 weeks. They were intermittent in nature, occurring every 2 to 3 days and lasting a couple of hours. However, over the past 5 days, her headaches have become constant and progressively worsened in their severity. They wake her up at night. They worsen in intensity with lying flat and she describes sitting up as the best position. Examination shows evidence of bilateral papilledema. Cranial imaging is obtained and shown below:

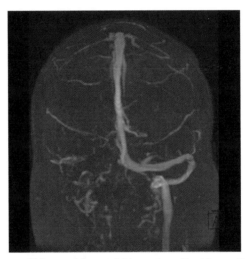

Courtesy of Dr. Omar Al-Louzi, Harvard Neurology Residency Program, Brigham and Women's & Massachusetts General Hospitals.

What would be the next best step in her management?

A. Administer mannitol 1 g/kg IV
B. Maintain BP <140 mmHg
C. Obtain blood cultures and start broad-spectrum IV antibiotics
D. Obtain lumbar puncture to rule out meningitis
E. Send thrombophilia workup and start therapeutic anticoagulation with heparin

32. A 56-year-old man with a history of hypertension and obesity presents with weakness and numbness in the right foot. He has trouble fully flexing at the ankle and has noticed that he catches his toes when walking, causing him to trip. He also reports shooting pain from the low back down the right lateral thigh and calf into the great toe. His symptoms came on suddenly after he helped his friend move. Initially he thought he had a muscle strain but decided to seek medical attention given the difficulty walking. On physical examination, he has 4+/5 weakness in right ankle dorsiflexion, foot inversion, and foot eversion. He has decreased sensation to pinprick over the right lateral calf and great toe. Reflexes are normal. When the patient is in a supine position and right leg is raised to 60°, it elicits a shooting pain from the low back down the right leg.

What is the localization of his symptoms?

A. L4 nerve root
B. L5 nerve root
C. Peroneal nerve
D. S1 nerve root
E. Thoracic spinal cord

33. A 71-year-old woman with a history of hypertension, hyperlipidemia, and coronary artery disease presents for evaluation of leg pain. The pain starts in her back and radiates down to both legs. It is worse with walking and better with rest, although she notes that she is able to use a stationary bicycle without much pain. She also reports pain and cramping in her calves, as well as numbness and tingling in both feet. On examination, she has full strength throughout, 1+ patellar reflexes, and absent ankle jerks. Pulses are normal.

Which feature(s) of her presentation are less consistent with neurogenic claudication, as opposed to a vascular cause?

A. Absent ankle jerks
B. Calf cramping
C. Numbness and paresthesias in the feet
D. Radiating pain down the legs
E. Both A and B

34. A 51-year-old woman with a history of non–small cell lung cancer presents to the ED with bilateral lower extremity weakness and numbness. Two hours prior to presentation, she noted sudden onset of worsening of her thoracic back pain, in addition to new numbness and tingling in her thighs bilaterally. This was associated with difficulty in walking and bilateral leg weakness. She was still able to walk but felt her legs were wobbly. She did not notice any urinary or stool incontinence. On examination, strength was full in her upper extremities. There was mild weakness in hip flexion bilaterally (4+/5). She was hyperreflexic at the patellae bilaterally (3+) with crossed adduction. Her toes were upgoing bilaterally. She has altered sensation to pinprick at the level of the nipples anteriorly. Imaging of the spine was obtained and is shown below:

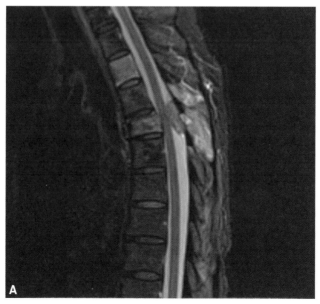

A: Sagittal view.

NEUROLOGY

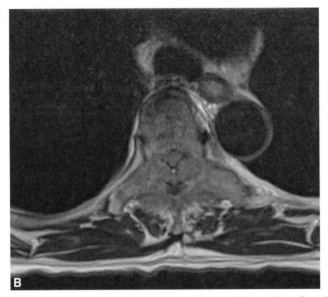

B: Axial view. Courtesy of Dr. Omar Al-Louzi, Harvard Neurology Residency Program, Brigham and Women's & Massachusetts General Hospitals.

What is the most appropriate next step in her management?

A. Administer dexamethasone 10 mg IV, with urgent evaluation for thoracic spine decompression

B. Administer mannitol 1 g/kg IV

C. Immobilize with a hard cervical collar

D. Obtain blood cultures and start broad-spectrum IV antibiotics

E. Supplement with vitamin B12

35. A 47-year-old man is found down after an out-of-hospital cardiac arrest. Bystander cardiopulmonary resuscitation is initiated in the field. On Emergency Medical Services (EMS) arrival, initial rhythm is ventricular tachycardia. The patient ultimately receives five rounds of chest compressions, two shocks, 2 mg total of epinephrine, and is intubated before return of spontaneous circulation (ROSC) is achieved. CT scan of the head is negative for acute intracranial hemorrhage. Active normothermia is maintained for the subsequent 24 hours. Clinical exam is notable for unequal and sluggishly reactive pupils; a weak corneal reflex on the left; intact vestibulo-ocular, cough, and gag reflexes. There is no motor response to noxious stimuli in any extremity. Neuron-specific enolase (NSE) 24 hours after ROSC is 110 ng/mL. Video EEG is pertinent for lack of reactivity to external stimuli. MRI brain 48 hours after ROSC reveals evidence of small-volume anoxic injury.

Which of the following prognostic indicators in combination suggests the possibility of a poor outcome?

A. Unequal pupils and NSE >33 ng/mL

B. Weak corneal reflex and anoxic injury on MRI

C. Unequal pupils and lack of reactivity on EEG

D. NSE >101 ng/mL and lack of reactivity on EEG

E. No motor response to noxious stimuli and anoxic injury on MRI

ANSWERS

1. **The correct answer is: B. Blood glucose fingerstick.** This patient presents with acute change in mental status, superimposed on chronic cognitive decline because of Alzheimer disease. The next best step in management is to check her blood glucose. She is at risk for hypoglycemia because she is on insulin, and this is a fast point-of-care test that can be done immediately at the bedside. Basic metabolic panel, complete blood count, and urinalysis should also be checked as part of the workup of encephalopathy, but would not be the next best test. Initial labs should also include liver function tests and a toxicology screen; the list can be expanded based on the clinical picture. Patients with Alzheimer disease are at increased risk of seizures because of encephalomalacia, so EEG may be appropriate for some patients. Noncontrast head CT is often indicated for acute change in mental status, particularly in patients on anticoagulation, but is not the next best test.

2. **The correct answer is: D. Symptoms are slowly progressive.** This patient has delirium secondary to a urinary tract infection. Patients have waxing and waning mental status changes, rather than slowly progressive symptoms. Inattention, as demonstrated by her inability to name days of the week backward, is a hallmark feature. Delirium is a symptom and should prompt a workup for underlying medical causes, including infection, metabolic abnormalities, toxin exposure/medications, and physiologic stressors (such as pain or constipation). An underlying dementia makes patients more vulnerable to delirium. Other risk factors include advanced age, medical and psychiatric comorbidities, poor functional baseline, and sensory impairment. Delirium is easier to prevent than to treat and is associated with increased mortality, so it is important to actively prevent delirium in hospitalized patients.

3. **The correct answer is: B. Behavioral variant of frontotemporal dementia.** The patient presents with a progressive behavioral syndrome manifested by disinhibition. His personality dramatically changed from calm and pleasant to inappropriate. The symptoms are clearly impairing both his social and occupational functioning. Frontotemporal dementia causes atrophy that typically involves the frontal and temporal lobes, as illustrated in the figure. This is a tauopathy, and, hence, pathology typically demonstrates rounded intracytoplasmic structures with immunoreactivity to tau immunostains. Alzheimer disease can certainly manifest with behavioral changes; this typically occurs during the later stages of the disease, and early frontal atrophy is not characteristic of this. Lewy body disease and corticobasal degeneration can manifest with psychosis but not dramatic behavioral changes without other Parkinsonian features. There is no language involvement in this patient to suggest primary progressive aphasia.

4. **The correct answer is: E. All of the above.** All of the above factors put the patient at risk for seizures. Generally, withdrawal and intoxications from medications and alcohol can put patients at risk for seizures. Laboratory abnormalities, particularly low glucose and sodium, are seizure risk factors. Bupropion is one of many medications known to lower the seizure threshold.

5. **The correct answer is: A. Family history of seizure.** The most consistently noted factors associated with an increased risk of seizure recurrence following an unprovoked first seizure include an EEG with epileptiform abnormalities, a prior brain lesion or insult causing seizure, a significant brain-imaging abnormality, and a nocturnal seizure. In contrast, clinical variables that were *not* consistently associated with an increased seizure recurrence

risk after an unprovoked first seizure in adults include the patient's age, sex, family history of seizures, seizure type, and presentation with status epilepticus or multiple (two or more) discrete seizures within 24 hours with recovery between them.

6. **The correct answer is: D. Ensure proper oxygenation.** The first step in managing seizure activity is to ensure the patient's ABCs (airway, breathing, and circulation) are addressed. Secondary testing, including head CT and lumbar puncture, may be considered to understand the etiology of the seizures, but the first step is to ensure the patient is protecting their airway. Lorazepam is the first medication to be given in status epilepticus, not phenytoin. Naloxone is typically given to reverse opioid withdrawal.

7. **The correct answer is: A. A normal routine EEG excludes the possibility of an underlying seizure disorder.** An interictal EEG (an EEG obtained when a patient is not manifesting symptoms of a possible seizure) has roughly 50% sensitivity for an underlying seizure disorder. Therefore, an abnormal EEG can rule in a seizure disorder if epileptiform discharges are seen, but a normal EEG cannot rule out the possibility of seizure disorder. If suspicion remains high for seizures after an inconclusive workup, further investigation with long-term EEG monitoring can be pursued in an effort to capture a clinical event during EEG monitoring and assess for an electrographic correlate. The remainder of the answer choices are all true for the workup of patients presenting with syncope versus seizure.

8. **The correct answer is: C. History of major depression.** In 10% to 20% of patients, levetiracetam causes mood symptoms ranging from depression to irritability and, in severe cases, rage and agitation. Given the patient's history of major depressive disorder with a prior suicide attempt, this medication should be avoided. Thrombocytopenia and hepatic disease are relative contraindications to valproic acid. First-degree heart block is a contraindication to lacosamide. Hyponatremia is a contraindication to carbamazepine and oxcarbazepine.

9. **The correct answer is: E. Thiamine.** Ataxia, ophthalmoparesis, and altered mental status compose the hallmark triad of Wernicke encephalopathy. Wernicke encephalopathy is an acute life-threatening condition from thiamine deficiency. Many vitamin deficiencies can occur in patients with alcohol use disorder; however, riboflavin deficiency typically causes stomatitis. Pyridoxine deficiency typically causes skin findings, neuropathy, and sometimes somnolence or confusion. Cyanocobalamin deficiency typically causes anemia and/or neurologic symptoms, including subacute combined degeneration of the spinal cord.

10. **The correct answer is: A. Delirium tremens.** The patient's history of alcohol abuse puts him at risk for alcohol withdrawal. Delirium tremens is usually seen around 3 days after the patient's last alcoholic drink. It typically manifests with hallucinations, hypertension, shivering, sweating, and tachycardia. Schizoaffective disorder, posttraumatic stress disorder, and depression would not be expected to have these vital sign abnormalities.

11. **The correct answer is: A. Alprazolam.** Alprazolam is a short-acting benzodiazepine, and because of its short half-life and potential for causing rebound seizures, it should not be used for the management of alcohol withdrawal. The remainder of the answer choices are all appropriate to consider.

12. **The correct answer is: D. Vestibular neuritis.** This patient has all the examination features of a peripheral cause of her dizziness (positive head thrust, no skew, and unilaterally beating nystagmus). Given that she has been experiencing symptoms for hours, with no reported association with head movement, this is unlikely to be benign paroxysmal positional vertigo. Given that hearing is normal, this is not labyrinthitis. Generally, central nystagmus is direction-changing and the patient also has no other localizing symptoms to suggest a posterior circulation stroke.

13. **The correct answer is: A. Benign paroxysmal positional vertigo.** Benign paroxysmal positional vertigo causes brief (seconds to minutes long) episodes of dizziness that are often noticed when changing head position. This is unlikely to be vestibular neuritis given how brief the episodes are. This is unlikely to be migraine given no reported associated headache. There is no trauma history and the episodic nature makes concussion less likely. Though vertigo can occur with vertebrobasilar insufficiency, there are typically other neurologic symptoms and signs on examination.

14. **The correct answer is: A. Diminished hearing.** Diminished hearing accompanying dizziness suggests an otologic etiology and is unlikely to be due to a central lesion. The remainder of the response choices are all concerning for a possible lesion in the brainstem or cerebellum, and any of these would warrant brain MRI to assess for an acute stroke in the posterior circulation.

15. **The correct answer is: A. Finger-to-nose coordination test.** The HINTS test consists of the Head Impulse test, Nystagmus, and Test of Skew. The head impulse test involves rapid, passive head turns while the patient maintains visual fixation. The test of skew involves alternately covering and uncovering each eye to assess for vertical misalignment of the eyes. If the HINTS test reveals absence of a correctional saccade on head impulse testing, presence of direction-changing nystagmus, or presence of a vertical skew deviation, MRI of the brain should be pursued to assess for a central etiology. The finger-to-nose coordination test assesses ipsilateral cerebellar function and may be abnormal in a posterior circulation stroke, but is not a component of the HINTS test.

16. **The correct answer is: A. Left middle cerebral artery (MCA).** The left MCA supplies the area of the brain responsible for language in the majority of people. The left MCA also supplies the left motor strip, which is responsible for controlling the right side of the body, which explains why the patient is unable to move the right side. In strokes, the eyes deviate toward the lesion, when compared to seizures, in which the eyes deviate away from the lesion. The right anterior cerebral artery would present with predominantly left leg more than left arm weakness, would not typically have an impact on language, and would have gaze deviation in the opposite direction. A right MCA infarction would present with weakness of the left side, not the right side, and also would have evidence of neglect on further testing. A left posterior cerebral artery infarction would predominantly cause visual symptoms, in particular, right homonymous hemianopia. A right posterior inferior cerebellar artery stroke is also known as a lateral medullary syndrome and would typically cause vertigo, ipsilateral (in this case right-sided) hemiataxia, dysarthria, ptosis, and miosis (ie, ipsilateral Horner syndrome).

17. **The correct answer is: D. A 68-year-old woman with a history of hypertension and diabetes who presents to the hospital with sudden onset of left face and arm weakness that started 4 hours ago.** The patient in answer D is presenting within 4.5 hours of last known well time and does not have any exclusion criteria. Choices A and E are incorrect because the patients are presenting outside the 4.5-hour tissue plasminogen activator window. Choice B is incorrect because the patient's recent surgery is a relative contraindication. Choice C is incorrect because the patient's recent intracerebral hemorrhage is a contraindication.

18. **The correct answer is: C. Determine the extent of an acute infarct.** Although CT is highly sensitive for acute intracranial hemorrhage, radiographic changes are typically absent for up to 6 hours following an ischemic stroke. As such, it is a poor tool for determining the infarct burden within 6 to 24 hours following an ischemic stroke. MRI is the preferred imaging modality for determining the extent of an acute infarct. CT perfusion is another option for visualizing the extent of stroke. CT angiography is an important

component of the acute stroke assessment for two reasons. First, it can detect the presence of a proximal large-vessel occlusion that would be an indication for endovascular thrombectomy. Second, it can detect atherosclerotic disease in the aortic arch or cervical and intracranial vessels that could contribute to the underlying stroke etiology. Though patients with ESRD or allergy to iodine cannot receive CT contrast, they may have vessel imaging with time-of-flight magnetic resonance angiography (MRA), which does not require IV contrast with gadolinium or a carotid duplex ultrasound.

19. **The correct answer is: E. Hypertension.** Hemorrhages of the deep gray matter structures such as the basal ganglia and pons are typically the result of hypertension. This is due to rupture of small perforator lenticulostriate arteries that arise from the MCAs. Most perforator arteries originate from the MCAs, but not necessarily the large arteries of the circle of Willis. Hemorrhage of an underlying neoplastic lesion is possible but less likely in a patient with no known history of malignancy. Arteriovenous malformations and cerebral amyloid angiopathy typically give rise to more peripheral lobar hemorrhages. Aneurysm rupture typically results in subarachnoid hemorrhage.

20. **The correct answer is: B. They are both one single bolus.** One advantage of TNK is that it is a single bolus compared to alteplase. Alteplase is a bolus followed by a drip (infusion). Multiple trials have now showed that TNK is noninferior to alteplase. As of now, they both have the same time window for use, and they both carry a small risk of bleeding.

21. **The correct answer is: C. Intravenous immunoglobulin (IVIG).** This patient has acute inflammatory demyelinating polyneuropathy or Guillain-Barré syndrome. Symptoms of symmetric proximal and distal limb weakness, areflexia, and distal paresthesias/sensory loss develop over a few days, with peak severity at 2 to 4 weeks. Up to two-thirds of patients can also present with back pain. Lumbar puncture shows cytoalbuminologic dissociation or elevated protein without cerebrospinal fluid (CSF) pleocytosis. These patients are at high risk for respiratory compromise (neck flexion weakness is a proxy for respiratory muscle involvement), and so require very close monitoring, including tests of respiratory mechanics. The clinical history, examination, and CSF are sufficient to begin treatment for acute inflammatory demyelinating polyneuropathy with either IVIG or plasmapheresis. EMG/nerve conduction studies can be helpful, but may be normal early in the disease course and is not required for diagnosis. MRI of the spine may show nerve root enhancement but is not a sensitive sign. Steroids have not been shown to have benefit in acute inflammatory demyelinating polyneuropathy and are not recommended. Although acute inflammatory demyelinating polyneuropathy is often preceded by an infection, this patient does not have signs of active infection or meningitis/encephalitis requiring antibiotics or antivirals.

22. **The correct answer is: C. Heavy metals screening including mercury, arsenic, and lead.** The American Academy of Neurology recommends three essential tests for initial screening of patients with a presumed diagnosis of a distal (length-dependent), symmetric, painful, sensory predominant polyneuropathy. This includes testing for hyperglycemia (eg, fasting glucose, hemoglobin A1c, or oral glucose tolerance test), vitamin B12 deficiency (serum vitamin B12 level, methylmalonic acid, with or without homocysteine), and evaluation for paraproteinemia (SPEP and immunofixation electrophoresis). Testing for additional etiologies should be targeted based on a careful history and review of systems.

23. **The correct answer is: A. Nonsteroidal anti-inflammatory drugs (NSAIDs).** First-line agents for treating neuropathic pain include gabapentin, pregabalin, tricyclic antidepressants (nortriptyline or amitriptyline), and serotonin and norepinephrine reuptake

inhibitors (duloxetine and venlafaxine). Second-line agents include tramadol and topical agents, such as lidocaine and capsaicin. Third-line options include opiates and botulinum toxin A. NSAIDs are not recommended for the treatment of neuropathic pain.

24. **The correct answer is: A. 3,4-Diaminopyridine (3,4-DAP).** The symptoms described in the vignette reflect Lambert-Eaton myasthenic syndrome. This presynaptic neuromuscular junction disorder is caused by autoantibodies against voltage-gated calcium channels, most commonly associated with small cell lung cancer. Lambert-Eaton myasthenic syndrome is characterized by proximal limb weakness, preferentially involving the lower extremities, and fatigability. Hyporeflexia or areflexia is also observed. Autonomic nervous system abnormalities, in particular dry mouth but also pupillary abnormalities, decreased sweating and lacrimation, and impotence are other important characteristics. The weakness and hyporeflexia tend to improve temporarily with brief, repeated muscle contractions. Diffusely reduced motor amplitudes on motor nerve conduction studies, often $<50\%$ of the laboratory's lower limits of normal, are commonly encountered at baseline in Lambert-Eaton myasthenic syndrome. Electrophysiologic tests of particular importance are repetitive nerve stimulation studies that, when performed at a slow rate (3 Hz), show a decremental response similar to myasthenia gravis (MG). After rapid repetitive nerve stimulation (30-50 Hz) or brief (10 sec), intense contractions, a marked increase of the compound muscle action potential amplitude by $>200\%$ is seen.

The most effective symptomatic treatment in Lambert-Eaton myasthenic syndrome is 3,4-DAP. Through blocking voltage-gated potassium channels on presynaptic motor neurons, 3,4-DAP prolongs nerve terminal depolarization and increases acetylcholine release. In theory, pyridostigmine should be synergistic with 3,4-DAP, but many patients with Lambert-Eaton myasthenic syndrome have no benefit from pyridostigmine, either on its own or in combination with 3,4-DAP.

25. **The correct answer is: E. Both B and C.** This woman has a probable diagnosis of MG based on history and examination. Brain MRI is not necessary to confirm a diagnosis of MG. ESR and CRP would be important if there is high suspicion for giant cell arteritis, which can also present with vision abnormalities, but typically also presents with jaw claudication and headache. It is important to send anti-AChR and anti-MuSK antibodies to confirm a diagnosis of antibody positive MG (though sensitivity is 80%) as well as a chest CT to determine if a thymoma is present. Recent studies suggest that patients with a thymoma or antibody positive patients with thymic tissue should undergo thymectomy to improve outcomes.

26. **The correct answer is: B. Perifascicular atrophy and perivascular inflammation.** The symptoms experienced in this case suggest a pattern of proximal muscle weakness. Difficulty going up and down stairs and difficulty getting out of low chairs are symptoms characteristic of proximal lower extremity weakness. On examination, proximal weakness in both upper and lower extremities, as well as mild weakness in the neck flexors, was found. In combination with the erythematous papules over the extensor surfaces (Gottron papules) and the skin rash over the upper back (shawl sign), the clinical picture is suggestive of dermatomyositis. The characteristic pathologic findings of dermatomyositis on muscle biopsy are perifascicular atrophy, in which atrophic fibers are present at the edges of fascicles that are otherwise composed of relatively normal-sized myofibers and perivascular inflammation composed primarily of macrophages, B cells, and plasma cells.

27. **The correct answer is: A. Cluster headache.** This patient's history is classic for cluster headache. Patients often describe an excruciating stabbing, boring, or burning pain that is unilateral and periorbital. Ipsilateral autonomic symptoms, including lacrimation, conjunctival injection, and rhinorrhea, are common. Patients often report a feeling of restlessness or panic associated with the headaches. The headaches often come on at the same time of day, with the evening being most common. Attacks can last 15 minutes to 3 hours, and patients can have up to eight attacks per day. The attacks often occur in clusters lasting weeks to months, and patients can be headache-free between clusters. Like cluster headache, short-lasting unilateral neuralgiform pain with conjunctival injection and tearing syndrome is classified as a trigeminal autonomic cephalalgia. Pain quality is similar, but pain is much briefer and more frequent, with attacks lasting 5 seconds to 4 minutes and happening up to 200 times per day. His symptoms are not typical for trigeminal neuralgia (shooting pain in the face) or tension headache (bilateral, mild-to-moderate pressure pain). Evaluation of new headaches should always include review of red flag symptoms and signs that could indicate a secondary headache. These include explosive onset (or "worst headache of life"), signs of increased intracranial pressure (including worse with lying down), vision symptoms (including eye pain, diplopia, and blurred vision), abnormal neurologic examination, age >50 years, and immunosuppressed state.

28. **The correct answer is: A. Indomethacin.** This patient's presentation is consistent with hemicrania continua—a chronic headache syndrome of severe attacks with autonomic features superimposed on a continuous headache of at least 3 months' duration. Brain imaging is usually indicated to exclude a structural lesion and dedicated venous imaging should also be considered to exclude venous sinus thrombosis in patients with risk factors for hypercoagulability. Hemicrania continua should resolve completely with indomethacin; this treatment response is part of the diagnostic criteria. An indomethacin trial is typically done over several days with incremental dose increases. After a successful trial, the headache resolves and indomethacin is stopped. If the headache does not completely resolve, an alternative diagnosis should be considered. Tricyclic antidepressants and topiramate are treatments for many headache types, but not for hemicrania continua. Verapamil is particularly effective in cluster headache. Triptans are used as abortive medications for migraines.

29. **The correct answer is: D. Start topiramate.** The patient's migraine is significantly debilitating her quality of life, making her miss work multiple times a month. Therefore, the best course of action is to start a migraine medication rather than to manage conservatively. She also needs something more than just breakthrough at this time, given that she has frequent migraine attacks every week. Out of the medications listed, given her weight gain, topiramate would be the best option, which has weight loss as a side effect.

30. **The correct answer is: D. *NOTCH3*.** This patient's presentation is highly suggestive of cerebral autosomal dominant arteriopathy with subcortical infarcts and leukoencephalopathy (CADASIL). This is based on her history of subcortical infarcts without the typical risk factors associated with vascular disease (eg, hypertension, diabetes mellitus, dyslipidemia), her history of migraine with aura, and her family history of migraines, stroke, and early cognitive impairment. Imaging in CADASIL shows diffuse white matter hyperintensities on T2-weighted imaging, often including the anterior temporal region and the external capsule (also known as the O'Sullivan sign). CADASIL is an autosomal dominant disorder caused by a *NOTCH3* gene mutation. It is the most common cause of inherited stroke and vascular dementia in adults. The *NOTCH3* gene encodes a transmembrane receptor that contains 34 epidermal growth factor repeats—a large transmembrane protein necessary for vascular smooth muscle differentiation and development.

31. **The correct answer is: E. Send thrombophilia workup and start therapeutic anticoagulation with heparin.** The patient has several red flags in her history that suggest a secondary cause of headaches, such as worsening in frequency and persistence, worsening with recumbent position, and awakening from sleep. Her examination is notable

for bilateral papilledema, suggesting that her intracranial pressure might be elevated. The cranial imaging depicted in the figure is a magnetic resonance venogram showing nonvisualization of the right transverse, sigmoid, and jugular venous system consistent with venous sinus thrombosis. The correct management in this case would be to send thrombophilia workup and start the patient on therapeutic anticoagulation as soon as possible.

32. **The correct answer is: B. L5 nerve root.** This patient's symptoms are consistent with an L5 radiculopathy causing foot drop, likely because of herniation of the L4 to L5 disk. Radiculopathy can present with shooting pain down the affected extremity, sensory loss, and motor weakness. The L5 nerve root innervates the tibialis anterior, which dorsiflexes the foot; weakness of this muscle causes foot drop. Sensory loss is over the lateral calf and great toe, with paresthesias shooting from the low back down the lateral thigh into the same distribution. Reflexes are typically normal, as the patellar reflex is mediated by L4 and the Achilles reflex is mediated by S1. L4 radiculopathy presents with quadriceps weakness (knee extension) and numbness over the anteromedial lower leg and inner foot. S1 radiculopathy presents with gastrocnemius weakness (ankle plantar flexion) and sensory loss over the lateral foot and sole of the foot. A thoracic spinal cord lesion would be more likely to present with a sensory level and upper motor neuron signs and would not cause radicular pain. Peroneal neuropathy is another common cause of foot drop, most often because of compression at the fibular head, but can be distinguished from L5 radiculopathy by the sparing of foot inversion, which is in the L5 myotome but innerved by the tibial nerve.

33. **The correct answer is: B. Calf cramping.** Both lumbar spinal stenosis and peripheral vascular disease with limb ischemia can cause lower extremity pain with certain activities. In lumbar spinal stenosis (neurogenic claudication), patients typically report radicular pain that is worse with walking, standing, or lying prone and better with bending forward or sitting. Sitting forward can help relieve mechanical compression of the nerve roots. There may also be associated focal weakness, sensory changes, and decreased reflexes. In peripheral artery disease (vascular claudication), the pain is a cramping that is predominantly in the calves and can radiate up the legs. It is worse with activity and better with rest, but there is no change between sitting and standing. On examination, there may be pale, cool extremities with diminished pulses, but neurologic findings would not be expected.

34. **The correct answer is: A. Administer dexamethasone 10 mg IV, with urgent evaluation for thoracic spine decompression.** This patient presents with symptoms of rapidly progressing weakness and numbness of her bilateral lower extremities. On examination, she has evidence of a thoracic myelopathy based on her pattern of weakness (involving the lower but sparing the upper extremities), hyperreflexia, upgoing toes, and T4 sensory level to pinprick. Her imaging reveals an epidural mass lesion compressing the spinal cord at the level of the T5 vertebra concerning for metastatic disease. The next step in management would involve administration of steroids and evaluation for urgent spinal cord decompression.

35. **The correct answer is: D. NSE >101 ng/mL and lack of reactivity on EEG.** Factors associated with poor outcome (dependence on others for daily support) following cardiac arrest include absent brainstem reflexes, treatment-resistant myoclonus, EEG with absent background or reactivity, and MRI with diffuse hypoxic injury. An NSE cutoff of 33 ng/mL is associated with a high false-positive rate for predicting poor outcome. False-positive rate can be further reduced when two or more negative prognostic indicators are present in combination. The high NSE in this patient and lack of reactivity on EEG together predict a poor outcome.

5-FU	fluorouracil		**CNS**	central nervous system
ABG	arterial blood gas		**COPD**	chronic obstructive pulmonary disease
ABPA	allergic bronchopulmonary aspergillosis		**CPR**	cardiopulmonary resuscitation
ACE	angiotensin-converting enzyme		**CRP**	C-reactive protein
ACTH	adrenocorticotropic hormone		**CSF**	cerebrospinal fluid
ADH	antidiuretic hormone		**CT**	computed tomography
AF	atrial fibrillation		**CTA**	CT angiography
AFB	acid-fast bacilli		**CVVH**	continuous veno-venous hemofiltration
AFP	α-fetoprotein		**CXR**	chest x-ray
AKI	acute kidney injury		**DDAVP**	desmopressin
AL	amyloid light chain		**DLBCL**	diffuse large B-cell lymphoma
ALL	acute lymphoblastic leukemia		**DMARD**	disease-modifying antirheumatic drug
ALT	alanine aminotransferase		**dsDNA**	double stranded DNA
AML	acute myelogenous leukemia		**DST**	dexamethasone suppression test
ANA	antinuclear antibody			
ANC	absolute neutrophil count		**DTR**	deep tendon reflex
ANCA	antineutrophilic cytoplasmic antibody		**DVT**	deep vein thrombosis
APLS	antiphospholipid syndrome		**ECG**	electrocardiogram
ARB	angiotensin receptor blocker		**ED**	emergency department
ARNI	angiotensin receptor neprilysin inhibitor		**EEG**	electroencephalogram
			EF	ejection fraction
ASCVD	atherosclerotic cardiovascular disease		**EGD**	esophagogastroduodenoscopy
AST	aspartate aminotransferase		**eGFR**	estimated glomerular filtration rate
ATN	acute tubular necrosis		**EGFR**	epidermal growth factor receptor
ATO	arsenic trioxide		**EGPA**	eosinophilic granulomatosis with polyangiitis
ATRA	all-*trans*-retinoic acid		**ELISA**	enzyme-linked immunosorbent assay
BAL	bronchoalveolar lavage			
BiPAP	bilevel positive airway pressure		**EMG**	electromyography
BMI	body mass index		**EMS**	Emergency Medical Services
BMP	basic metabolic panel		**ER**	emergency room
BP	blood pressure		**ERCP**	endoscopic retrograde cholangiopancreatography
BPH	benign prostatic hyperplasia			
BUN	blood urea nitrogen		**ESR**	erythrocyte sedimentation rate
CABG	coronary artery bypass grafting		**ESRD**	end-stage renal disease
CAD	coronary artery disease		**ET**	essential thrombocythemia
CAR-T	chimeric antigen receptor T-cell		**EUS**	endoscopic ultrasound
CBC	complete blood count		**FDG**	fluorodeoxyglucose
CCB	calcium channel blocker		**FEV$_1$**	forced expiratory volume
CCP	cyclic citrullinated peptide		**FNA**	fine needle aspiration
CHB	complete heart block		**FOBT**	fecal occult blood test
CI	confidence interval		**fT4**	free thyroxine
CKD	chronic kidney disease			
CMV	cytomegalovirus			

G6PD	glucose-6-phosphate dehydrogenase		**LFT**	liver function test
G-CSF	granulocyte-colony stimulating factor		**LP**	lumbar puncture
GCA	giant cell arteritis		**LVEF**	left ventricular ejection fraction
GDMT	guideline-directed medical therapy		**mAb**	monoclonal antibody
GERD	gastroesophageal reflux disease		**MAHA**	microangiopathic hemolytic anemia
GI	gastrointestinal		**MALT**	mucosa-associated lymphoid tissue
GLP-1 RA	glucagon-like peptide-1 receptor agonist		**MAP**	mean arterial pressure
GVHD	graft-versus-host disease		**MCV**	mean corpuscular volume
HbA$_{1c}$	hemoglobin A$_{1c}$		**MELD**	Model for End-Stage Liver Disease
HBV	hepatitis B virus		**MEN1**	multiple endocrine neoplasia type 1
HCC	hepatocellular carcinoma		**MET**	metabolic equivalent
HCV	hepatitis C virus		**MGUS**	monoclonal gammopathy of unknown significance
HF	heart failure		**MI**	myocardial infarction
HFrEF	heart failure with reduced ejection fraction		**MRA**	magnetic resonance angiography
HIT	heparin-induced thrombocytopenia		**MRI**	magnetic resonance imaging
HIV	human immunodeficiency virus		**MRSA**	methicillin-resistant *Staphylococcus aureus*
HLA	human leukocyte antigen		**MSSA**	methicillin-sensitive *Staphylococcus aureus*
hpf	high-power field		**NAFLD**	nonalcoholic fatty liver disease
HR	heart rate		**NHL**	non-Hodgkin lymphoma
HSCT	hematopoietic stem cell transplantation		**NSAID**	nonsteroidal anti-inflammatory drug
HSV	herpes simplex virus		**NSCLC**	non-small cell lung cancer
HTN	hypertension		**NSTEMI**	non–ST-elevation myocardial infarction
HUS	hemolytic uremic syndrome		**NT-proBNP**	N-terminal pro B-type natriuretic peptide
IBD	inflammatory bowel disease		**PA**	pulmonary artery
ICD	implantable cardioverter-defibrillator		**PAD**	peripheral arterial disease
ICS	inhaled corticosteroid		**PAH**	pulmonary arterial hypertension
ICU	intensive care unit		**PAN**	polyarteritis nodosa
Ig	immunoglobulin		**PARP**	poly (ADP-ribose) polymerase
IGF	insulin-like growth factor		**PCP**	primary care physician
ILD	interstitial lung disease		**PCR**	polymerase chain reaction
IM	intramuscular		**PCWP**	pulmonary capillary wedge pressure
INR	international normalized ratio		**PD-1**	programmed cell death protein 1
IV	intravenous		**PEEP**	positive end-expiratory pressure
IVC	inferior vena cava		**PET**	positron emission tomography
IVIG	intravenous immunoglobulin		**PFT**	pulmonary function testing
JVD	jugular venous distention		**PMH**	past medical history
JVP	jugular venous pressure		**PMN**	polymorphonuclear
LABA	long-acting β2-agonist		**PMR**	polymyalgia rheumatica
LAD	left anterior descending			
LAMA	long-acting muscarinic antagonist			
LBBB	left bundle branch block			
LDH	lactate dehydrogenase			

PSA	prostate-specific antigen	**SVR**	systemic vascular resistance
PT	prothrombin time	**T1DM**	type 1 diabetes mellitus
PTH	parathyroid hormone	**T2DM**	type 2 diabetes mellitus
RA	rheumatoid arthritis	**TB**	tuberculosis
RBBB	right bundle branch block	**TEE**	transesophageal echocardiogram
RBC	red blood cell	**TFT**	thyroid function test
RF	rheumatoid factor	**TIBC**	total iron binding capacity
RHC	right heart catheterization	**TMP-SMX**	trimethoprim-sulfamethoxazole
RR	respiratory rate	**TNF**	tumor necrosis factor
RUQ	right upper quadrant	**TSH**	thyroid-stimulating hormone
SBP	spontaneous bacterial peritonitis	**TTE**	transthoracic echocardiogram
SC	subcutaneous	**UA**	urinalysis
SGLT2i	sodium-glucose cotransporter 2 inhibitor	**UPEP**	urine protein electrophoresis
		UTI	urinary tract infection
SI	sacroiliac	**VATS**	video-assisted thoracoscopic surgery
SIADH	syndrome of inappropriate antidiuretic hormone		
		VBG	venous blood gas
SLE	systemic lupus erythematosus	**VT**	ventricular tachycardia
SPEP	serum protein electrophoresis	**vWF**	von Willebrand factor
STEMI	ST-elevation myocardial infarction	**WBC**	white blood cell

NOTES

NOTES

NOTES

NOTES

NOTES

NOTES